Cardiovascular Risk Factors: Recent Developments

Cardiovascular Risk Factors: Recent Developments

Edited by **Janice Hunter**

New Jersey

Published by Foster Academics,
61 Van Reypen Street,
Jersey City, NJ 07306, USA
www.fosteracademics.com

Cardiovascular Risk Factors: Recent Developments
Edited by Janice Hunter

International Standard Book Number: 978-1-63242-072-5 (Hardback)

Contents

Preface

It is often said that books are a boon to mankind. They document every progress and pass on the knowledge from one generation to the other. They play a crucial role in our lives. Thus I was both excited and nervous while editing this book. I was pleased by the thought of being able to make a mark but I was also nervous to do it right because the future of students depends upon it. Hence, I took a few months to research further into the discipline, revise my knowledge and also explore some more aspects. Post this process, I begun with the editing of this book.

Amongst non-communicable diseases, cardiovascular disorders are the leading cause of fatality in both developed and developing nations. The range of risk factors is extensive, and their consideration is crucial to avoid the first and recurring episodes of myocardial infarction, stroke or peripheral vascular disease which may prove fatal or disabling. This book presents researches recently undertaken regarding cardiovascular factors covering major issues such as hypertension - a risk factor among adult population, hostility and other forms of negative effects, theoretical identification of behavioral risk factors and the effects of dietary fiber. This book will be a valuable source of information for medical students and practitioners.

I thank my publisher with all my heart for considering me worthy of this unparalleled opportunity and for showing unwavering faith in my skills. I would also like to thank the editorial team who worked closely with me at every step and contributed immensely towards the successful completion of this book. Last but not the least, I wish to thank my friends and colleagues for their support.

Editor

Blood Pressure Regulation During Bathing: Is There a Cardiovascular Risk?

Takeshi Otsuki and Yasuko Okuda
Ryutsu Keizai University & Hiroshima Bunka Gakuen University,
Japan

1. Introduction

Water immersion-induced augmentations of external hydrostatic pressure increase central venous and atrial volume and pressure (Arborelius et al., 1972; Gabrielsen et al., 1993; Onodera et al., 2001). The increased left ventricular preload results in the elevation of stroke volume and cardiac output (Arborelius et al., 1972; Ueno et al., 2005). In Poiseuille's law, an elevated stroke volume should increase blood pressure. Therefore, it is reasonable to predict that blood pressure increases during bathing. However, previous studies have reported contradictory results. Ohnaka et al. (1995) have demonstrated that 10-min bathing (40 °C) decreased systolic blood pressure (SBP) in young and middle-aged subjects. Additionally, Nagasawa et al. (2001) have reported that SBP decreased during hot-water immersion (40 °C, 10 min) in young subjects, but increased at the onset of immersion and recovered during the latter phase of immersion in older subjects. Furthermore, Allison & Reger (1998) have reported that SBP in young and middle-aged men showed initial decrease, followed by a gradual increase back toward the baseline during 21-min bathing (40.0 °C). Taken together, the vasopressor effects of bathing are less likely to be marked. Blood pressure during bathing may be maintained by some facilitated regulatory mechanisms.

Blood pressure is regulated mainly by autonomic nervous, endocrine, and renal body-fluid modulation systems. Particularly, the autonomic nervous system rapidly responds to changes in blood pressure. The cardiovagal baroreflex is one of the autonomic functions that regulate blood pressure. Arterial baroreceptors, stretch receptors in the carotid arterial and aortic bodies, detect any blood pressure-associated strain of arterial walls and send afferent signal to increase or decrease heart rate (HR). In this way, the cardiovagal baroreflex regulates blood pressure. Since the baroreceptor firing rate is proportional to changes in arterial circumference at a physiological blood pressure (Aars, 1969), cardiovagal baroreflex sensitivity (BRS) is considered to be affected by carotid arterial or aortic stiffness (Kingwell et al., 1995; Monahan et al., 2001; Rowe, 1987). Additionally, *in vitro* diameter-pressure curves at different temperatures, illustrated using harvested human common carotid arteries, have suggested that hyperthermia may have softening effects on the carotid artery (Guinea et al., 2005). Therefore, bathing-induced hyperthermia may reduce carotid arterial stiffness and consequently increase cardiovagal BRS. Evidence demonstrating that short-term heat stress (5 min, 46.0-48.0 °C) increases skeletal muscle sympathetic BRS (Keller et al., 2006), may support this hypothesis. However, it has remained unclear whether cardiovagal BRS increases during bathing.

We hypothesized that cardiovagal BRS increases during bathing to attenuate bathing-induced blood pressure changes. To test this hypothesis, cardiovagal BRS and hemodynamics in women were measured before, during, and after bathing. Cardiovagal BRS was evaluated using the sequence method (Bertinieri et al., 1988; Hayashi et al., 2006). As a control experiment, a showering session was performed according to the protocol for the bathing session. Body temperature before and after showering/bathing and carotid arterial pulse wave velocity (PWV; an index of arterial stiffness) at rest were also investigated.

2. Methods

2.1 Subjects

Twelve women [age, 35.5±6.6 (19-69) years; height, 157±2 (147-169) cm; weight, 52.4±2.1 (39.3-62.7) kg; and BMI, 21.2±0.7 (16.2-25.4) kg/m²] volunteered to participate in this study. All subjects were free of signs and symptoms of cardiac diseases, diabetes, and hypertension. None of the participants were currently taking any medications. Premenopausal women were tested at least 3 days before or 3 days after menses. All subjects provided written informed consent before inclusion in the study. This study conformed to the principles outlined in the Helsinki Declaration.

2.2 Experimental protocol

Two testing sessions, showering and bathing sessions, were performed in a randomized order on the same day, at least 2 h apart, in a quiet and temperature-controlled room. First, carotid arterial PWV was measured at supine position after a rest period (formPWV/ABI; Omron Colin, Tokyo, Japan). Second, radial arterial pulse waveforms were continuously recorded for 5 min by applanation tonometry in a seated position (BP-508SD, Omron Colin). At the onset of waveforms recording, brachial arterial pressure was measured by oscillometry (BP-508SD, Omron Colin). Skin temperature was measure at the end of the rest period using an electronic axillary thermometer (CT513, Citizen Systems, Tokyo, Japan). Also, tympanic temperature was measured via an infrared ear thermometer (CT820, Citizen Systems). Third, subjects were showered with hot water (40 °C, 12.5 L/min) or immersed in hot water (40 °C) up to the axillae for 10 min in a sitting position. The radial arterial waveforms and brachial blood pressure waveforms were investigated as previously mentioned. Finally, subjects underwent a 10-min recovery period after the cessation of showering/bathing in the same position as in the pre-showering/bathing period. Again, radial pressure waveforms, brachial blood pressure, and body temperatures were measured in this period.

2.3 Carotid arterial PWV

Carotid arterial PWV was measured using a device to investigate PWV (formPWV/ABI; Omron Colin), as previously described with minor modifications (Kimoto et al., 2003; Kobayashi et al., 2004). Briefly, subjects assumed a supine position with a cardiac sound microphone placed at the right sternal margin at the second intercostal level, with an applanation tonometer on the common carotid artery. The pulse wave transit time between the aortic valve and carotid artery was determined based on the time delay between the beginning of the second heart sound and notch of the carotid artery pulse wave. The distance traveled by the pulse waves was estimated according to the height of subjects using the following equation: 0.2437 x height - 18.999 (Kimoto et al., 2003; Kobayashi et al., 2004). Carotid arterial PWV was calculated as the distance divided by the transit time.

2.4 Cardiovagal BRS

Cardiovagal BRS was assessed according to previous studies with minor modifications (Bertinieri et al., 1988; Hayashi et al., 2006). Under all recording conditions, an applanation tonometer (BP-508SD, Omron Colin) was placed at the forth intercostal level. The applanation tonometer sampled the radial arterial pressure waveforms and stored data in a computer. HR was calculated from pulse intervals. We identified baroreflex sequences (three or more beats relating to pulse intervals and progressively and spontaneously changing SBP at the same detection points). Next, we determined the slope of the linear relationship between the pulse intervals and SBP at these points. The minimum changes observed were 1 mmHg for SBP and 1 ms for the pulse interval. Linear regressions relating SBP to the pulse interval were plotted for each sequence; only those sequences with linear r values > 0.85 were accepted. For the latter 5-min of respective period, the results were averaged to provide a single data set.

2.5 Statistical analysis

Data are expressed as means±SE. Statistical analysis was carried out using repeated-measures two-way ANOVA followed by Scheffe's test for multiple comparisons. Linear correlation analysis was used to examine the relationship between carotid arterial PWV and cardiovagal BRS. $P<0.05$ was regarded as significant.

3. Results

Respective temperatures of shower/bath water were 40.6±0.2/40.6±0.1 °C. Bathroom temperature in showering and bathing sessions was 27.3±0.1 and 27.8±0.1 °C, and room humidity was 66.7±0.9 and 62.3±1.7 %, respectively.

Cardiovagal BRS before, during, and after showering/bathing is indicated in Fig. 1. Two-way ANOVA revealed an interaction between session (showering or bathing) and time in cardiovagal BRS. In multiple comparisons, cardiovagal BRS did not change during showering but increased during bathing compared to the baseline. Also, cardiovagal BRS was greater during bathing than during showering. The elevated cardiovagal BRS recovered to the baseline after the cessation of bathing.

Hemodynamics during sessions are summarized in Table 1. We did not identify interactions (session x time) in all measures. Again, there were no main effects of session in all indices. Main effects of time were detected in SBP, mean blood pressure (MBP), HR, and double-product (DP, i.e., product of SBP and HR). In details, SBP was higher during and after showering and bathing than the baseline. MBP increased after showering and bathing compared to at rest. HR was higher during showering and bathing in comparison to before showering and bathing. Increased DP was observed during and after showering and bathing. Time was not associated with diastolic blood pressure and pulse pressure.

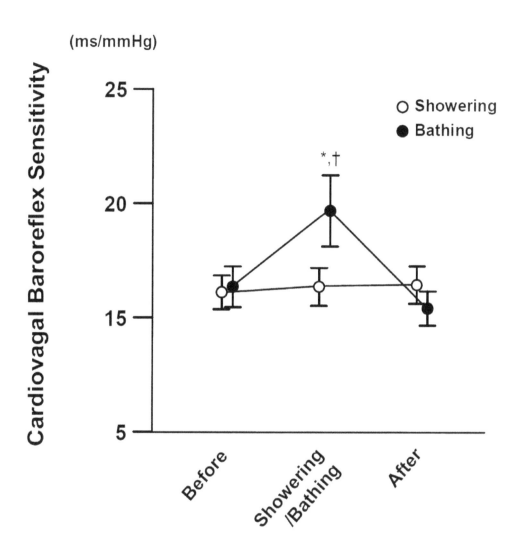

Fig. 1. Cardiovagal baroreflex sensitivity (BRS) before, during, and after showering/bathing. Data are expressed as means±SE. Repeated-measures two-way ANOVA (session x time) revealed an interaction in cardiovagal BRS ($F=6.4$, $P<0.01$). On multiple comparisons, showering was not associated with cardiovagal BRS, but bathing increased it compared to the baseline. The increased BRS during bathing recovered to the baseline after the cessation of bathing. *$P<0.05$ vs. before bathing; †$P<0.05$ vs. showering.

		Before			Showering /Bathing			After			Interaction
SBP, mmHg	Showering	100	±	2	103	±	2	105	±	2	F=0.3
	Bathing	99	±	3	103	±	2	102	±	3	P=0.73
MBP, mmHg	Showering	67	±	2	71	±	2	73	±	3	F=0.7
	Bathing	70	±	2	71	±	2	72	±	2	P=0.49
DBP, mmHg	Showering	55	±	2	55	±	2	56	±	2	F=1.3
	Bathing	52	±	3	56	±	4	58	±	3	P=0.28
PP, mmHg	Showering	45	±	2	48	±	2	49	±	3	F=1.4
	Bathing	46	±	2	47	±	4	44	±	2	P=0.27
HR, bpm	Showering	68	±	1	70	±	2	68	±	2	F=2.2
	Bathing	68	±	2	72	±	3	71	±	2	P=0.12
DP, AU	Showering	68.4	±	1.7	71.5	±	1.6	71.3	±	1.4	F=1.6
	Bathing	66.5	±	2.7	73.7	±	3.3	72.0	±	3.0	P=0.20

Table 1. Hemodynamics before, during, and after showering/bathing. Values are means±SE. SBP, systolic blood pressure; MBP, mean blood pressure; DBP, diastolic blood pressure; PP, pulse pressure; HR, heart rate; DP, double product; AU, arbitrary unit.

The relationship between carotid arterial PWV and cardiovagal BRS at rest is demonstrated in Fig. 2. Carotid arterial PWV was correlated with cardiovagal BRS.

Table 2 shows body temperatures before and after showering/bathing. There was no interaction between session and time in skin temperature. However, two-way ANOVA identified the main effect of time; skin temperature increased after showering and bathing. No differences in skin temperature between showering and bathing were present. On the other hand, we observed an interaction (session x time) in tympanic temperature. In multiple comparisons, showering did not change tympanic temperature but bathing increased it.

4. Discussion

Spontaneous cardiovagal BRS, hemodynamics, and body temperature in women were measured before, during, and after showering/bathing. Carotid arterial PWV, an index of arterial stiffness, was also measured at rest. We demonstrated for the first time that spontaneous cardiovagal BRS increased during bathing compared to the baseline. There were no differences in the changes from the baseline in blood pressure, HR, and DP between showering and bathing sessions. Tympanic temperature did not change after showering but increased after bathing in comparison to the baseline. Cardiovagal BRS was negatively correlated with carotid arterial PWV. We concluded that cardiovagal BRS increases during bathing. Increased cardiovagal BRS may attenuate the blood pressure changes during bathing, resulting in comparable hemodynamics responses between showering and bathing. We would like to propose that it may be unreasonable to withhold bathing by reason of cardiovascular risk. Taking into consideration the slight but significant hyperthermic effects, bathing may be more beneficial to humans in comparison to showering, although caution may be required for humans with stiffened carotid arteries.

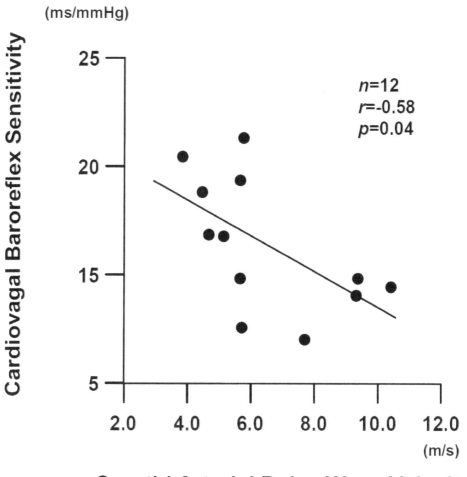

Fig. 2. Relationship between carotid arterial pulse wave velocity (PWV), an index of arterial stiffness, and cardiovagal baroreflex sensitivity (BRS) at rest. Carotid arterial PWV was correlated with cardiovagal BRS.

		Before			After			Interaction
Skin temperature, °C	Showering	36.4	±	0.1	36.6	±	0.2	F=0.3
	Bathing	36.3	±	0.2	36.6	±	0.1	P=0.57
Tympanic temperature, °C	Showering	37.0	±	0.1	36.9	±	0.1	F=7.4
	Bathing	37.0	±	0.1	37.1	±	0.1*	P=0.01

Values are means±SE. *$P<0.05$ vs.

Table 2. Body temperature before and after showering/bathing.

Water immersion increases venous return and ventricular preload (Arborelius et al., 1972; Gabrielsen et al., 1993; Onodera et al., 2001). Consequently, stroke volume and cardiac output increases in the water-immersed subjects (Arborelius et al., 1972; Ueno et al., 2005). Therefore, theoretically, arterial SBP and pulse pressure are speculated to be elevated during bathing. However, the reported effects of bathing on blood pressure are not consistent (Allison & Reger, 1998; Nagasawa et al., 2001; Ohnaka et al., 1995). Also in this study, we did not observe differences in blood pressure changes between showering and bathing periods. It is reasonable to consider that the effects of bathing on blood pressure are not marked. The mechanisms underlying the paradox (i.e., bathing increases blood flow but not arterial blood pressure) have, up to now, remained unclear. This study demonstrated that cardiovagal BRS increases during bathing. This enhanced cardiovagal BRS may participate in the regulation of blood pressure and reduce cardiovascular risks during bathing.

Cardiovagal BRS is regulated via arterial baroreceptors, stretch receptors in arterial tissue. The baroreceptors are located in carotid arterial and aortic bodies. Baroreceptors sense arterial wall strain caused by blood pressure changes and send afferent signals corresponding to the strain level to the cardiovascular center. The stiffness of baroreceptor-containing arteries such as the carotid artery has been hypothesized to be one of the key factors determining cardiovagal BRS (Kingwell et al., 1995; Monahan et al., 2001; Rowe, 1987). Indeed, Monahan et al. (2001) have demonstrated that age-related carotid arterial stiffening, evaluated using echo tracking, was closely associated with decreased cardiovagal BRS, investigated using the Oxford technique. Again, we demonstrated a linear relationship between carotid arterial PWV and cardiovagal BRS. It is well-established that arterial stiffness increases with advancing age (Avolio et al., 1985; Otsuki et al., 2006a; Otsuki et al., 2006b; Vaitkevicius et al., 1993). Central arterial stiffness are also associated with daily physical activities (Iemitsu et al., 2006; Sugawara et al., 2006). Although the present subjects did not experience a marked blood pressure increase during bathing [e.g., maximal SBP increase was 16 mmHg (from 98 at rest to 114 mmHg)], humans with markedly stiff arteries may need to take precautions.

Body temperature was measured before and after showering/bathing at two sites. The skin temperature increased after both showering and bathing. On the other hand, the effects on tympanic temperature were different between showering and bathing. Showering did not change the tympanic temperature, bathing slightly but significantly increased it. The tympanic temperature is closer to the core temperature than skin temperature. It is possible that bathing elevated not only the surface but also internal temperature. At least, the hyperthermic effects are likely to be greater in bathing compared to showering.

We showed that cardiovagal BRS increased on short-term (*i.e.*, 10 min, 40.6 °C) bathing. Also, Keller et al. (2006) have demonstrated that skeletal muscle sympathetic BRS is enhanced by short-term heat stress (5 min, 46.0-48.0 °C). On the other hand, prolonged bathing may be counterproductive. Lee et al. (2003) have reported that hot-water (44.0 °C) immersion of the lower legs for 30 min reduced spontaneous cardiovagal BRS. Prolonged hot-water bathing should be refrained from.

The mechanisms responsible for bathing-induced increases in cardiovagal BRS remain unclear. One explanation for this response may be hyperthermia-related reduction of arterial stiffness. Guinea et al. (2005) have reported that hyperthermia shifts the carotid arterial diameter-pressure curve to the right, suggesting that hyperthermia reduces carotid arterial stiffness. Carotid arterial baroreceptors are stretch receptors. A compliant carotid artery is easily stretched and would be sensitive to changes in blood pressure. Indeed, the present and previous (Monahan et al., 2001) studies have showed a negative relation between cardiovagal BRS and carotid arterial stiffness. We observed that showering increased only the skin temperature, but bathing increased both the skin and tympanic temperature. Collectively, it may be possible that a hyperthermia-induced reduction of carotid arterial stiffness is associated with increased cardiovagal BRS during bathing. Another possible explanation for the changes in cardiovagal BRS is the direct effect of an elevated core temperature on central baroreflex pathways. Previous findings have demonstrated that an increased temperature enhances the neuronal firing rate of thermosensitive neurons (Boulant, 1998). While these findings were limited to the hypothalamic region of the brain, it is a possibility that neurons involved in the pathways of baroreflex control are also thermosensitive and are responsible for the changes in cardiovagal BRS with bathing.

In conclusion, cardiovagal BRS appears to increase during bathing. It may attenuate the bathing-induced blood pressure changes.

5. References

Aars, H. (1969). Relationship between aortic diameter and aortic baroreceptor activity in normal and hypertensive rabbits, *Acta Physiol Scand* 75 (3):406-414.

Allison, T. G. & Reger, W. E. (1998). Comparison of responses of men to immersion in circulating water at 40.0 and 41.5 degrees c, *Aviat Space Environ Med* 69 (9):845-850.

Arborelius, M., Jr., Ballidin, U. I., Lilja, B. & Lundgren, C. E. (1972). Hemodynamic changes in man during immersion with the head above water, *Aerosp Med* 43 (6):592-598.

Avolio, A. P., Deng, F. Q., Li, W. Q., Luo, Y. F., Huang, Z. D., Xing, L. F. & O'Rourke, M. F. (1985). Effects of aging on arterial distensibility in populations with high and low prevalence of hypertension: Comparison between urban and rural communities in china, *Circulation* 71 (2):202-210.

Bertinieri, G., Di Rienzo, M., Cavallazzi, A., Ferrari, A. U., Pedotti, A. & Mancia, G. (1988). Evaluation of baroreceptor reflex by blood pressure monitoring in unanesthetized cats, *Am J Physiol* 254 (2 Pt 2):H377-383.

Boulant, J. A. (1998). Cellular mechanisms of temperature sensitivity in hypothalamic neurons, *Prog Brain Res* 115: 3-8.

Gabrielsen, A., Johansen, L. B. & Norsk, P. (1993). Central cardiovascular pressures during graded water immersion in humans, *J Appl Physiol* 75 (2):581-585.

Guinea, G. V., Atienza, J. M., Elices, M., Aragoncillo, P. & Hayashi, K. (2005). Thermomechanical behavior of human carotid arteries in the passive state, *Am J Physiol Heart Circ Physiol* 288 (6):H2940-2945.

Hayashi, K., Miyachi, M., Seno, N., Takahashi, K., Yamazaki, K., Sugawara, J., Yokoi, T., Onodera, S. & Mesaki, N. (2006). Fluctuations in carotid arterial distensibility during the menstrual cycle do not influence cardiovagal baroreflex sensitivity, *Acta Physiol* 186 (2):103-110.

Iemitsu, M., Maeda, S., Otsuki, T., Sugawara, J., Tanabe, T., Jesmin, S., Kuno, S., Ajisaka, R., Miyauchi, T. & Matsuda, M. (2006). Polymorphism in endothelin-related genes limits exercise-induced decreases in arterial stiffness in older subjects, *Hypertension* 47 (5):928-936.

Keller, D. M., Cui, J., Davis, S. L., Low, D. A. & Crandall, C. G. (2006). Heat stress enhances arterial baroreflex control of muscle sympathetic nerve activity via increased sensitivity of burst gating, not burst area, in humans, *J Physiol* 573 (Pt 2):445-451.

Kimoto, E., Shoji, T., Shinohara, K., Inaba, M., Okuno, Y., Miki, T., Koyama, H., Emoto, M. & Nishizawa, Y. (2003). Preferential stiffening of central over peripheral arteries in type 2 diabetes, *Diabetes* 52 (2):448-452.

Kingwell, B. A., Cameron, J. D., Gillies, K. J., Jennings, G. L. & Dart, A. M. (1995). Arterial compliance may influence baroreflex function in athletes and hypertensives, *Am J Physiol* 268 (1 Pt 2):H411-418.

Kobayashi, K., Akishita, M., Yu, W., Hashimoto, M., Ohni, M. & Toba, K. (2004). Interrelationship between non-invasive measurements of atherosclerosis: Flow-mediated dilation of brachial artery, carotid intima-media thickness and pulse wave velocity, *Atherosclerosis* 173 (1):13-18.

Lee, K., Jackson, D. N., Cordero, D. L., Nishiyasu, T., Peters, J. K. & Mack, G. W. (2003). Change in spontaneous baroreflex control of pulse interval during heat stress in humans, *J Appl Physiol* 95 (5):1789-1798.

Monahan, K. D., Tanaka, H., Dinenno, F. A. & Seals, D. R. (2001). Central arterial compliance is associated with age- and habitual exercise-related differences in cardiovagal baroreflex sensitivity, *Circulation* 104 (14):1627-1632.

Nagasawa, Y., Komori, S., Sato, M., Tsuboi, Y., Umetani, K., Watanabe, Y. & Tamura, K. (2001). Effects of hot bath immersion on autonomic activity and hemodynamics: Comparison of the elderly patient and the healthy young, *Jpn Circ J* 65 (7):587-592.

Ohnaka, T., Tochihara, Y., Kubo, M. & Yamaguchi, C. (1995). Physiological and subjective responses to standing showers, sitting showers, and sink baths, *Appl Human Sci* 14 (5):235-239.

Onodera, S., Miyachi, M., Nishimura, M., Yamamoto, K., Yamaguchi, H., Takahashi, K., In, J. Y., Amaoka, H., Yoshioka, A., Matsui, T. & Hara, H. (2001). Effects of water depth on abdominal [correction of abdominails] aorta and inferior vena cava during standing in water, *J Gravit Physiol* 8 (1):P59-60.

Otsuki, T., Maeda, S., Kesen, Y., Yokoyama, N., Tanabe, T., Sugawara, J., Miyauchi, T., Kuno, S., Ajisaka, R. & Matsuda, M. (2006a). Age-related reduction of systemic arterial compliance induces excessive myocardial oxygen consumption during sub-maximal exercise, *Hypertens Res* 29 (2):65-73.

Otsuki, T., Maeda, S., Sugawara, J., Kesen, Y., Murakami, H., Tanabe, T., Miyauchi, T., Kuno, S., Ajisaka, R. & Matsuda, M. (2006b). Age-related reduction of systemic arterial compliance relates to decreased aerobic capacity during sub-maximal exercise, *Hypertens Res* 29 (10):759-765.

Rowe, J. W. (1987). Clinical consequences of age-related impairments in vascular compliance, *Am J Cardiol* 60 (12):68G-71G.

Sugawara, J., Otsuki, T., Tanabe, T., Hayashi, K., Maeda, S. & Matsuda, M. (2006). Physical activity duration, intensity, and arterial stiffening in postmenopausal women, *Am J Hypertens* 19 (10):1032-1036.

Ueno, L. M., Miyachi, M., Matsui, T., Takahashi, K., Yamazaki, K., Hayashi, K., Onodera, S. & Moritani, T. (2005). Effect of aging on carotid artery stiffness and baroreflex sensitivity during head-out water immersion in man, *Braz J Med Biol Res* 38 (4):629-637.

Vaitkevicius, P. V., Fleg, J. L., Engel, J. H., O'Connor, F. C., Wright, J. G., Lakatta, L. E., Yin, F. C. & Lakatta, E. G. (1993). Effects of age and aerobic capacity on arterial stiffness in healthy adults, *Circulation* 88 (4 Pt 1):1456-1462.

Sagittal Abdominal Diameter as the Anthropometric Measure of Cardiovascular Risk

Edita Stokić[1], Biljana Srdić[2], Vladimir Brtka[3] and Dragana Tomić-Naglić[1]
[1]Department of Endocrinology,
Institute of Internal Disease, Clinical Centre Vojvodina, Novi Sad,
[2]Department of Anatomy, Medical Faculty, Novi Sad, Medical Faculty Novi Sad,
[3]Technical Faculty "Mihajlo Pupin" Zrenjanin,
Serbia

1. Introduction

Obesity has a profound impact on the cardiovascular disease development, and is associated with a reduced overall survival. There is a strong correlation between the central (abdominal) type of obesity and the cardiovascular and metabolic diseases. Among a variety of anthropometric measurements of the abdominal fat size, sagittal abdominal diameter has been proposed as the valid measurement of the visceral fat mass and cardiometabolic risk level. Many studies have analyzed the relationship between sagittal abdominal diameter (SAD), visceral fat area, and different markers of cardiometabolic disturbances with respect to age, gender and ethnicity. Some of them have offered the cut-off values that could be useful in clinical practice, in identifying individuals who are at higher risk of comorbidities of the obesity. Using the principles of rough set theory, based on producing *If-Then* rules, we have developed a model that allows better applicability of SAD in identifying patients at higher cardiovascular risk. In this chapter, we describe the basic principles of the proposed model. Furthermore, we give a broad overview of the main concerns regarding the significance of SAD and its use in diagnosing the abdominal obesity and predicting the adverse cardiometabolic outcomes.

2. Obesity as a cardiovascular risk factor

The prevalence of obesity has increased dramatically worldwide during the past few decades. Obesity is recognized as an independent factor for the development of the cardiovascular diseases. It also predisposes to the development of other cardiovascular risk factors.

Obesity implies increased body weight due to the enlargement of the adipose tissue to the extent that impairs health. Regional obesity appears to be an important indicator of the risk level. Thus, the diagnosis of obesity depends on three main aspects: relative weight (total body mass with relation to body height), total body fat, and fat distribution.

Body mass index (BMI) has been widely accepted as a simple and the most practical measure of fatness in clinical and epidemiological surveys, eventhough it doesn't distinguish fat from lean body mass. In fact, it is an indicator of the nutritional status, not a measure of body fat mass. It has been shown that BMI≥25 kg/m² is associated with increased morbidity, while BMI≥30 kg/m² carries increased risk for both morbidity and mortality, primarily from diabetes and cardiovascular diseases (Irribaren et al., 1995). However, recent studies showed that BMI can be a reliable predictor of cardiovascular mortality only in severe obesity (Romero-Corral et al., 2006). The category of overweight people (BMI: 25-29.9 kg/m²) seems to be the most confusing, especially from the aspect of the therapeutic approach.

BMI doesn't provide sufficient information about fat mass. Therefore, body composition assessment is necessary for the diagnosis of obesity and prediction of its comorbidities. It discriminates individuals with true excess body fat from those with "normal weight obesity", as well as from overweight individuals with normal body fat mass. Using a cut-off value of 30% body fat, Marques-Vidal et al. (2008) reported prevalence of "normal weight obesity" of 10.1% in women, and 3.2% in men, with increasing prevalence with aging.

Specific fat distribution determines the risk level more accurately than the total body fatness *per se*. Excess adipose tissue in the abdominal region is more hazardous than the overall obesity, due to higher visceral fat deposition. Furthermore, it is associated with greater risk of cardiovascular diseases, metabolic disorders and type 2 diabetes mellitus (Després et al., 1990; Molarius & Seidell, 1998). Central or abdominal obesity (firstly assigned as android type of obesity) has been identified as a risk factor for the cardiovascular diseases, as well as a symptom of metabolic syndrome. Normal weight subjects with higher visceral fat mass are at a higher risk (metabolically obese normal weight subjects). In addition, obese subjects with normal visceral fat mass can present with normal metabolic profile (metabolically healthy obese subjects) (Ruderman et al., 1998; Sims, 2001).

2.1 Abdominal obesity

It is well known that the risk of cardiovascular and metabolic abnormalities is determined by specific distribution of the adipose tissue. Abdominal (central) obesity is associated with dyslipidemia, impaired fasting glucose, insulin resistance and hypertension, which result in increased risk of cardio- and cerebrovascular diseases, and consequently premature death (Guzzaloni, 2009).

Adverse effects of the abdominal obesity have been supported by many studies of the metabolism and endocrine activity of adipocytes from different regions of the abdominal adipose tissue. Abdominal fat includes two morphologically and functionally different depots: subcutaneous (superficial) and deep, visceral (intraabdominal). The latter is located in the abdominal cavity and includes intraperitoneal (omental and mesenterial) adipose tissue, which makes 80% of the intraabdominal fat mass, and retroperitoneal adipose tissue, which makes 20% of the intraabdominal fat mass (Misra&Vikram, 2003). Abdominal obesity can reflect expansion of either subcutaneous or visceral depot, or a combination of excess fat in both depots. However, visceral adipose tissue compartment has been considered more important in pathogenesis of the obesity complications. It is responsible for the development of insulin resistance, glucose intolerance and type 2 diabetes mellitus. According to Brochu et al. (2000), visceral fat depot explains 10% of variability of insulin resistance and 16% of blood glucose. Visceral adipose tissue enlargement is mainly associated with lower values of HDL-cholesterol, elevated tryglicerides, apolipoprotein B (Couillard et al., 1996), as well as with elevated atherogenic lipoprotein subfractions and reduced concentration of HDL particles (Nakata et al., 2010). It positivly correlates with glucose intolerance and hyperinsulinemia (Wajchenberg, 2000), as well as the markers of the proinflammatory and prothrombotic state.

Visceral adipose tissue function plays a crucial role in the development of metabolic abnormalities and insulin resistance, mainly due to the direct access of intraperitoneal adipose tissue to the liver through the portal circulation (Matsuzawa et al. 1995, Bosello & Zamboni, 2000). In comparison to the subcutaneous adipose tissue, visceral adipose tissue contains higher number of adipocytes per unit mass, higher number of endothelial cells in the stromal vascular fraction, higher β_3-adrenoreceptor and α_2-adrenergic receptor sensitivity, and it is better vascularized (Misra & Vikram, 2003; van Harmelen et al., 2004). Visceral adipocytes are more metabolically active, have higher lipolytic activity when stimulated by catecholamines, and are poorly responsive to the antilipolythic action of insulin. In addition, they secrete more proinflammatory (interleukin-6, interleukin-8, interleukin-1β) and prothrombotic (plasminogen-acivator inhibitor-1) adipokines. Obesity is characterized by an increased number of β_3- and decreased number of α_2-adrenergic receptors, decreased insulin activity, increased activity of lipoprotein-lipase and acylation-stimulating protein, with higher upload of triglycerides and lower postprandial suppression of lipolysis (Wajchenberg, 2000; van Herpen & Schrauwen-Hinderling, 2008). All of the above mentioned changes in the visceral adipose tissue provide increased release of free fatty acids and their flux towards the liver, where they induce gluconeogenesis, synthesis of triglycerides and apolipoprotein-B rich lipoproteins, as well as impairment of insulin action (Lonnquist et al., 1995, Freedland, 2004). Free fatty acids also exhibit proarrhythmic properties which explains association between the visceral fat and sudden death (Empana et al. 2004). On the other hand, obese adipose tissue is characterized by impairment of blood flow, development of hypoxia and local inflammation, infiltration by macrophages, and by disturbances in secretion of adipokines, which all together result in insulin resistance and systemic inflammation (Berg & Scherer, 2005; Coppack, 2005; Goossens, 2008).

Computerized tomography (CT) and magnetic resonance imaging (MRI), performed at the L_4-L_5 level, are the most reliable anatomical methods for abdominal fat assessment, since they discriminate between the subcutaneous and the visceral fat depots (van der Kooy et al., 1993). However, these methods are expensive, not feasible and unportable, which makes their use in clinical and epidemiological practice limited. Anthropometric parameters are more suitable as they are inexpensive, non-invasive and simple. Besides, most of them show a strong correlation with visceral abdominal fat size.

2.1.1 Anthropometric parameters of abdominal obesity

Several anthropometric indicators of abdominal obesity have been developed to measure abdominal adipose tissue mass. Some of them are presented in the form of ratios, especially the ones that incorporate body height, which gives more realistic picture of body proportions. On the other hand, it is difficult to interpret them biologically (Bouchard et al., 1990). Many studies have compared them in order to demonstrate advantages of a particular parameter in predicting the risk and visceral fat mass. As a rule, an ideal anthropometric measure of abdominal adiposity should predict individual cardiometabolic risk and clearly show effects of different preventative and therapeutic approaches.

Waist-to-hip and waist-to-thigh ratios (WHR and WTR, respectively) were originally proposed as the key determinants of android and gynoid obesity (Krotkiewski et al., 1983; Molarius & Seidell, 1998). WHR has been most commonly used in identifying abdominal fat distribution. Waist circumference alone has received more attention in management of obesity since it requires only one measurement. It showed to be a better predictor of visceral fat volume and related cardiovascular risk profile than WHR (Després et al., 1991; Pouilot et al., 1994; Vissher et al., 2001; Wajchenberg, 2000; Logfren et al., 2004). Moreover, changes in waist circumference better reflect changes in cardiovascular risk factors. It is widely accepted as a surrogat marker of abdominal fat. On the other hand, waist circumference has been criticized for measuring both visceral and subcutaneous adipose tissues (Molarius & Seidell, 1998). Other studies suggest waist-to-height ratio (WHTR) as the better marker because it correlates highly with cardiometabolic risk factors (Hsieh & Yoshinaga, 1995; Ashwell, 2005). Conicity index, which is based on cylindrical shape of the body, has also been introduced as a potentially useful measure of abdominal adiposity (Valdez, 1991). However, it is considered to be very complex because it requires calculations from several different anhropometric values (Molarius & Seidell, 1998).

Sagittal abdominal diameter (SAD), or abdominal height was first demonstrated by Kvist et al. (1988) to be a good correlate of visceral adipose tissue volume, observed by CT. Sjöstrom et al. (1994) proposed the use of sagittal abdominal diameter in the assessment of visceral fat mass. Soon after, Richelsen and Pedersen (1995) confirmed its value in assessing the abdominal fatness and prediction of the metabolic risk profile.

3. Sagittal abdominal diameter – Visceral fat measure and cardiovascular risk predictor

First measures of SAD were done on CT images and showed good predictive values in the assessment of visceral adipose tissue volume (Kvist et al., 1988). SAD, thus, may be a reliable represent of the visceral fat size. Moreover, two recent studies confirmed that SAD was a stronger predictor of metabolic syndrome than the whole visceral fat area (Valsamakis et al., 2008; Hoenig, 2010), which could pointed to functionally different adipose tissue in the midline.

External, anthropometric measurement of SAD is usually done using Holtain-Kahn abdominal caliper, at the level of the iliac crest, which approximates to the L_4-L_5 interspace (Figure 1). Since it has been proposed, SAD has been considered as more closely related to visceral fat mass than the other anthropometric measures beacuse it is measured in a supine position, when a subcutaneous fat is moved to the sides of the waist (van der Kooy et al., 1993; Mukunddem-Petersen, 2006; Sampaio et al., 2007). Measuring SAD in that position reflects the width of intraabdominal fat in the antero-posterior plane, like on CT or MRI images. At the same value of SAD, an increase of waist circumference may reflect increase of subcutaneous adipose tissue size.

Many studies confirmed strong association between anthropometrically assessed SAD and visceral adipose tissue area. Anjana et al. (2004), Sampaio et al. (2007) and Yim et al. (2010)

reported stronger correlation between SAD and visceral fat area, comparing to waist circumference. Zamboni et al. (1998) found better association between SAD and visceral fat area in lean and moderately overweight subjects than in the obese. Regarding to gender, some studies have found better correlation in men, ranged between 0.61 and 0.82 (van der Kooy et al., 1993; Zamboni et al., 1998), while others have reported stronger relationship in women, with the range between 0.52 and 0.87 (Pouilot et al., 1994, Sampaio et al., 2007). Some studies demonstrated that SAD is a better predictor of visceral fat than waist circumference in men (Després et al., 1991; van der Kooy et al., 1993), while others gave opposite results in women (Sampaio et al., 2007). In the MRI study, van der Kooy et al. (1993) showed that SAD was superior to waist circumference and WHR in assessing visceral fat mass changes in men, while waist circumference and WHR were better measures in women.

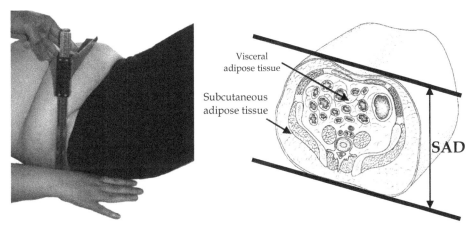

Fig. 1. Measurement of sagittal abdominal diameter (horizontal section of abdomen)

Comparing to other anthropometric measures, like waist circumference or WHR, SAD has been showed to have better correlation with biochemical and hemodynamic parameters associated with cardiovascular diseases and metabolic syndrome in both, lean and obese subjects:

- Higher values of SAD correlate with **atherogenic lipid profile** including elevated triglycerides, reduced HDL-cholesterol, elevated apolipoprotein B levels, and atherogenic lipoprotein subfractions (Pouilot et al., 1994; Sjöström, 1994; Richelsen & Pedersen, 1995; Öhrvall et al., 2000; Turcato et al., 2000; Sampaio et al., 2007; Petersson et al., 2007; Nakata et al., 2010).
- SAD is an important factor in prediction of **glucose intolerance and insulin resistance** (Pouliot et al., 1994; Öhrvall et al., 2000; Gustat et al., 2000; Risérus et al., 2004; Mazzali et al., 2006; Vasques et al., 2009a). Risérus et al. (2004) found that SAD was a strong predictor of hyperproinsulinemia, higher values of C-peptide and lower levels of insulin-like growth factor (IGF) binding protein-1.
- SAD highly correlates with **inflammatory and prothrombotic markers**, like CRP (Mazzali et al., 2006; Petersson et al. 2007; Nakata et al., 2010) or PAI-1 (Öhrvall et al., 2000). According to Petersson et al. (2007), every one-centimetre increase in SAD is followed by an increase of C-reactive protein (CRP) by 0.41 mg/L. The same authors

suggested that SAD may carry information concerning inflammatory status and possibly insulin resistance beyond that of other measures of obesity and fat distribution.

• SAD is associated with **blood pressure** and predicts hypertension (Öhrvall et al., 2000; Strazzulo et al., 2001). Gustat et al. (2000) highlight that SAD can predict blood pressure when other measures cannot.

• Among **adipokines**, SAD correlates with leptin and adiponectin blood levels (Mazzali et al., 2006); it also correlates with 11β-hydroxysteroid dehydrogenase-type 1 (11β-HSD-1) mRNA expression in visceral adipose tissue, which is known to be associated with features of metabolic syndrome (Desbriere et al., 2006).

Our previous results showed significantly higher values of SAD in obese women who displayed lipid and lipoprotein disturbances and hyperinsulinemia, comparing to healthy normal-weight women (Stokić et al, 1996, Stokić & Ivković-Lazar, 1996). According to our unpublished results (a group of 1090 men and 1231 women of different BMI-values, aged 18-79 years), SAD showed a significant correlation with sistolic and diastolic blood pressure and glycaemia in both genders, and with total cholesterol and triglycerides in men. In both, men and women, SAD showed best correlation with diastolic blood pressure (men: r=0.340, women:r=0.198). By discriminative analysis we determined range of SAD that correspond with lowest risk (men: 20.12-24.97 cm; women: 19.85-24.75 cm), while extremely high values were in the following ranges: 32.58-34.65 cm (men) and 29.87-31.80 cm (women).

In the large longitudinal study, Iribarren et al. (2006) confirmed utility of SAD in prediction of cardiovascular risk, independently of body mass index. Reed et al. (2003) found association between SAD and carotid artery intima-media thickness.

Empana et al. (2004) established that age-adjusted risk of sudden death increases linearly with SAD increasement in both, normal-weight and overweight men. SAD has been shown to be an independent risk factor for death and morbidity in patients in the intensive care unit (Paolini et al., 2010).

There are also two indexes derived from SAD:

• SAD-to-body height ratio (SAD/H) has been showed as slightly better predictor than SAD alone. Kumlin et al. (1997) reported that SAD/H is a strong predictor of Framingham coronary risk score.

• SAD to mid-thigh circumference ratio, or abdominal diameter index (ADI), has been proposed by Kahn (1993) as even better predictor of cardiovascular risk, which was confirmed by Smith et al. (2005).

3.1 Application of sagittal abdominal diameter in elderly

Aging process is characterized by body composition changes that could not be captured by standard anthropometric measures like BMI. Increasing of total body fat occurs in both genders, which is followed by decreasing of muscle mass (sarcopenic obesity) and body fat redistribution in terms of changes from peripheral to central (abdominal) pattern (Prentice & Jebb, 2001; Greenlund & Nair, 2003; Davidson & Getz, 2004). In women, menopause plays important role in transitioning from a premenopausal gynoid (gluteo-femoral) to a postmenopausal central (visceral) pattern of body fat distribution and increase in total body fat (Movsesyan et al., 2003). Even in early menopause women have a 49% greater visceral fat mass comparing with premenopausal women (Toth et al., 2000). Together with other physiological and life style changes caused by aging, age-associated central fat distribution contributes to cardiovascular morbidity and mortality. That is why is highly recommended to assess central adiposity in older persons (Dorner & Rieder, 2011).

Some evidences pointed to better predictive value of SAD in younger individuals (Iribarren et al., 2006, Mukuddem-Petersen et al., 2004). However, SAD could be also very useful indicator in the elderly. According to Turcato et al. (2000), SAD and waist circumference are the anthropometric parameters which are the most closely related to cardiovascular risk factors in women and men aged from 67 to 78 years, independently of BMI. Harris et al. (2000) and Snijder et al. (2002) found that SAD was even better predictor of visceral fat area in subjects older than 70 years, comparing to waist circumference, while Mukuddem-Petersen et al. (2004) indicated that SAD had no advantages over simpler and more commonly used anthropometric measures such as waist circumference, regarding to their associations with components of the metabolic syndrome in older subjects.

3.2 Gender and ethnic specific usage of sagittal abdominal diameter

Men and women have different adipose tissue topography. Fat deposition is gluteo-femoral region is more typical for women, while men show preferential abdominal fat accumulation. Within abdominal region, visceral fat compartment is more predominant in men, while women have higher size of subcutaneous fat compartment (Anjana et al., 2004). Men and women also have different dynamics of losing visceral and subcutaneous fat during weight loss - men lose more visceral, and women lose more subcutaneous fat (van der Kooy et al., 1993).

It is assumed that SAD has a stronger capacity to predict visceral fat area, insulin resistance, and cardiometabolic risk in men, because they have higher visceral fat mass (Risérus et al., 2004). Vasques et al. (2009b) confirmed its greater ability to identify insulin resistance in men. However, according to the results given by Mukuddem-Petersen et al. (2004) SAD is a stronger predictor of cardiovascular risk in women, while Duarte-Pimentel et al. (2010) recommend SAD as a marker of central adiposity preferentially in women.

Some ethnic groups show different pattern of body fat distribution and different susceptibility to insulin resistance. For example, Asian Indians have greater abdominal fat mass than Europeans of the same nutrition level (Anjana et al., 2004), while middle-aged and older African-American men and women have lower visceral fat than Hispanic and white men and women (Carroll et al., 2008). There are race and ethnical differences in the relationship between body fat distribution and health risk factors; thus, anthropometric measures could differ regarding the predictive capacity of cardiovascular risk factors. However, according to the results of several studies, SAD seems to be an excellent marker of metabolic and cardiovascular risk factors, irrespectively of national origin or ethnic background (Hwu et al., 2003; Valsamakis et al., 2004; Petersson et al., 2007, Iribarren et al., 2006).

3.3 Treshold values for sagittal abdominal diameter – Reflection of critical visceral fat mass or cardiometabolic risk

In spite of many evidences that SAD is very good in capturing the cardiometabolic risk, its use in clinical practice is limited due to a lack of specific cut-offs. Some authors have proposed cut-off values for SAD using different criteria, usually its correlation with cardiometabolic parameters and visceral fat area (Table 1). These results were mostly obtained using Receiver Operating Characteristics (ROC) curves, or linear regression analysis, and vary from 19.3 cm (Sampaio et al., 2007) to 27.6 cm (Valsamakis et al., 2004). Our results were obtained using the principles of rough set theory that will be described below. They were derived from evaluation of relationship between SAD and cardiovascular risk factors.

We produced "transparent", semantic model which can be easily analyzed. The most important information which can be extracted from semantic models is concerned with the meaning and importance of its elements, as well as with the relations between them. Data were represented in the form of a table with rows containing the objects and columns containing the attributes, and model was produced in the multiple sets containing *If – Then* rules.

SAD (cut-offs)	Population	Criterion	Author
≥25 cm	Men/Women	Association with multiple metabolic disorders	Pouliot et al., 1994
≥22.8 cm ≥25.2 cm	Men Women	Corresponds to 130 cm² of visceral fat area	Lemieux et al., 1996
≥27.6 cm	Men	Predictive value for metabolic syndrome	Valsamakis et al., 2004
≥23 cm	Men	Predictive value for sudden death	Empana et al., 2004
≥20.5 cm ≥19.3 cm	Men Women	Corresponds to 100 cm² of visceral area	Sampaio et al., 2007
≥20 cm	Men	Predictive value for insulin resistance	Vasques et al., 2009a
≥22.2 cm ≥20.1 cm	Men Women	Predictive value for an elevated cardiometabolic risk score	Risérus et al., 2010
≥23.1 cm ≥20.1 cm	Men Women	Corresponds to altered waist circumference (>102 cm for men and >88 cm for women)	Duarte Pimentel et al., 2010
≥24.3 cm	Men/Women	Corresponds to increased cardiovascular risk in overweight and obese individuals	Stokić et al., 2010

Table 1. Recommended cut-off values for SAD

4. Model for the better applicability of SAD in identifying patients at higher cardiovascular risk

Modern healthcare and computer science are fields that are interlaced to form the field of medical informatics. As mentioned by Øhrn (1999), Blois and Shortliffe define medical informatics as "the rapidly developing scientific field that deals with the storage, retrieval and optimal use of biomedical information, data, and knowledge for problem solving and decision making." In its broadest sense, medical informatics can be said to concern itself with the management of information in the context of modern healthcare. According to Øhrn (1999) current research in the field of medical informatics covers a wide array of topics, including:

- **Data acquisition:** Capturing and recording of the medical data usually include things that are not easily recorded or precisely defined.
- **Medical vocabularies:** Medical data has to be represented in machine-readable form.
- **Electronic medical records:** An electronic medical record has to be searchable. Its content should be structured internally.
- **Decision support systems:** These are computer programs that help clinicians make clinical decisions.
- **Deployment barriers:** The barriers of deployment may be technical, operational, organizational and legal nature. Often, systems that may prove successful in research settings do not make it into clinical use.
- **Confidentiality issues:** Medical information is often sensitive and with a potential for misuse by third-parties.

Obviously, as a main prerequisite there is a existence of medical dataset or database. Medical datasets are often described as incomplete, sparse, vague, fuzzy, etc. According to Greco et al. (1998), the rough sets theory has often proved to be an excellent mathematical tool for the analysis of a vague description of objects.

On the base of the table-organized data it is possible to produce semantic model which provides information about meaning and importance of its elements, as well as the relationship between them (Brtka et al., 2008; Stokić et al., 2010). In order to investigate relationship between SAD and anthropometric and cardiovascular risk factors, we used methodology based on rough set theory (Pawlak et al, 1995, Pawlak & Skowron, 2007) applied to table–organized data with producing decision rules in the *If -Then* form.

Our study included 1334 subjects (700 women and 634 men), aged 43.49±10.43 years. Following parameters were analyzed: age (years), body mass index (kg/m^2), SAD (cm), body fat mass (%), systolic and diastolic blood pressure (mmHg), total-, LDL- and HDL-cholesterol (mmol/L), triglycerides (mmol/L), fasting plasma glucose (mmol/L), fibrinogen (g/L), uric acid (μmol/L), and 10-year Framingham Risk Score. The experiments were conducted by software system *Rosetta - A Rough Set Toolkit for Analysis of Data*. All numerical attributes were discretized using a simple "equal frequency binning" technique. The attribute SAD was chosen to be the decision attribute while all remaining attributes were chosen to form the set of condition attributes and the set of rules containing rules in the *If – Then* form was generated. The decision attributes (SAD) were classified into three classes:

- 13.00-24.2 cm,
- 24.3-31.6 cm and
- 31.7-36.2 cm.

4.1 Rough-set theory principles

As the mathematical basis of the rough set theory there is the indiscernibility relation. Every object of the universe is described by certain amount of information expressed by means of some attributes used for that object description. The objects characterized by the same information are indiscernible in view of the available information about them.

As in Greco et al. (1998), Øhrn (1999) and Pawlak & Skowron (2007), let U be a universe (finite set of objects), $Q=\{q_1,q_2,...,q_m\}$ is a finite set of attributes, V_q is the domain of attribute q (attribute values) and V is the union of V_q for every $q \in Q$. An information system is the 4-tuple $S=(U,Q,V,f)$ where f is a function such that $f(x,q) \in V_q$ for each $q \in Q$, $x \in U$, called information function.

Let $x,y \in U$ (x and y are two objects e.g. patients), f is an information function and $q \in Q$. Every non–empty subset of attributes P determines an indiscernibility relation on U, denoted by

$$I_P = \{(x,y) \in U \times U : f(x,q) = f(y,q), \forall q \in P\} \tag{1}$$

The I_P is an equivalence relation. The family of all the equivalence classes of the I_P is denoted by U/I_P and the equivalence class containing an element x by $I_P(x)$.

Let us consider a simple example of an information system based on the example from Greco et al. (1998), see Table 2.

Object	Age	Body Mass (BM)	Systolic blood pressure	SAD
x_1	young	good	low	low
x_2	middle-age	medium	low	high
x_3	middle-age	medium	low	low
x_4	old	medium	low	high
x_5	middle-age	good	high	high
x_6	young	medium	high	low

Table 2. Simple example of an information system

In the given table, there is a universe of six objects $U=\{x_1,...,x_6\}$ and each object is described by means of four attributes: *Age, Body Mass, Systolic Blood Pressure (SBP)* and *SAD*.

If $P=\{Age,BM,SBP\}$ then, by (1), we have: $I_P=\{(x_1,x_1),\ (x_2,x_2),\ (x_2,x_3),\ (x_3,x_2),\ (x_3,x_3),\ (x_4,x_4),\ (x_5,x_5) (x_6,x_6)\}$, $U/I_P=\{\{x_1\},\ \{x_2,x_3\},\ \{x_4\},\ \{x_5\},\ \{x_6\}\}$.

4.1.1 The definition of the rough set

The rough set theory proved to be an excellent mathematical tool for the analysis of data in various domains. The information about the real world is given in a form of a decision system. The next definitions are based on Pawlak et al. (1995), Greco et al. (1998), Øhrn (1999) and Pawlak & Skowron (2007).

Let $C \subset Q$ and $D \subset Q$ so that $C \cap D = \varnothing$, where Q is a set of attributes. The attributes from C are called the condition attributes and the attributes from D are called the decision attributes. An information system where the set of condition attributes and the set of decision attributes are defined is called the decision system.

In most cases there is usually one binary decision attribute, while the other attributes are the condition attributes. In the previous example P might be the set of the condition attributes, and the set of decision attributes contains one element: $D = \{SAD\}$.

Let X be a non-empty subset of U and $\varnothing \neq P \subseteq Q$. The set X is approximated by means of P-lower (2) and P-upper (3) approximations of X:

$$\underline{P}(X) = \{x \in U : I_P(x) \subseteq X\} \tag{2}$$

$$\overline{P}(X) = \bigcup_{x \in X} I_P(x) \tag{3}$$

The P-boundary region $Bn(X)$ of X is defined by:

$$Bn(X) = \overline{P}(X) - \underline{P}(X) \tag{4}$$

For example, let us consider a case when the set X contains only those elements where the value of the decision attribute SAD is low: $X = \{x_1, x_3, x_6\}$ (Table 2). Now, we can approximate the set X using only the information contained in P by constructing the P-lower (2) and P-upper (3) approximations of X:

$$\underline{P}(X) = \{x_1, x_6\},$$

$$\overline{P}(X) = \{x_1, x_2, x_3, x_6\}.$$

The P-boundary region (4) of X is:

$$Bn(X) = \{x_2, x_3\}.$$

The reader may notice that the objects x_2 and x_3 have exactly the same values of the condition attributes but different value of the decision attribute. So, they constitute boundary region. We can say that the rough sets can be defined as follows (Pawlak et al., 1995; Pawlak & Skowron, 2007):

The set X is rough (inexact) with respect to I_P, if the boundary region of X is nonempty. The set X is crisp (exact) with respect to I_P, if the boundary region of X is empty.

4.1.2 Data reduction

If we manage to identify equivalence classes then some savings (reductions) are to be made since only one element of the equivalence class is needed to represent the entire equivalence class. An issue of practical importance in reduction is to keep only those attributes that preserve the indiscernibility relation and consequently, the set approximation. The rejected attributes are redundant (superfluous) since their removal cannot worsen the classification (Greco et al., 1998).

Let $\varnothing \neq P \subseteq Q$ and $a \in P$. Attribute a is superfluous in P if $I_P = I_{P-\{a\}}$.

For example, if $R = \{Age, BM\}$, $S = \{Age, SBP\}$, and $T = \{BM, SBP\}$ (Table 2), then it is obvious that $I_R = I_P$ and $I_S = I_P$ while $I_T \neq I_P$. This means that R and S are reducts of P, while T is not. The attribute Age is indispensable, but the attributes BM and SBP may be mutually exchanged. This means that it is enough to use reduct $\{Age, BM\}$ to estimate the value of the decision attribute SAD. In the analog case we can use the reduct $\{Age, SBP\}$ to estimate the value of decision attribute SAD, but we can not use the reduct $\{BM, SBP\}$.

The calculation of all reducts is very complex but in many practical applications it is not necessary to calculate all the reducts, but only some of them.

4.1.3 Discretization

If we want numerical attributes to be properly incorporated into the classification rules, we should to discretize them. This enables the numerical attributes to be treated as categorical ones, and several algorithms for this purpose are available (Greco et al., 1998; Øhrn, 1999). The goal of the discretization process is to search for intervals or bins, where all cases that fall within the same interval are grouped together. This process can be also seen as the process of classification of the attributes' value set to some classes. The discretization is not specific to the rough set approach but is a pre – required step and is often performed implicitly, behind the scene, using human expert knowledge.

4.1.4 Decision rules

The expression $a = v$, where a is an attribute and v is an attribute value is called the descriptor. Now, it is possible to investigate the rules of the form: *If α Then β*. Here α denotes a conjunction (AND logical operator) of descriptors that only involve attributes of some reduct (rule's antecedent) and β (rule's consequent) denote a descriptor $d = v$, where d is a decision attribute and v is the allowed decision value.

For example, if we use the reduct $R = \{Age, BM\}$ from Table 2 and SAD as a decision attribute, then it is possible to generate the rules with two descriptors in the antecedent part and one descriptor in the consequent part of the rule. It is important to notice that a shorter reduct set means shorter decision rules in the rule set generated from that reduct.

4.2 Application of rough-set theory in identification of patients at higher cardiovascular risk using SAD

Our results showed that SAD could be a clinically useful marker for identification of combination and structure of risk factors by applying different rules in individuals of different BMI-categories.

Lower values of SAD in normal-weight individuals younger than 50 years always corresponded with Framingham risk score <9. However, in normal-weight subjects older than 50 years, SAD couldn't identify those at lower risk. SAD values between 24.3 and 31.6 cm, or even lower, between 13.0 and 24.2 cm, corresponded with Framingham risk score between 9 and 14 (Table 3). It is in agreement with observations which indicate a centralization of adipose tissue with aging, irrespective of BMI. This would represent a category of metabolically obese normal weight individuals.

According to these results, measurement of SAD is not enough for identification of cardiovascular risk in normal-weight individuals. In that regard, it is necessary to include other methods of fat mass assessment, like CT or MRI.

					IF							THEN SAD (cm)
Age (years)	Body fat mass (%)	Systolic blood pressure (mmHg)	Diastolic blood pressure (mmHg)	Total cholesterol (mmol/L)	Triglycerides (mmol/L)	LDL-cholesterol (mmol/L)	HDL-cholesterol (mmol/L)	Glycaemia (mmol/L)	Fibrinogen (g/L)	Acidum uricum (µmol/L)	Framingham risk score	
<41	<28.92	<123	>88	<5.37	1.4-2.19	<3.24	1.01-1.21	<4.7	3.06-3.76	273-344	<9	
	<28.92	123-141	>88	>6.51	<1.4	<3.24	<1.01	4.7-5.4	>3.76	<273	<9	
41-50	<28.92	<123	78-88	<5.37	<1.4	3.24-4.0	<1.01	<4.7	<3.06	<273	<9	13.0-24.2
	<28.92	123-141	>88	<5.37	>2.19	<3.24	<1.01	4.7-5.4	>3.76	<273	<9	
	<28.92	<123	78-88	>6.51	1.4-2.19	>4.00	>1.21	>5.4	3.06-3.76	<273	<9	
>50	<28.93	123-141	>88	>6.51	>2.19	3.24-4.0	>1.21	4.7-5.4	3.06-3.76	273-344	9-14	13.0-24.2 OR 24.3-31.6

Table 3. Obtained rules for normal-weight subjects (BMI<26.43 kg/m²)

By examining the decision rules, SAD could point out a group of overweight patients with high level of visceral fat with different combination and composition of cardiovascular risk factors (Table 4). Thus, in overweight individuals aged 41-50 years, with higher fat mass, and SAD between 24.3 and 31.6 cm, we could expect higher values of diastolic blood pressure, total- and LDL-cholesterol, triglycerides, uric acid, as well as Framingham risk score over 14. The same range of SAD in older overweight individuals (>50 years) with higher fat mass, include higher systolic blood pressure, fasting plasma glucose and fibrinogen. On the other side, in younger overweight subjects with lower SAD (<24.3 cm) we could expect lower values of all atherogenic parameters, higher values of HDL-cholesterol and Framingham risk score <9, even if they have higher fat mass.

It means that SAD could identify metabolically healthy overweight individuals.

IF												THEN SAD (cm)
Age (years)	Body fat mass (%)	Systolic blood pressure (mmHg)	Diastolic blood pressure (mmHg)	Total cholesterol (mmol/L)	Triglycerides (mmol/L)	LDL-cholesterol (mmol/L)	HDL-cholesterol (mmol/L)	Glycaemia (mmol/L)	Fibrinogen (g/L)	Acidum uricum (μmol/L)	Framingham risk score	
<41	>39.71	<123	<78	<5.37	<1.4	<3.24	>1.21	4.7-5.4	>3.76	>344	<9	13.0-24.2
41-50	>39.71	<123	>88	>6.51	>2.19	<3.24	1.01-1.21	>5.4	>3.76	>344	9-14	13.0-24.2 OR 24.3-31.6
41-50	28.92-39.71	<123	>88	>6.51	<1.4	>4.0	1.01-1.21	<4.7	>3.76	>344	9-14	
>50	<28.92	123-141	>88	5.37-6.51	>2.19	<3.24	>1.21	4.7-5.4	>3.76	<273	9-14	
>50	<28.92	<123	78-88	>6.51	1.4-2.19	>4.00	1.01-1.21	>5.4	>3.76	273-344	9-14	
<41	<28.92	123-141	78-88	<5.37	<1.4	<3.24	>1.21	4.7-5.4	3.06-3.76	>344	<9	24.3-31.6
41-50	28.92-39.71	<123	>88	>6.51	>2.19	>4.00	1.01-1.21	4.7-5.4	<3.06	>344	>14	
41-50	>39.71	123-141	>88	>6.51	<1.4	>4.00	>1.21	<4.7	3.06-3.76	<273	9-14	
>50	28.92-39.71	>141	>88	>6.51	>2.19	>3.24	1.01-1.21	>5.4	3.06-3.76	273-344	9-14	
>50	28.92-39.71	>141	>88	>6.51	>2.19	>4.00	>1.21	<4.7	<3.06	<273	9-14	

Table 4. Obtained rules for overweight subjects (BMI: 26.43-32.52 kg/m²)

As it is displayed in the Table 5, SAD values above 31.7 cm in obese subjects always correspond to Framingham risk score >14. Younger obese individuals (<41 years) with lower values of SAD usually are at the lower cardiovascular risk (metabolically healthy obese individuals).

IF												THEN SAD (cm)
Age (years)	Body fat mass (%)	Systolic blood pressure (mmHg)	Diastolic blood pressure (mmHg)	Total cholesterol (mmol/L)	Triglycerides (mmol/L)	LDL-cholesterol (mmol/L)	HDL-cholesterol (mmol/L)	Glycaemia (mmol/L)	Fibrinogen (g/L)	Acidum uricum (μmol/L)	Framingham risk score	
	>39.71	<123	<78	<5.37	>2.19	<3.24	1.01-1.21	4.7-5.4	3.06-3.76	<273	<9	13.0-24.2
<41	>39.71	<123	>88	<5.37	<1.4	3.24-4.00	1.01-1.21	<4.7	3.06-3.76	>344		
	28.92-39.71	123-141	>88	>6.51	1.4-2.19	>4.00	>1.21	>5.4	>3.76	>344	>14	
41-50	>39.71	123-141	>88	>6.51	>2.19	3.24-4.00	>1.21	4.7-5.4	<3.06	>344	9-14	
<41	>39.71	<123	78-88	5.37-6.51	<1.4	>4.00	>1.21	4.7-5.4	>3.76	>344	<9	24.3-31.6
	>39.71	<123	<78	<5.37	<1.4	<3.24	<1.01	<4.7	3.06-3.76	<273		
	>39.71	123-141	>88	<5.37	<1.4	<3.24	>1.21	4.7-5.4	3.06-3.76	>344		
	>39.71	<123	<78	<5.37	<1.4	<3.24	<1.01	<4.7	3.06-3.76	<273		
	>39.71	123-141	>88	>6.51	1.4-2.19	3.24-4.00	<1.01	4.7-5.4	3.06-3.76	273-344	9-14	
>50	>39.71	123-141	78-88	5.37-6.51	1.4-2.19	<3.24	1.01-1.21	4.7-5.4	3.06-3.76	>344	>14	
41-50	>39.71	>141	>88	5.37-6.51	>2.19	3.24-4.00	<1.01	>5.4	3.06-3.76	273-344	>14	24.3-31.6 OR 31.7-36.2
>50	28.92-39.71	123-141	>88	>6.51	<1.4	3.24-4.00	>1.21	>5.4	>3.76	273-344	9-14	
<41	>39.71	123-141	78-88	>6.51	>2.19	3.24-4.00	<1.01	>5.4	>3.76	>344	>14	31.7-36.2
>50	>39.71	>141	>88	>6.51	>2.19	>4.00	>1.21	>5.4	>3.76	>344	>14	

Table 5. Obtained rules for obese subjects (BMI>32.52 kg/m²)

5. Conclusion

Many studies have proved that SAD is a good predictor of abdominal, especially visceral, fat mass, as well as of cardiometabolic risk. Several authors have suggested specific cut-off values for SAD that corresponded with cardiovascular and metabolic risk or with visceral fat area obtained by CT. Using the concept of a rough set, proved as a formal tool for modeling and processing information systems, we developed a useful model for identification of individuals with multiple cardiovascular risk factors using SAD.

Our results revealed connection between SAD and cardiovascular risk factors which showed dependence on age and nutrition level. We primarily recommend application of SAD in the assessment of the cardiovascular risk in overweight and obese individuals. SAD values ≥24.3 cm in overweight and obese subjects older than 41 years should correspond to increased risk, while values <24.3 cm in overweight subjects younger than 41 years could point to healthy metabolic profile.

6. References

Anjana, M.; Sandeep, S.; Deepa, R.; Vimaleswaran K.S.; Farooq, S. & Mohan, V. (2004). Visceral and central abdominal fat and anthropometry in relation to diabetes in Asian Indians. *Diabetes Care*, Vol.27, No.12, pp. 2948-2953

Ashwell, M. (2005). Waist to height ratio and the Ashwell shape chart could predict the health risks of obesity in adults and children in all ethnic groups. *Nutrition&Food Science*, Vol.35, No.5, pp. 359-64

Berg, A.H. & Scherer, P.E. (2005). Adipose tissue, inflammation, and cardiovascular disease. *Circulation Research*, Vol.96, pp. 939-949

Bosello, O. & Zamboni, M. (2000). Visceral obesity and metabolic syndrome. *Obesity Reviews*, Vol.1, pp. 47-56

Bouchard, C.; Bray, G.A. & Hubbard, V.S. (1990). Basic and clinical aspects of regional fat distribution. *American Journal of Clinical Nutrition*, Vol.52, pp.946-950

Brochu, M.; Starling, R.D.; Tchernof, A.; Matthews, D.E.; Garcia-Rubi, E. & Poehlman, E.T. (2000). Visceral adipose tissue is an independent correlate of glucose disposal in older obese postmenopausal women. *The Journal of Clinical Endocrinology & Metabolism*, Vol.85, pp. 2378-2384

Brtka, V.; Stokić, E. & Srdić, B. (2008). Automated extraction of decision rules for leptin dynamics--a rough sets approach, *Journal of Biomedical Informatics*, Vol.41, No.4, pp. 667-674

Carroll, J.F.; Chiapa, A.L.; Rodriquez, M.; Phelps, D.R.; Cardarelli, K.M.; Vishwanatha, J.K.; Bae, S. & Cardarelli, R. (2008). Visceral fat, waist circumference, and BMI: impact of race/ethnicity. *Obesity*, Vol.16, No.3, pp. 600–607

Coppack, S.W. (2005). Adipose tissue changes in obesity. *Biochemical Society Transactions*, Vol.33, pp. 1049-1052

Couillard, C.; Lamarche, B.; Tchernof, A.; Prud'homme, D.; Tremblay, A.; Bouchard, C.; Moorjani, S.; Nadeau, A.; Lupien, P.J. & Després J-P. (1996). Plasma high-density lipoprotein cholesterol but not apolipoproetin A-I is a good correlate of the visceral obesity-insulin resistance dyslipidemic syndrome. *Metabolism*, Vol.45, pp.882-888

Davidson, J. & Getz, M. (2004). Nutritional risk and body composition in free-living elderly participating in congregate meal-site programs. *Journal of Nutrition for the Elderly*, Vol.24, No.1, pp. 53-68

Desbriere, R.; Vuaroqueaux, V.; Achard, V.; Boullu-Ciocca, S. Labuhn, M.; Dutour, A. & Grino, M. (2006). 11β-Hydroxysteroid Dehydrogenase Type 1 mRNA is Increased in Both Visceral and Subcutaneous Adipose Tissue of Obese Patients. *Obesity*, Vol.14, pp. 794-798

Després, J-P.; Moorjani, S.; Lupien, P.J.; Tremblay, A.; Nadeau, A. & Bouchard C. (1990). Regional distribution of body fat, plasma lipoproteins, and cardiovascular disease. *Arteriosclerosis*, Vol.10, No.4, pp. 497-511

Després, J-P.; Prud'homme, D.; Pouiliot, M.C.; Tremblay, A. & Bouchard C. (1991). Estimation of deep abdominal adipose-tissue accumulation from simple anthropometric measurements in men. *American Journal of Clinical Nutrition*, Vol.54, pp. 471-477

Dorner, T.E. & Rieder, A. (2011). Obesity paradox in elderly patients with cardiovascular diseases. *International Journal of Cardiology*, doi: 10.1016/j.ijcard.2011.01.076

Duarte Pimentel, G.; Portero-McLellan, K.C.; Maestá, N.; Corrente, J.E. & Burini, R.C. (2010). Accuracy of SAD as predictor of abdominal fat among Brazilian adults: a comparation with waist circumference. *Nutrición hospitalaria*, Vol.25, No.4, pp. 656-661

Empana, J.P.; Ducimetiere, P.; Charles, M.A. & Jouven, X. (2004). SAD and risk of sudden death in asymptomatic middle-aged men – the Paris prospective study. *Circulation*, Vol.110, pp. 2781-2785

Freedland, E.S. (2004). Role of a critical visceral adipose tissue threshold (CVATT) in metabolic syndrome: implications for controlling dietary carbohydrates: a review. *Nutrition&Metabolism*, Vol.1, (November 2004), doi: 10.1 186/1743-7075-1-12

Goossens, G.H. (2008). The role of adipose tissue dysfunction in the pathogenesis of obesity-related insulin resistance. *Physiology&Behaviour*, Vol.94, pp. 206-218

Greco, M.; Benedetto, R.; Slowinski, R. (1998). New developments in the rough set approach to multi–attribute decision analysis, *Proceedings of 16th European Conference on Operational Research*, Brussels, July 1998

Greenlund, LJ.S. & Nair K.S. (2003). Sarcopenia – consequences, mechanisms, and potential therapies. *Mechanisms of Aging and Development*, Vol.124, pp. 287-299

Gustat, J., Elkasabany, A., Srinivasan, S. & Berenson, G.S. (2000). Relation of abdominal height to cardiovascular risk factors in young adults. *American Journal of Epidemiology*, Vol.151, No.9, pp. 885-891

Guzzaloni, G.; Minocci, A.; Marzullo, P. & Liuzzi, A. (2009). SAD is more predictive of cardiovascular risk than abdominal fat compartments in severe obesity. *International Journal of Obesity*, Vol.33, pp. 233-238

Harris, T.B.; Visser, M ; Everhart, J.; Caulcy, J.; Tylavsky, F., Fuerst, T.; Zamboni, M.; Taatte, D.; Resnick, H.E.; Scherzinger, A. & Nevitt, M. (2000). Waist circumference and sagittal diameter reflect total body fat better than visceral fat in older men and women. The Health, Aging and Body Composition Study. *Annals of the New York Academy of Sciences*, Vol.904, pp. 462-473

Hoenig, M.R. (2010). MRI sagittal diameter is a stronger predictor of metabolic syndrome than visceral fat area or waist circumference in a high-risk vascular cohort. *Vascular Health and Risk Management*, Vol.6, pp. 629-633.

Hsieh, S.D. & Yoshinaga, H. (1995). Abdominal fat distribution and coronary heart disease risk factors in men – waist/height ratio as a simple and useful predictor. *International Journal of Obesity and Related Metabolic Disorders*, Vol.19, pp. 585-589

Hwu, C.M.; Hsiao, C.F.; Sheu, W.H.H.; Pei, D.; Tai, T.Y.; Quertermous, T.; Rodriguez, B.; Pratt, R.; Chen, Y.DI, Ho, L.T. (2003). SAD is associated with insulin sensitivity in Chinese hypertensive patients and their siblings. *Journal of Human Hypertension*, Vol.17, pp. 193-198

Iribarren, C.; Darbinian, J.A.; Lo, J.C.; Fireman, B.H. & Go, A.S. (2006). Value of the SAD in coronary heart disease risk assessment: cohort study in a large, multiethnic population. *American Journal of Epidemiology*, Vol.164, No.12, pp. 1150–1159

Iribarren, C.; Sharp, D.S.; Burchfiel, D.M. & Petrovich, H. (1995). Association of weight loss and weight fluctuation with mortality among Japanese men. *New England Journal of Medicine*, Vol.333, pp. 686-692

Kahn, H.S. (1993). Choosing an index for abdominal obesity: an opportunity for epidemilogical clarification. *Journal of Clinical Epidemiology*, Vol.46, pp. 491-494

Krotkiewski, M.; Björntorp, P.; Sjöström, L. & Smith, U. (1983). Impact of obesity on metabolism in men and women. Importance of regional adipose tissue distribution. *Journal of Clinical Investigation*, Vol.72, pp. 1150-1162

Kumlin, L.; Dimberg, L. & Mårin, P. (1997). Ratio of abdominal sagittal diameter to heigh is strong indicator of coronary risk (letter). *British Medical Journal*, Vol.314, p. 830

Kvist, H.; Chowdhury, B.; Grangard, U.; Tylen, U. & Sjostrom L. (1988). Total and visceral-adipose tissue volumes derived from measurements with computed tomography in adults man and women: predictive equations. *American Journal of Clinical Nutrition*, Vol.48, No.6, pp. 1351-1361

Lemieux, S.; Prud'homme, D.; Bouchard, C.; Tremblay, A. & Despres, A. (1996). A single threshold value of waist girth identifies normal-weight and overweight subjects with excess visceral adipose tissue. *American Journal of Clinical Nutrition*, Vol.64, pp.685-693

Lofgren, I.; Herron, K.; Zern, T.; West, K.; Partalay, M.; Shachter, N.S.; Koo, S.I. & Fernandez, M.L. (2004). Waist circumference is a better predictor than body mass index of coronary heart disease risk in overweight premenopausal women. *Journal of Nutrition*, Vol.134, pp. 1071–1076

Lonnqvist, F.; Thorne, A.; Large, V. & Arner, P. (1995). Sex differences in visceral fat lipolysis and metabolic complications of obesity. *Atherosclerosis, Thrombosis, and Vascular Biology*, Vol.17, No.7, pp. 1472-1480

Marques-Vidal, P.; Chiolero, A. & Paccaud, F. (2008). Large differences in the prevalence of normal weight obesity using various cut-offsfor excess body fat. *e-SPAN, the European e-Journal of Clinical Nutrition and Metabolism*, Vol.3, pp. e159-e162

Matsuzawa, Y.; Shimomura, I.; Nakamura, T.; Keno, Y.; Kotani, K. & Tokunaga, K. (1995). Pathophysiology and pathogenesis of visceral fat obesity. *Obesity Research*, Vol.3, No.2, pp.187-194S.

Mazzali, G.; Di Francesco, V.; Zoico, E.; Fantin, F.; Zamboni, G.; Benati, C.; Bambara, V.; Negri, M.; Bosello, O. & Zamboni M. (2006). Interrelations between fat distribution, muscle lipid content, adipocytokines, and insulin resistance: effect of moderate weight loss in older women. *American Journal of Clinical Nutrition*, Vol.84, No.5, pp. 1193-1199

Misra, A. & Vikram, N.K. (2003). Clinical and patophysiological consequences of abdominal adiposity and abdominal adipose tissue depots. *Nutrition*, Vol.19, pp. 457-66

Molarius, A. & Seidell, J.C. (1998). Selection of anthropometric indicators for classification of abdominal fatness: A critical review. *International Journal of Obesity and Related Metabolic Disorders*, Vol.22, No.8, pp. 719-727

Movsesyan, L.; Tanko, L.B.; Larsen, P.J.; Christiansen, C. & Svendsen, O.L. (2003). Variations in percentage of body fat within different BMI groups in young, middle-aged and old women. *Clinical Physiology and Funcional Imaging*, Vol.23, pp.130-133

Mukuddem-Petersen, J.; Snijder, M.B.; van Dam, R.B.; Dekker, J.M.; Bouter, L.M.; Stehouwer, C.D.A.; Heine, R.J.; Nijpels, G. & Seidell, J.C. (2004). SAD: no advantage compared with other anthropometric measures as a correlate of components of the metabolic syndrome in elderly from the Hoorn Study. *American Journal of Clinical Nutrition*, Vol.84, pp.995-1002

Nakata, K.; Choo, J.; Hopson, M.S.J.; Ueshima, H.; Curb, D.; Shin, C.; Evans, R.W.; Kadowaki, T.; Otake, T.; Kadota, A.; Kadowaki, S.; Miura, K.; El-Saed, A.; Edmudowicz, D.; Sutton-Tyrell, K.; Kuller, L.H. & Sekikawa, A. (2010). Stronger associations of SAD with atherogenic lipoprotein subfractions than waist circumference in middle-aged US white and Japanese men. *Metabolism Clinical and Experimental*, Vol.59, pp.1742-1751

Øhrn, A. (1999). Discernibility and Rough Sets in Medicine: Tools and Applications. PhD thesis. Department of Computer and Information Science (Norwegian University of Science and Technology, Trondheim, Norway)

Öhrvall, M.; Berglund, L. & Vessby, B. (2000). SAD compared with other anthropometric measurements in relation to cardiovasular risk. *International Journal of Obesity and Related Metabolic Disorders*, Vol.24, No.4, pp.497-501.

Paolini, J.B.; Mancini, J.; Genestal, M.; Gonzalez, H.; McKay, R.E.; Samii, K. & Fourcade, O.A. (2010). Predictive value of abdominal obesity vs. body mass index for determining risk of intensive care unit mortality. *Critical Care Medicine*, Vol.38, No. 5, pp. 1308-1314

Pawlak, Z. & Skowron, A. (2007). Rudiments of rough sets. *An International Journal of Information Sciences*, Vol.177, pp. 3–27

Pawlak, Z.; Grzymala-Busse, J.; Slowinski, R. & Ziarko, W. (1995). Rough sets. *Communications of the ACM*, Vol.38, No.11, pp. 89–95R.

Petersson, H.; Daryani, A. & Risérus, U. (2007). SAD as a marker of inflammation and insulin resistance among immigrant women from the Middle East and native Swedish women: a cross-sectional study. *Cardiovascular Diabetology*, Vol.6, pp. 10.

Pouliot, M.C.; Despres, J.P.; Lemieux, S., Mourjani, S.; Bouchard, C. & Tremblay, A. (1994). Waist circumference and abdominal sagittal diameter: best simple anthropometric indexes of abdominal visceral adipose tissue accumulation and related cardiovascular risk in men and women. *American Journal of Cardiology*, Vol.73, No.7, pp. 460-468

Prentice, A.M. & Jebb, S.A. (2001). Beyond body mass index. Obesity Reviews, *Vol.2, No.3, pp. 141-147*

Reed, D.; Dwyer, K.M. & Dwyer, J.H.; (2003). Abdominal obesity and carotid artery wall thickness. The Los Angeles Atherosclerosis Study. *International Journal of Obesity and Related Metabolic Disorders*, Vol.27, pp. 1546-1551

Richelsen, B. & Pedersen, S.B. (1995). Associations between different anthropometric measurements of fatness and metabolic risk parameters in non-obese, healthy, middle-aged men. *International Journal of Obesity*, Vol.19, No.3, pp. 169-174

Risérus, U.; Ärnlöv, J.; Brismar, K.; Zethelius, B.; Berglund, L. & Vessby, B. (2004). SAD is a strong anthropometric marker of insulin resistance and hyperinsulinemia in obese men. *Diabetes Care*, Vol.27, No.8, pp. 2041-2046

Risérus, U.; de Faire, U.; Berglund, L. & Hellénius, M.L. (2010). SAD as a screening tool in clinical research: cutoffs for cardiometabolic risk. *Journal of Obesity*, doi:10.1155/2010/757939

Romero-Corral, A.; Montori, V.M.; Somers, V.K.; Korinek, J.; Thomas, R.J.; Allison, T.G.; Mookadam, F. & Lopez-Jimenez, F. (2006). Association of bodyweight with total mortality and with cardiovascular events in coronary artery disease: a systematic review of cohort studies. *Lancet*, Vol.368, No.9536, pp.666-678

Ruderman, N.; Chisholm, D., Pi-Sunyer, X. & Schenider, S. (1998). The metabolically obese, normal-weight individual revisited. *Diabetes*, Vol.47, pp.699-713

Sampaio, L.R.; Simões, E.J.; Assis, A.M.O. & Ramos, L.R. (2007). Validity and reliability of the SAD as a predictor of visceral abdominal fat. *Arquivos Brasileiros de Endocrinologia & Metabologia*, Vol.51, No.6, pp. 980-986

Sims, E.A. (2001). Are there persons who are obese, but metabolically healthy? *Metabolism*, Vol.50, pp. 1499-1504

Sjöstrom, L. (1994). The sagittal diameter is valid marker of visceral adipose tissue. *International Journal of Obesity*, Vol.18, No.2, pp. 46-52

Smith, D.A.; Ness, E.M.; Herbert, R.; Schechter, C.B.; Phillips, R.A.; Diamond, J.A. & Landrigan, P.J. (2005). Abdominal diameter index: a more powerful anthropometric measure for prevalent coronary heart disease risk in adult males. *Diabetes, Obesity and Metabolism*, Vol.7, pp.370-380.

Snijder, M.B.; Visser, M.; Dekker, J.M.; Seidell, J.C.; Fuerst, T.; Tylavsky, F.; Cauley, J.; Lang, T.; Nevitt, M. & Harris, T.B. (2002). The prediction of visceral fat by dual-energy X-ray absorptiometry in the elderly: a comparison with computed tomography and anthropometry. *International Journal of Obesity*, Vol.26, pp. 984-993

Stokić, E. & Ivković-Lazar, T. (1996). Relation between the abdominal sagittal diameter, fat tissue distribution and metabolic complications. *Medicinski Pregled*, Vol.49, No. 9-10, pp. 365-368

Stokić, E.; Brtka, V. & Srdić, B. (2010). The synthesis of the rough set model for the better applicability of SAD in identifying high risk patients. *Computers in Biology and Medicine*, Vol. 40, pp. 786-90

Stokić, E.; Đureković-Katona, A. & Ivković-Lazar, T. (1996). The role and significance of SAD in the determination of adipose tissue distribution. *Medicinski Pregled*, Vol.49, No.5-6, pp. 217-220

Strazzullo, P.; Barba, G.; Cappuccio, F.P.; Siani, A.; Trevisan, M.; Farinaro, E.; Pagano, E.; Barbato, A.; Iacone, R. & Galletti, F. (2001). Altered renal sodium handling in men with abdominal adiposity: a link to hypertension. *Journal of Hypertension*, Vol.19, No.12, pp. 2157-2164.

Toth, M.J.; Tchernof, A.; Sites, C.K. & Poehlman, E.T. (2000). Effect of menopausal status on body composition and abdominal fat distribution. *International Journal of Obesity*, Vol.24, pp. 226-231

Turcato, E.; Bosello, O.; Di Francesco, V.; Harris, T.B.; Zoico, E.; Bissolo, L; Fracassi, E. & Zamboni, M. (2000). Waist circumference and abdominal sagittal diameter as surogates of body fat distribution in the elderly: their relation with cardiovascular risk factors. *International Journal of Obesity*, Vol.24, pp. 1005-1010

Valdez, R. (1991). A simple model-based index of abdominal adiposity. *Journal of Clinical Epidemiology*, Vol.44, pp. 955-956

Valsamakis, G.; Chetty, R.; Anwart, A.; Banerjee, A.K.; Barnett, A. & Kumar, S. (2004). Association of simple anthropometric measures of obesity with visceral fat and the metabolic syndrome in male Caucasion and Indo-Asian subjects. *Diabetic Medicine*, Vol.21, pp. 1339-1345

Valsamakis, G.; Jones, A.; Chetty, R.; McTernan,P.G.; Boutsiadis, A.; Barnett, A.H.; Banerjee, A.K. & Kumar, S. (2008). MRI total SAD as a predictor of metabolic syndrome compared to visceral fat at L4-L5 level. *Current Medical Research&Opinion*, Vol.28, pp. 1853-1860

van der Kooy, K.; Leenen, R.; Seidell, J.C.; Deurenberg, P. & Visser M. (1993). Abdominal diameters as indicators of visceral fat: comparison between magnetic resonance imaging and anthropometry. *British Journal of Nutrition*, Vol.70, No.1, pp. 47-58

van Harmelen, V.; Röhrig, K. & Hauner, H. (2004). Comparison of proliferation and differentation capacity of human adipocyte precursor cells from the omental and subcutaneous adipose tissue depot of obese subjects. *Metabolism*, Vol.53, No.5, pp.632-7

van Herpen, N.A, & Schrauwen-Hinderling, V.B. (2008). Lipid accumulation in non-adipose tissue and lipotoxicity. *Physiology&Behaviour*, Vol.94, pp. 231-41

Vasques, A.C.; Rosado, L.E.; Rosado, G.P.; Ribeiro R. de C.; Franceschini S. do C.; Geloneze, B.; Priore, S.E. & Oliveira, D.R. (2009a). Predictive ability of anthropometric and body composition indicators in the identification of insulin resistance. *Arquivos Brasileiros de Endocrinologia & Metabologia*, Vol.53, No.1, pp.72-79

Vasques, A.C.; Rosado, L.E.; Rosado, G.P.; Ribeiro R. de C.; Franceschini, S. do C.; Geloneze, B.; Priore, S.E. & Oliveira, D.R. (2009b). Different measurements of the SAD and waist perimeter in the prediction of HOMA-IR. *Arquivos Brasileiros de Endocrinologia & Metabologia*, Vol.93, No.5, pp. 511-518

Visscher, T.I.; Seidell, J.C.; Molarius, A.; van der Kuip, D.; Hofman, A. & Witteman, J.C. (2001). A comparison of body mass index, waist-hip ratio and waist circumference as predictors of all-cause mortality among the elderly: the Rotterdam study. *International Journal of Obesity and Related Metabolic Disorders*, Vol.25, No.11, pp. 1730–1735

Wajchenberg, B.L. (2000). Subcutaneous and visceral adipose tissue: their relation to the metabolic syndrome. *Endocrine Reviews*, Vol.21, No.6, pp. 697-738

Yim, J.Y.; Kim, D.; Lim, S.H.; Park, M.J.; Choi, S.H.; Lee, C.H.; Kim, S.S. & Cho, S.H. (2010). SAD is a strong anthropometric measure of visceral adipose tissue in the Asian general population. *Diabetes Care*, Vol.33, No.12, pp. 2665-2670

Zamboni, M.; Turcato, E.; Armellini, F.; Kahn, H.S.; Zivelonghi, A.; Santana, H.; Bergamo-
    Andreis, I.A. & Bosello, O. (1998). SAD as a practical predictor of visceral fat.
    Interantional Journal of Obesity, Vol.22, pp. 655-660

3

The Assessment of Prevalence of Hypertension as Cardiovascular Risk Factors Among Adult Population

Aida Pilav
Federal Ministry of Health,
Faculty of Health Studies, University of Sarajevo,
Bosnia and Herzegovina

1. Introduction

Significant increase in noncommunicable diseases, in particular cardiovascular disease, in the past few decades worldwide represents one of the major health challenges in the overall global and social development of society. Cardiovascular conditions have the highest impact on lost years of life, lost quality of life, but also on the differences in longevity in different population groups. Global statistics show that cardiovascular conditions are responsible for one third of global deaths, while coronary heart conditions are the leading cause of death worldwide. (1,2) Many population research studies corroborated that high blood pressure is an independent and significant risk factor of cardiovascular disease and coronary heart disease and most significant determinant of morbidity and mortality in developed countries. (2,3)

Constant increase in morbidity and mortality caused by cardiovascular disease, in particular high blood pressure as one of the most significant public health problem, evaluation of prevalence of high blood pressure and evaluation of control of high blood pressure in the population, including the distribution of cardiovascular risk factors altogether represent the basis for the modeling of an integrated risk and disease prevention program – an integrated management of hypertension in the community (4), which is effectively a step further in providing efficient, effective and high-quality health care.

Globally health care is becoming more complex and more expensive and countries are now faced with various problems that need to be addressed in order to ensure sustainability of their health care systems. With the advance in technology, clinical treatment is also becoming more complex and more expensive so that countries are now more and more focused on preventive programs and controls of conditions which entail less direct costs. Key argument for introduction of preventive public health programs is that such programs have much bigger potential for long-term improvement of the population's health status and also involve much lower costs than clinical medicine. (1,3)

2. Cardiovascular diseases and leading risk factors

A number of research studies clearly showed that cardiovascular disease can be attributed to unhealthy life styles and poor social and physical environment. Unhealthy diet, smoking, physical inactivity and psychosocial stress are the leading risk factors for cardiovascular disease, as well as consequential manifestations of such life styles: hypertension, glucose intolerance and hyperlipidemia. These risk factors also reflect major preventable health problems. (5-12))

In the world the issue of cardiovascular disease became very pressing in early 1970s. At that time many health intervention program were planned at the level of the community and their purpose was to promote health and reduce detrimental life style changes. The basic starting premise was that the use of measures to reduce risk factors in population with clinically identified risk factors has only a limited effect on prevention of cardiovascular risk factor at the national level; on the other hand, global public health actions have more effects altogether.

The first implemented program that was based on these ideas was the North Karelia Project carried out in Finland in 1972. This project achieved significant results, in particularly through the hypertension control programs. It started off as a pilot but after significant net reductions in both risk factors and cardiovascular disease-caused mortality rate, the project was rolled out to the national level. Over the next 25 years, smoking prevalence in men was significantly reduced and so was serum cholesterol and blood pressure levels. Over this period, mortality rate caused by cardiovascular disease in men aged 35-64 years dropped by 68%, coronary heart disease mortality rate by 73%, cancer mortality rate by 44%, and mortality rate for all samples effectively dropped by 49%. (13-15)

Building on this success, many projects have been implemented since then in the form of demonstrational projects under different WHO programs: CINDI (WHO/EURO), CARMEN (WHO/AMRO), and INTERHEALTH (WHO/HQ). Apart from clinical trials, all these projects involved different design, intervention approach, method, intensity, goals in reducing the risk factors, evaluation measurements and timeline. Major role of projects implemented in community is to demonstrate and stimulate health policies of non-contagious disease prevention. (16)

In their recommendations for 2003, the WHO and the International Society of Hypertension (ISH) defined three sets of risk factors required for monitoring in management of hypertension. *(Table 1.)* (28)

Based on this, a stratification of overall cardiovascular risk factors was provided. Three major risk categories - low, medium and high risk - were calibrated to effectively indicate absolute likelihood of developing a cardiovascular disease in the next 10 years as follows: (1) low risk – less then 15%; (2) medium risk – 15-20%; and (3) high risk – over 20%. *(Table 2.)*

3. Hypertension as a cardiovascular risk factor

Nearly 1 billion of people worldwide are suffering from hypertension. Population research studies showed that 15-37% of adult global population is stricken by hypertension. The WHO statistics in 2002 showed that hypertension is the third leading cause of the global burden of disease. Untreated and non-controlled hypertension as highly prevalent risk factor for cardiovascular disease results in cerebrovascular accidents, myocardial infarction, heart failure and dementia, kidney failure and blindness. (2,3,4).

Cardiovascular disease risk factors	Target organ damage (TOD)	Associated clinical condition (ACC)
1. SBP/DBP values (level 1-3) 2. Man > aged 55 years 3. Women > aged 65 years 4. Smoking 5. Total cholesterol > 6.1 mmol/l or LDL - cholesterol > 4.0 mmol/l 6. HDL - cholesterol Males < 1.0 mmol/l Females < 1.2 mmol/l 7. History of cardiovascular disease in the first degree relatives before the age of 50 8. Obesity, physical inactivity	1. Left ventricular hypertrophy 2. Microalbuminuria (20-300 mg/daily) 3. Radiological or ultrasound evidenced extensive atherosclerotic plaque (aorta, carotids, coronary, iliac or femoral arteries) 4. Grade 3 or 4 hypertensive retinopathy	1. Diabetes mellitus 2. Cerebrovascular conditions: • Stroke • Cerebral hemorrhage • Transitory ishemic attack (TIA) • Heart disease • Myocardial infarction • Angina pectoris • Coronary revascularization • Congestive coronary insufficiency 3. Kidney diseases • Plasma creatinine concentrations • Females > 1.4 mg/dl • Males > 1.5mg/dl (120, 133 μmol/l) • Albuminuria >300mg/dnevno 4. Peripheral arterial disease

Source: 2003 World Health Organization (WHO)/International Society of Hypertension (ISH) statement on management of hypertension

Table 1. Risk factors required for monitoring in hypertension management

Other risks and history of disease	Blood pressure (mmHg)		
	Grade 1 mild hypertension SBP 140-159 or DBP 90-99	Grade 2 medium hypertension SBP 160-179 or DBP 100-109	Grade 3 severe hypertension SBP ≥180 or DBP ≥110
No other risk factors	LOW	MEDIUM	HIGH
1-2 risk factors	MEDIUM	MEDIUM	HIGH
3 or more risk factors or damaged target organs or diabetes mellitus	HIGH	HIGH	HIGH

Source: 2003 World Health Organization (WHO)/International Society of Hypertension (ISH) statement on management of hypertension

Table 2. Stratification of risk in quantification of prognosis

Hypertension is estimated to cause 7.1 million of deaths worldwide or roughly 13% of total global morality. Significance of high blood pressure is becoming increasingly higher when it comes to disability caused by stroke and coronary ischemia, which expressed in DALY (Disability-Adjusted Life Year) that is 64.3 million DALYs of lost life or 4.5% of the total burden of disease. Each year globally there are 12 million fatal and approximately 20 million non-fatal myocardial infarctions, mostly in developing countries. Research showed that treated hypertension reduces risk of cerebrovascular accidents by 40% and risk of myocardial infarctions by 15%. (2,3,4)

Even with extensive knowledge about the pathophysiology and the epidemiology of hypertension, simple diagnostics, availability of efficient drugs, hypertension still has high prevalence and as a result introduction of an effective hypertension control represents considerable public health challenge. (18,19) Public health systems worldwide continue to cope with inadequate management of hypertension and there is a need to ensure constant improvement of management by health professionals in order to make sure that at least two thirds of treated patients suffering from hypertension reach adequate control of blood pressure.

In doing so it is necessary to perform control of major risk factors, such as smoking, obesity, increased total serum cholesterol and diabetes mellitus. (18,19) All this creates necessary prerequisites for setting up different methods of controlling hypertension that basically prevent continuation of costly cycle of clinical management of hypertension and the related complications.

Definitions of hypertension, in particular in public health sense, are essentially pragmatic. They can be used and they were also defined to characterize a group of individuals who potentially may benefit from specific treatment regimes – non-pharmacological and pharmacological. Definition of hypertension which is more then 30 years old and which says that "*Hypertension should be defined as the level of blood pressure which requires investigation and treatment to improve the condition*" indicates that any numerical definition and categorization should be flexible and based on evidenced risk and availability of effective and well-tolerated drugs. (20-24) Also clinically used definitions are rather arbitrary because of the nature of blood pressure distribution in the population. (25-27) Researchers have long discussed about threshold values of high blood pressure in different populations, in particular those threshold values that warrant therapeutic interventions. There is also variability in deciding the threshold values for evaluation of cardiovascular disease risk factor in individuals.

Problem-based approach to hypertension is twofold: (i) it is described as a separate clinical entity/condition and is classified as a prevalent cardiovascular disease. Also hypertension is a very important factor in development of morbidity and mortality that are caused by cardiovascular disease; or (ii) it is described as intermediary (biological) factor in development of cardiovascular disease and conditions of circulatory system. In both cases hypertension is recognized as "an entry point" for the management of cardiovascular disease.

The World Health Organization/International Society of Hypertension issued in 1999 and 2003 guides for the management (diagnostics and treatment) of hypertension. The European Society of Hypertension (ESH) and the European Society of Cardiology (ESC) did not develop their own guides but simply endorsed the WHO/ISH guides. As the number of population research studies and clinical trials in Europe increased and their results brought to light the new evidence, the European Society of Hypertension and the European Society of Cardiology developed for the first time in 2003 their own guides for the management of hypertension as a response to a suggestion by the WHO/ISH that regional experts should develop recommendations for the management of the disease based on regional conditions, depending on the degree of their health care and health care availability and their economic resources. (25) In 2007 these guides were updated based on the new clinical evidence. (28) As a result, a classification of blood pressure levels was made on the basis of the adopted definitions.(Table 3.)

Category*	Systolic pressure	Diastolic pressure
Optimal blood pressure	<120	<80
Normal blood pressure	120-129	80-84
High normal blood pressure	130-139	85-89
Grade 1 hypertension – mild	140-159	90-99
Grade 2 hypertension – medium	160-179	100-109
Grade 3 hypertension – severe	≥180	≥110
Isolated systolic hypertension	≥140	<90

Isolated systolic hypertension should be graded (1,2,3) according to systolic blood pressure values in the ranges indicated, provided that diastolic values are < 90mmHg. Grades 1, 2 and 3 correspond to classification in mild, moderate and severe hypertension, respectively. These terms have been now omitted to avoid confusion with quantification of total cardiovascular risk.

Source: 2007 Guidelines for the Management of Arterial Hypertension. The Task Force for the Management of Arterial Hypertension of the European Society of Hypertension (ESH) and of the European Society of Cardiology (ESC)

Table 3. Definitions and classification of blood pressure levels (mmHg)

4. Situational analysis in the Federation of Bosnia and Herzegovina

The Federation of Bosnia and Herzegovina is a part of Bosnia and Herzegovina. In April 1992, Bosnia and Herzegovina was internationally recognised as a new independent country and became a member of the United Nations. War broke out in 1992 and ended with the signing of the Dayton Peace agreement in December 1995. The Peace Agreement established Bosnia and Herzegovina as a country of two entities and one district - the Federation of Bosnia and Herzegovina, Republika Srpska and District Brcko. The war 1992-1995 caused drastically demographic and epidemiological changes in Bosnia and Herzegovina. (29,30)

The Federation of Bosnia and Herzegovina is currently going through a period of considerable political and economical transition which altogether has evident implications on the population's health status. Changed lifestyles are result of transitional socioeconomic changes. Over the past two decades health reports have constantly showed high mortality and morbidity rates for noncommunicable diseases, in particular cardiovascular disease.

Hospital discharge rate statistics for these diseases is not analyzed at the Federation of Bosnia and Herzegovina level. (32)

As the Federation of Bosnia and Herzegovina is currently going through a strong transitional and reform period of its socioeconomic development, its health system should be responsive to health and social needs of its population, especially at times when such needs turbulently change. Health system of the Federation of Bosnia and Herzegovina should be flexible and prompt to provide adequate and timely response to demographical and social changes, changes in epidemiological patterns of diseases, expectations of health care users for quality and their role in decision-making, inequity in health care system, and scientific an technological progress. (32,33)

According to the official statistics of the Federation BiH Statistics Office, population of the Federation of Bosnia and Herzegovina in 2009 reached 2,327,318 with average population density at 89 people per square kilometer. Population of the Federation of Bosnia and Herzegovina falls under the category of stationary/regressive population with 14% of people over 65+ years of age. In the overall structure of the population, female population accounts for 51%. (34) According to the World Health Organization (WHO) estimates, life expectancy at birth for males is 73 and for female 78.

The Federation of Bosnia and Herzegovina hypertension morbidity rate reported for 2009 was almost 12% increase compared to the time before 1992 when practically started the period of strong political and socio-economic transition. The hypertension morbidity rates are not reliable, primary as a result of inconsistency of the health statistics system. Statistics available on morbidity rates originate from the primary health care and as such they are simply tip of an iceberg. In fact the statistics is based on the patient-requested health care, not on actual health needs of population. Assessment of actual health needs of the population requires additional sensitive research, such as cross-sectional research population studies. (31) This was the original idea in designing this particular research and assessment of the health needs. (30)

In recent years, there have been several isolated population research studies in tthe Federation of Bosnia and Herzegovina which used different samples. Findings of one such study based on the CINDI methodology showed that unhealthy life habits have slightly increased in the population as a result of exposure to bad life habits such as smoking, unhealthy diet, physical inactivity, etc). (35) Wider public health implications of growingly unhealthy lifestyles are reflected in increased morbidity rates for chronic conditions and early disability, in particular those caused by cardiovascular disease. Statistics on awareness, treatment and control of hypertension in adult population of the Federation of Bosnia and Herzegovina are completely unreliable.

5. The case study

In order to effectively evaluate the prevalence of cardiovascular risk factors (overweight and obesity, smoking, history of hypercholesterolemia and diabetes mellitus) and also blood pressure values, a cross-sectional population study was carried out in the Federation of Bosnia and Herzegovina on a sample of adult population (aged 25-64 years), which was representative for the Federation of Bosnia and Herzegovina. (30)

The households were selected using the random sample method, following the survey conducted in the field. From each household one individual aged 25 to 64 years was selected. Stratified sampling allowed inclusion of both urban and rural areas within the selected municipalities.

Original size of the sample was 3,020 households/respondents, which is effectively the internationally recommended sample size for evaluation of noncommunicable diseases risk factors in adult population. The survey was carried out in the autumn of 2002. Compared to the original sample (3,020 people), response rate was very high (91.5 %). Female respondents made 59 % of the total sample.

Methodology of the survey fully complied with the international recommendations for survey protocol. (36-39) The survey involved interviews with and physicals measurements of individual respondents in their homes. The physicals measurements actually included blood pressure measurements.

Hypertension awareness in the respondents was evaluated through a question listed on the survey questionnaire about whether the respondents being informed on high blood pressure by health professionals.

Drug treatment of hypertension was evaluated by another question listed on the survey questionnaire. The term "treated" included the respondents who at that point were using antihypertensive drugs.

Control of hypertension was evaluated by the question on awareness of their hypertension, use of antihypertensive drugs and measured value of blood pressure.

The survey used a criterion for evaluation of hypertension prevalence which is normally used in population research studies. This criterion was based on the blood pressure threshold values and values of actual treatment by antihypertensive drugs. The respondents were hypertensive if they were using antihypertensive drugs and/or if their systolic blood pressure (SBP) was ≥ 140 mmHg and/or diastolic blood pressure (DBP) was ≥ 90 mmHg.

In addition to the above definitions, the research study also used the WHO/ISH definitions which categorize hypertension into three grades: mild, medium and severe. Following these definitions, **mild hypertension** included respondents who reported SBP of 140-159 mmHg and/or DBP of 90-99 mmHg; **medim hypertension** included respondents who reported SBP of 160-179 mmHg and/or DBP of 100-109 mmHg; and **severe hypertension** included respondents who reported SBP of > 180 mmHg and/or DBP of > 110mmHg. *(see Table 3)*

Limitation of the survey is reflected in the categorization of hypertensive respondents based on one off blood pressure measurement, which in fact may lead to overrated hypertension levels, especially in patients who reported threshold values of SBP of 140mmHg and/or DBP of 90mmHg.

Although cross-sectional research studies are not ideal tools for evaluation, they are necessary to obtain information about individuals who have no contact with health professionals in health care institution, individuals who are not aware of their hypertension, level of treatment and control of hypertension in different countries. Description of blood pressure patterns in the population and the underlying trends classified by age, sex, education and other socioeconomic variables, actually allows development of strategies for reduction of morbidity and mortality caused by high blood pressure.

5.1 Blood pressure

Mean value of SBP was under 140 mmHg, while the DBP mean value was above 80 mmHg in both male and female respondents. Reported values were higher in female respondents.

Age and gender structure showed that the lowest percentage of the respondents was from the youngest age group 25-34 years, males in particular. The highest number of respondents was from the age group 35-44 years, which proportionally included the highest number of females and males. *(See Figure 1.)*

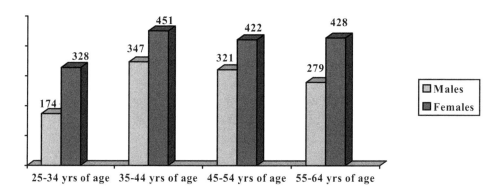

Fig. 1. Number of respondents by age and gender

$$\chi^2(3)=12.5, p<.006$$

Mean value of SBP in male respondents was 132 mmHg and in female respondents it was 135 mmHg. The difference was statistically significant (p < 0.001) *(See Table 4.)*. Mean value of DBP was 84 mmHg in both genders. As with the SBP, mean value of DBP also increased with the age of the respondents.

5.2 Prevalence of hypertension

Following the definition of hypertension whereby the respondents were hypertensive if they were using antihypertensive drugs and/or if their SBP was ≥ 140 mmHg and/or DBP was ≥ 90 mmHg. Total of 41% respondents were hypertensive *(Table 5.)*

Prevalence of hypertension was 36% in male and 45% in female respondents. Proportion of the respondents with hypertension statistically increased to a significant degree in both female and male respondents (p < 0.0001), but slightly higher in female respondents in elderly age group (aged 45 to 64 years). *(See Table 6.)*.

In addition to the above definitions, as already mentioned, the research study also used the WHO/ISH definitions which categorize hypertension into three grades: mild, medium and severe. Following these definitions, **mild hypertension** included respondents who reported

SBP of 140-159 mmHg and/or DBP of 90-99 mmHg; m**edim hypertension** included respondents who reported SBP of 160-179 mmHg and/or DBP of 100-109 mmHg; and **severe hypertension** included respondents who reported SBP of > 180 mmHg and/or DBP of > 110mmHg. *(See Table 3.)*

Age (years)	Males			Females		
	Mean value	(SD)	N	Mean value	(SD)	N
Systolic blood pressure						
25-34	124	(10.8)	172	119	(12.8)	325
35-44	128	(13.2)	346	126	(17.8)	450
45-54	134	(16.5)	320	141	(24.5)	419
55-64	142	(23.7)	279	150	(25.1)	426
Total	*132*	*(18.1)*	*1117*	*135*	*(24.2)*	*1620*
Diastolic blood pressure						
25-34	79	(8.2)	172	77	(8.6)	325
35-44	83	(8.0)	346	81	(10.1)	450
45-54	85	(9.1)	320	87	(12.3)	419
55-64	87	(10.9)	279	90	(12.9)	426
Total	*84*	*(9.4)*	*1117*	*84*	*(12.3)*	*1620*

Table 4. Systolic and diastolic blood pressure (mean value and SD), by age and gender

Age (Years)	Normotensive		Hypertensive	
	N	%	N	%
Grade 1 hypertension				
25-34	422	88	58	12
35-44	572	73	213	27
45-54	372	50	365	50
55-64	220	31	482	69
Total	*1586*	*59*	*1118*	*41*

Table 5. Prevalence of hypertension by age

Prevalence of mild hypertension was equally distributed in both female and male respondents. Proportion of respondents suffering from mild hypertension statistically increased significantly with the age of both female and male respondents ($p < 0.0001$). Prevalence of moderate and severe hypertension was higher in female respondents. *(See Table 7.)*.

Prevalence of hypertension on the threshold value of 140 and/or 90 mmHg among the adult population of the Federation of Bosnia and Herzegovina was higher than in some countries in this part of Europe, including Albania and Hungary. Cross-sectional research studies carried out in Albania and Hungary in recent years showed much lower prevalence of hypertension which in Albania was reported at 32% and in Hungary at 37%. (40,41)

Furthermore, compared to findings of research studies carried out in developed European counties (e.g. UK, Germany) in the past 10 years, where prevalence of hypertension was 38% and 32% respectively (and it was much lower in female respondents), prevalence of hypertension in the Federation of Bosnia and Herzegovina is quite high. (42,43) This altogether should be a challenge for public health of the Federation of Bosnia and Herzegovina in order to effectively identify potential additional risk factors.

Age (Years)	Normotensive		Hypertensive	
	N	%	N	%
Males				
25-34	145	88	20	12
35-44	254	75	86	25
45-54	190	60	129	40
55-64	120	43	158	57
Total	709	64	393	36
Females				
25-34	277	88	38	12
35-44	318	71	127	29
45-54	182	43	236	57
55-64	100	24	324	76
Total	877	55	725	45

* The respondent were classified as hypertensive if they were using antihypertensive drugs and/or if their systolic blood pressure was > 140 mmHg and/or diastolic blood pressure was > 90 mmHg
Males $\chi^2(3)$=113.3, p<.0001; Females $\chi^2(3)$=377.6, p<.0001

Table 6. Prevalence of hypertension by age and gender

Age (Years)	Normotensive		Grade 1 Mild hypertension		Grade 2 Moderate hypertension		Grade 3 Severe hypertension	
	N	%	N	%	N	%	N	%
Males*								
25-34	151	88	18	10	2	1	1	1
35-44	261	75	73	21	9	3	3	1
45-54	196	61	91	28	27	9	6	2
55-64	131	47	88	32	37	13	23	8
Total	739	66	270	24	75	7	33	3
Females**								
25-34	290	89	32	10	3	1	0	0
35-44	330	73	92	20	19	5	9	2
45-54	193	46	126	30	59	14	41	10
55-64	123	29	134	31	109	26	60	14
Total	936	58	384	24	190	12	110	6

*$\chi^2(9)$=128.6, p < .0001
** $\chi^2(6)$=394.2, p < .0001

Table 7. Prevalence of hypertension by age and gender (clinical classification of hypertension)

5.3 Awareness of hypertension, treatment and control of hypertension

Almost 54% of hypertensive respondents were not aware of their hypertension. Very high 79% of the hypertensive respondents who are aware of their hypertension were pharmacologically treated, which indicates relatively good availability of antihypertensive drugs. Of the total number of respondents who were pharmacologically treated, the condition was adequately controlled in only 13%. Generally female respondents were more aware of their hypertension and they were more regularly treated and controlled then male respondents.

In the hypertensive respondents there was a statistically significant difference between the genders with respect to the degree of awareness, treatment and control of hypertension. There were 63% of hypertensive male respondents who were not aware of their hypertension as opposed to 50% of females in this particular category of respondents. Hypertension treated but not controlled respondents included 24% male and 34% female respondents. Percentage of the hypertensive respondents who were both treated and controlled was relatively low - 5% in male and 6% in female respondents. *(See Figure 2.)*

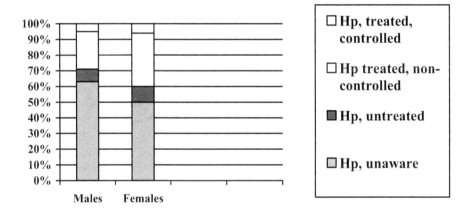

Fig. 2. Awareness, treatment and control in hypertensive respondents, by gender

In genders there was a statistically significant difference among the age groups with regards the degree of awareness of hypertension, treatment and control of hypertension. The degree of awareness of hypertension in both genders significantly increases with the age of the respondents. There were more hypertensive, treated, and non-controlled respondents in older age groups (45 to 64 years) and the portion significantly increased with the age of the respondents. Percentage of hypertensive, treated, and controlled respondents was low at males 5% and females 6%). *(Table 8.)*

The low rate of detection and control of hypertension in hypertensive respondents can be attributed to the lack of standardized integrated programs for reduction of hypertension or at least developed screening programs at the Primary health care (PHC) level. The degree of detection, treatment and control of hypertension increased with the age of the respondents as prevalence of hypertension increased.

	Hypertensive, Unaware		Hypertensive, untreated		Hypertensive, treated, non-controlled		Hypertensive, treated, controlled	
	N	%	N	%	N	%	N	%
Males								
25-34	19	95	0	0	1	5	0	0
35-44	75	87	6	7	1	1	4	5
45-54	81	63	15	12	28	22	5	4
55-64	74	47	11	7	63	40	10	6
Total	*249*	*63*	*32*	*8*	*93*	*24*	*19*	*5*
Females								
25-34	29	77	6	16	0	0	3	8
35-44	80	63	16	13	23	18	8	6
45-54	126	53	27	11	72	30	11	5
55-64	123	38	26	8	153	47	22	7
Total	*358*	*50*	*75*	*10*	*248*	*34*	*44*	*6*

Table 8. Awareness, treatment and control in hypertensive respondents by age and gender

6. Control of hypertension

Experiences of good practice exercised in various countries have showed that significant progress in health can be made through a well organized and focused approach to prevention, treatment and control of the disease, which should be a part of any health system. This is possible to achieve in social environments which support intervention programs in community. In order to make this happen, major changes need to be made in the areas of health policies, organization of health, training/academic education of health professional who also need to be properly equipped. Ultimately, such approaches do not require considerable resources compared to highly complex clinical interventions. (2,3,4)

Following the general managerial approach, the World Health Organization introduced in mid 1980s a number of integrated programs for prevention and control of disease that were defined as *"programs that combine resources and approaches to prevention and control of selected diseases and related conditions and programs that will allow managerial unification of activities that will lead to prevention and control of diseases and promotion of health in overall community."* (4)

Integrated management of disease and risk factors is particularly recommended in countries with limited financial resources for health care. Mechanisms of such integrated approach can be used to evaluate actual health needs, develop manuals to be used at all levels of management, supervision, adequate treatment and mobilization of community in support of the population's health.

One of well-founded approaches and an example of good practice is Integrated Management of Childhood Illness (IMCI) which is very efficient and applicable in developing countries as more than 80 developing countries has adopted the IMCI as their national policy aimed at improving children's health. This approach allows provision of children's health care in an efficient and effective way. (2)

Since non-communicable diseases, in particular cardiovascular disease, are leading cause of global morbidity and mortality, defining an integrated management of cardiovascular disease, including risk factor management, represents a major challenge for the national health systems worldwide. The modeling of an integrated management of non-communicable diseases means improved supervision and monitoring, development and implementation of intervention prevention programs for different target population groups, implementation of intervention programs in the community and advocacy in public policies with considerable support for health care services. The model of integrated management should promote rational allocation of resources, evidence-based treatment, cost-effectiveness and self-management strategies aimed at achieving improved health outcomes through full involvement of the entire community. (44,45)

The integrated approach to control of hypertension is innovative in shifting the paradigm from "treatment of hypertension" to "management of hypertension" as an integrative program in control of risk factors such as high cholesterol, obesity and diabetes mellitus. This movement to an innovative approach is supported by evidence of cost-effectiveness of managerial approaches to the integrative control of hypertension in the population. Therefore the developing of an integrated hypertension management model at the level of the community should be supported in the country as the original, flexible approach and comprehensive package that combines different sustainable activities that will produce a synergic effect in fight against selected risk factors. (46-48)

Population approaches in dealing with the health needs of the population are the bigger challenge with the long-term results. Epidemiological theories confirmed by research studies have indicated that intensive treatment of individuals who are under a threat of high risk of developing a disease have actually yielded limited progress in reducing general risk in the population as opposed to the population approaches. (49-51)

This effectively corroborate the fundamental axiom of preventive medicine which says that a large number of people exposed to small risk can result in much bigger number of cases that the small number of people exposed to high risk.(2)

However, effective and efficient control of blood pressure in the population requires two approaches: *population approach and individual approach to high risk individuals.* Both approaches are necessary and complementary for effective control and management of hypertension in the community. It is important to specifically note that balanced combination of population preventive strategy and preventive strategy in dealing with the high risk individuals is vital for effective control of epidemic and growing burden of non-communicable in the community in general, in particular hypertension and cardiovascular disease. *(See Figure 3)* (2,4)

7. Strategies for reducing high blood pressure

Despite many efforts to diagnose and effectively treat hypertension, this condition is still the leading cause of cardiovascular morbidity and mortality. This is why it is very important to improve unsatisfactorily treatment and control of hypertension globally. According to the research studies published by the WHO, major barriers for adequate management of hypertension include lack of standardized clinical guides at the national level, inadequate training of health professionals in management of hypertension and poor availability of hypertension drugs at the Primary health care level. Development of management of hypertension in public health context represents the best way to introduce the management of cardiovascular risks. (52,53)

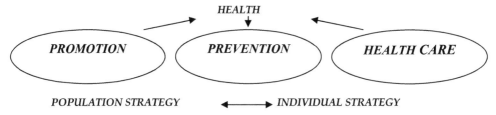

Fig. 3. Population vs. individual approach in improved health of the population

For the most part, successful implementation of guides and recommendations requires a multidisciplinary approach, from mass dissemination of recommendations, provision of public health education programs direction in the field, all the way to clinical treatment of ill patients. To achieve all this it is necessary to ensure involvement of lager number of stakeholders, from strategic to operational levels of management. Formal approval of guides essentially depends on national associations of hypertension and professional associations, in order to promote the proposed changes in behavior and improve prognosis for patients. (54-59)

Leading non-communicable diseases, including hypertension, are associated with common preventable risk factors – obesity, smoking and increased levels of fats in the blood. Better understanding of these risk factors and their determinants means better opportunities for prevention and control of the associated non-communicable diseases. Early detection and understanding of extent of this health issue, early warning and early response altogether allow timely prevention of future epidemic and "explosion" of risk factors. (60,61)

High rate of undetected hypertension and unsatisfactorily control of hypertension indicate that hypertension today is insufficiently and inadequately treated. This results in far reaching consequences in development of heart-, brains- and kidney-related conditions and eventually fatal outcomes. At this point the health system of the Federation of Bosnia and Herzegovina is treating adverse health outcome and the sequels. Number of complicated cardiac surgeries is on the rise and this in fact puts additional strain on already limited health sector budget allocations.

Lessons from many countries which developed the comprehensive policies showed that there is a significant reduction in mortality caused by cardiovascular disease. In Finland, for example, the comprehensive strategy that effectively combined prevention, promotion in the community and the approach to the treatment resulted in decrease of mortality rate by staggering 60%.

Two preventive strategies are described in the scientific literature: population and individual strategy.

Population strategy in reducing high blood pressure in countries throughout the world is very cost-effective – it is especially suitable for countries with limited resources such as Bosnia and Herzegovina. Population strategy allows potential control of incidence of disease in the population. With respect to hypertension, this approach includes reduction of mean value of blood pressure in the population by shifting the entire distribution towards the left lower values (*distributional transition* – a shift from the current values towards the desired value and planned scenario) and reduction of prevalence of high blood pressure and hypertension in adult population in elderly age as well. *(See Figure 4.)* Population approach strongly supports promotion and improvement of cardiovascular health of the population. INTERSALT study showed that population measures which can reduce mean value of systolic blood pressure by 2-3 mmHg can also reduce prevalence of hypertension in the population by one fifth at the age of 20 to 59 years. This means that organized, focused and controlled measures put in place in the population/community can successfully lead to distributional transition. (62)

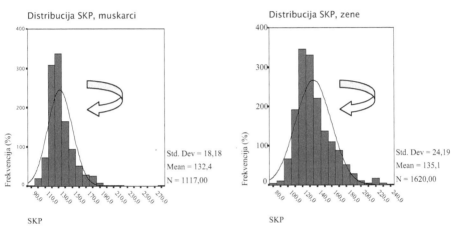

Fig. 4. Distribution of SBP in adult respondents and directions of distributional transition by gender

Population approach supports identification and modification of risk factors associated with different behaviors such as, for example, dietary habits, smoking and physical inactivity. Multiple interventions with regards the risk factors are possible by setting up health policies in the country through the multisectorial approaches in the community. Managerial approach to the population/community requires active involvement of large number of stakeholders from all three levels of management (strategic, tactical and operational) in health sector which is the primary public sector for the starting of such initiative.

It is described in the scientific literature that interventions aimed at changing the unhealthy lifestyles are very successful in reducing the absolute risk of development of hypertension in the population. (52,63,64) Preventive strategies implemented in young population, or rather in early stages of life, allow long-term potential for prevention of conditions which lead to development of hypertension and high blood pressure, as well as for reduction of overall morbidity and complications associated with conditions caused by high blood pressure. (53)

On the other hand, *individual approach* in prevention of disease does not provide a big picture of causes of diseases in the environment and projections of potential trends of the disease. However, it requires continuous and considerable screening of new highly risk individuals. Individual approach to high risk individuals with respect to hypertension includes detection, treatment and effective control of high blood pressure. Such approach requires effective treatment and both modification of lifestyle and pharmacological treatment.

It is necessary to create prerequisites necessary to study the approach to high-risk individuals which in fact primarily includes detection, early diagnosis and start of a treatment of hypertension. Changes to attitudes of health professionals in terms of the integrated hypertension management can be achieved through formal education of health professionals.

Based on the international recommendations, tables of cardiovascular risk stratification are recommended for management of hypertension at the level of an individual. Cardiovascular risk assessment systems have been for the most part developed on the findings of the Framingham Risk Score study. (65,66) Recent SCORE project developed the risk assessment tables to estimate the probability of developing fatal cardiovascular disease within the next 10 years, in particular for high-risk countries in the north of Europe and low-risk countries in the south of Europe.(67)) These categories can be used as indicators for assessment of relative risk in the population. It is recommended that the countries adapt the risk stratification tables and to introduce them in daily practice. The SCORE tables are based on risk assessment relative to values of cholesterol and blood pressure and age and gender.

8. Model of integrated hypertension management in community

Based on the survey results, it has become necessary to introduce a model of integrated management of hypertension in the Federation of Bosnia and Herzegovina at this point because of the relatively high prevalence of hypertension and leading cardiovascular risk factors.

In the countries with limited budgetary allocations for health, such as the Federation of Bosnia and Herzegovina, population prevention strategies are the most cost-effective solution. (2, 68) These strategies control incidence of risk factors in the population, their goal is to change health behavior and reduce exposure to risk factors and also to reduce risk in the entire population. Potential benefits are high but there are challenges as well because the community largely benefits from preventive measures while it seems that such measures produce limited benefits for an individual. This, on the other hand, may cause a negative motivation in the population and this is described as "preventive paradox." Therefore it is necessary to use the both approaches complementary. The key challenge is to find a suitable balance between the population approach and the approach to high-risk individuals. (69)

Managerial approach to the community (to the population) requires active involvement of large number of stakeholders from all three levels of management (strategic, tactical and operational) in health sector which is the primary public sector for the starting of such initiative.

Role of strategic management in the health sector (a country's government) in reduction of risk is significant. The government should act as an advisor in the initiative to reduce the risk factors – selected, highly prevalent in the population and widely distributed risks. One of potential instruments include the passing of legislation, which is more cost-effective as it is assumed that the legal regulations will more readily lead to changes in agreements rather than professional recommendations alone. Both approaches require consultations with a large number of active stakeholders and the multisectoral approach. *(See Table 9.,)* Unfortunately transition countries, such as the Federation of Bosnia and Herzegovina, have a poor regulatory structure and they are more dependable on the non-controlled market. Against such backdrop, it is necessary to select sustainable and implementable measures, including, for example, higher taxes on tobacco products, legislation on reduced salt content in industrially produced food products, use of mandatory content labeling of products, support for production of healthy food or subsidization of price of food produced by local producers.

Levels of management	Possible interventions	Responsible organizations	Theoretical coverage of population
Strategic management	1. Legal regulations on reduced content of salt in local industrially produced food products and mandatory food product content labeling	Government of the country	100%
Tactical management	1. Health education through mass media 2. Campaigns 3. Introduction of risk screenings 4. Development of diagnostics and therapeutic protocols 5. Training for health professionals 6. Development of reference programs such as the School of Hypertension in Community	Public health institutes, medical associations, professional associations, non-governmental organizations	60-80%
Operational management	1. Pharmacological treatment and patient education on lifestyles including dietary counseling for individuals with SBP over 160 mmHg or 140 mmHg. 2. Pharmacological treatment and patient education on lifestyles including dietary counseling for individuals with cholesterol serum concentration of over 5.7 mmol/l. 3. Nicotine replacement therapy with medical consultations by physician. 4. Triple therapy treatment for reduction of high blood pressure for individuals with absolute risk of cardiovascular events of 5% (15, 20, 25%) over the next 10 years. 5. Development of hypertension consultation facilities.	PHC Hospitals	26-41%

Table 9. Cost-effective interventions in reducing prevalence of hypertension

Role of tactical management in health sector, such as public health institutes, medical associations, professional physician associations, is reflected in designing, introducing and implementing intervention programs in the community through a series of mapped activities including preparation of culturally-sensitive promotional and preventive education messages, services aimed at supporting the changed lifestyles, introduction of risk screenings, development of diagnostic and therapeutic protocols, training for of health professionals and development of reference programs.

Role of operational management in the health sector, such as primary, secondary and tertiary health care levels (hospitals, clinics and health resorts) and non-governmental sector is reflected in the active implementation of recommendations, design and dissemination of written materials and active participation in the health training/education.

These interventions could be used as strategies in creation of population approach in management of hypertension.

Findings of this research study showed that prevalence of detection and prevalence of control of hypertension were relatively low, which further supports the importance of introducing the integrated management of hypertension.

Based on evaluation of prevalence of hypertension and distribution of major cardiovascular factors in the population research study, the managerial approach was assumed, through all developmental stages of the process (input, process and output) for for hypertension. *(See Figure 5.)*

Input included input variables (income) and resources (actual input).

Input variables (income) included:

1.   High prevalence of hypertension in the population (41%),
2.   High prevalence of selected major cardiovascular risk factors (27% in both genders)
3.   High prevalence of smoking in young males aged 25 to 44 years (56%)
4.   High prevalence of obesity in middle-aged women aged 35 to 54 years (35%).

Actual input included required resources:

1.   Staff
2.   Premises
3.   Equipment
4.   Time
5.   Money

Process included supervision, stakeholders and activities.

1.   **Supervision** included formal bodies such as steering committees of projects implemented in the community or intervention programs which targeted subgroups within the population.
2.   **Implementers** included predominantly the health sector experts from different implementation sites (Family Medicine Ambulantas, work places, schools).
3.   **Activities** were linked together through project cycles, with clearly defined goals, performance indicators and monitoring that was carried out. *(See Table10.)*

Output included output variables and outcome.

Output variables were:
1.   Process evaluation of the project (resources, process, monitoring)
Outcome and impact was:
1.   Degree of achieved value – achievement of the desired quantified goal.

GOAL – WHAT?	PROCESS - HOW?	LOCATION - WHERE?	TIME - WHEN?
1. Reduced prevalence of hypertension by 10% in adult population	Legal regulations on reduced content of salt in local industrially produced food products and mandatory food product content labeling	THE COMMUNITY **Coverage** 100% of the population	CONTINUOUSLY
2. Reduced mean value of blood pressure in the population (distributional transition) aimed at promoting and improving cardiovascular health of the population	Develop the reference program *the School of Hypertension in the Community*	THE COMMUNITY **Coverage** 100% of the population 1. Health professionals – Family Medicine teams (PHC) 2. Support groups – healthy population 3. Population under the risk 4. Representatives of mass media	ONE-YEAR CONTROLLED PROGRAM IN LOCAL DEMONSTRA-TIONAL AREAS
3. Reduced smoking by 10%, especially in young males	- Campaigns on possible use of nicotine replacement therapies with medical counseling by physician. - Health education through the mass media – TV shows on how to quit smoking	Big shopping centers, places which people of this age normally visit (entertainment and sports venues), sports non-governmental organizations, TV stations **Coverage** 55% of male population	ONE-YEAR CONTROLLED PROGRAM IN LOCAL DEMONSTRA-TIONAL AREAS
4. Reduced obesity by 10%, especially in middle-aged women	- Health education through the mass media – TV shows on importance of physical activity - On-the-job education - Promotion of recipes for low-calorie meals	TV stations big shopping centers, women's non-governmental organizations **Coverage** 40% of female population	ONE-YEAR CONTROLLED PROGRAM IN LOCAL DEMONSTRA-TIONAL AREAS

Table 10. Activities proposed in managerial process of intervention programs in the community – population approach

These interventions could be used as strategies in creation of population approach in management of hypertension. Findings of this research study showed that prevalence of detection and prevalence of control of hypertension were relatively low, which further supports the importance of introducing the integrated management of hypertension. The individual approach is better suited for high prevalence of hypertension. Compounded by the high prevalence of major cardiovascular factors, detection, adequate treatment and control are placed at (70)

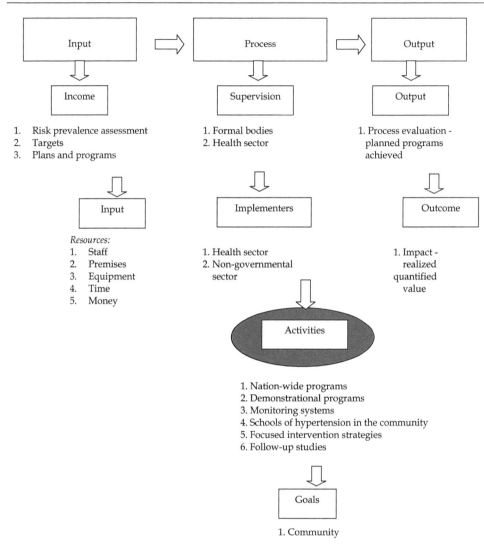

Fig. 5. Integrated management of blood pressure in the community (Intervention programs in the community)

9. Recommendations

1. Ensure support to healthy policies in the country by introducing a number of multisectorial approaches in the community that will allow multiple interventions in reducing the risk factors. The community is a significant partner and the vital point in achieving the goals that have been set.
2. It is necessary to develop a model of integrated management of hypertension and major cardiovascular risk factors as a comprehensive model introduced in the community that should be primarily directed towards modification of a detrimental lifestyle.

3. Health care should be restructured in order to effectively provide integrated health care through changed attitudes of health professionals, availability of technologies used for diagnostics and treatment of hypertension and improved quality of the referral system that will reduce inequities in the health.
4. With regards to the findings of the research study, purpose of the integrated hypertension program should be reduction of high blood pressure in adult population, with the following specific objectives –
    *   Raise awareness of hypertension in hypertensive individuals through efficient *detection* of hypertensive individuals by health professionals through improved monitoring, in particular at the level of Primary health care;
    *   Introduce standardized and suitable diagnostic and therapeutic protocols to be used by health professionals – efficient *monitoring and treatment of hypertension*;
    *   Improve *control of hypertension* in hypertensive individuals;
    *   Allow effective collection of data on epidemiology of hypertension.
5. Strong support to development of population approach in the managerial process of implementation of intervention programs of blood pressure control that will promote reduction of mean value of blood pressure in the population (distributional transition) in order to improve and advance cardiovascular health of the population.

In the light of the above recommendations, these activities should be focused on clear identification of health needs. Carefully planned, well designed and well implemented programs of disease control, either population or individual, represent a strong sole instruments to effectively deal with the problem of morbidity through the use of preventive measures. (71,72)

Prevention of disease is crucial to human development. Through such approach, it will be possible to reach different groups of the population, which will in turn facilitate equity in health. (31,33.)

10. References

[1] Health 21–Health for all in the 21.Century.WHO Regional Office for Europe.Copenhagen 1999.
[2] The World Health Report 2002:Reducing Risks, Promoting Healthy life. WHO 2002.
[3] The World Health Report 2003:Shaping the future.WHO 2003.
[4] Integrated management of cardiovascular risk: report of a WHO meeting Geneva, 9-12 July 2002. WHO 2002.
[5] Coca A. Actual blood pressure control: are we doing things right? J. Hypertension. 1998;16: S45-S51
[6] Kannel W.B. Elevated systolic blood pressure as a cardiovascular risk factor. American Journal of Cardiology. 2000;85:251-255.
[7] MacMahon B,Pugh T.F. Epidemiology:Principles and methods.Boston, 1970.
[8] Lilienfeld A.M, Lilienfeld D.E.Foundations of epidemiology.Oxford University Press 1980.
[9] Raljević E, Dilić M, Čerkez F. Prevencija kardiovaskularnih bolesti.Sarajevo 2003.
[10] Sholer C et all. Synthesis of findings and issues from community prevention trials.Annals of Epidemiology. 1997, S7:S54-S68.
[11] Winkleby MA, Jatulis DE, Frank E, Fortmann SP. Socioeconomic status and Health: How Education, Income, and Occupation Contribute to Risk Factors for Cardiovascular Disease.American Journal of Public Health. 1992;82(6):816-820.

[12] PREMIER Collaborative Research Group. Effects of comprehensive lifestyle modification on blood pressure control:Main results of the PREMIER Clinical Trial. JAMA.2003;289(16):2083-2093.

[13] Puska P, Tuomilehto J, Nissinen A, Vartiainen E. The North Karelia Project:20 year results and experiences. National Public Health Institute Finland KTL. Helsinki 1995.

[14] Puska P. Successful prevention of noncommunicable disease:25 year experiences with North Karelia Project in Finland. Public Health Medicine. 2002;4(1):5-7

[15] Puska P, Vartiainen E, Tuomilehto J. et all. Changes in premature deaths in Finland: successfull long-term prevention of cardiovascular diseases. Bulletin of the WHO. 1998;76(4):419-425.

[16] Nissinen A, Ximena B, Puska P. Community-based noncommunicable disease interventions:lessons from developed countries for developing ones. Bulletin of the World Health Organization. 2001, 79: 963-970.

[17] 2003 World Health Organization (WHO)/International Society of Hypertension (ISH) statement on management of hypertension. J. Hypertension.2003;21:1983-1992.

[18] He J, Muntner P, Chen J, Roccella EJ, Streiffer RH, Whelton PK Factors associated with hypertension control in the general population of the United States. Archives of Internal Medicine 2002;162:1051-1058.

[19] Coca A. Actual blood pressure control: are we doing things right? J. Hypertension. 1998;16:S45-S51

[20] Guibert R, Franco E.D. Choosing a definition of hypertension:impact on epidemiological estimates. J Hypertension. 1996;14(11):1275-1280

[21] Birkett N.J. The effect of alternative criteria for hypertension on estimates of prevalence and control. J. Hypertension.1997;15:237-244

[22] Le Pailleur C, Helft G, Landais P. Et all. The effects of talking, reading and silence on the «white coat» phenomenon in hypertensive patients.American Journal of Hypertension. 1998;11:203-207.

[23] Wilber JA, Barrow JG. Hypertension–a community problem. Am Journal of Medicine. 1972;52(5):653-663

[24] Bulpitt C.J. Epidemiology of hypertension. Elsevier 2000.

[25] 2003 European Society of Hypertension-European Society of Cardiology guidelines for the management of arterial hypertension – Guidelines Committee.J. Hypertension. 2003;21:1011-1053.

[26] 2003 World Health Organization (WHO)/International Society of Hypertension (ISH) statement on management of hypertension. J. Hypertension.2003;21:1983-1992.

[27] Chobanian A.V, Bakris G.L, Black H.R et all. The Seventh Report of the Joint National Committee on prevention, detection, evaluation and treatment oh high blood pressure–The JNC 7 Report. JAMA 2003; 289

[28] 2007 Guidelines for the Management of Arterial Hypertension. The Task Force for the Management of Arterial Hypertension of the European Society of Hypertension (ESH) and of the European Society of Cardiology (ESC). J. Hypertension 2007, 25:1105–1187

[29] Smajkic A et al. Social health consequences of the war in Bosnia and Herzegovina, Public Health Institute of BIH,Sarajevo 1995.

[30] Pilav A, Nissinen A, Haukkala A, Nikšić D, Laatikainen T. Cardiovascular Risk Factors in the Federation of Bosnia and Herzegovina. European Journal of Public Health 2006. 17:75-79

[31] Report on health status and organization of health care in the FBiH, Federal Public Health Institute, Sarajevo 2009.

[32] Strategic plan for Primary Health Care in the FBIH, Federal Ministry of Health, 2006.

[33] Strategic plan for health care development in the FBIH 2008-2018, Federal Ministry of Health
[34] Statistical Yearbook 2010. Federal Office for Statistics, Sarajevo 2010.
[35] Omanić A, Omanić J. Rezultati istraživačkog programa CINDI u Sarajevskom kantonu. Medicinski fakultet. Sarajevo 2002.
[36] WHO MONICA Project. Survey protocol.
        http://www.ktl.fi/publications/monica/index.html
[37] Prattala R, Helasoja V, Laaksonen M, Laatikainen T, Nikander P and Puska P. CINDI Health Monitor. Proposal for practical guidelines.WHO Regional Office for Europe. Publications of the National Public Health Institute,B14/2001.
[38] CINDI Protocol and Guidelines.WHO Regional Office for Europe Copenhagen.1996.
[39] Tolonen H, Kuulasmaa K, Laatikainen T et al. European Health Risk Monitoring Project. Recommendation for indicators, international collaboration, protocol and manual for operations for chronic disease risk factor surveys.
        http://www.ktl.fi/ehrm/
[40] Shapo L, Pomerleau J, McKee M. Epidemiology of hypertension and associated cardiovascular risk factors in a country in transition: a population based survey in Tirana City, Albania.J Epidemiol Community Health 2003; 57:734-739
[41] Jenei Z, Pall D, Katana E et al. The epidemiology of hypertension and its associated risk factors in the city of Debrecen, Hungary.Public Health 2002; 116:138-144.
[42] Primatesta P. Brookes M., Poulter NR. Improved hypertension management and control:results from the health survey for England 1998. Hypertension. 2001;38:827-832.
[43] Gasse C, Hense H-W, Stieber J. Et all. Assessing hypertension management in the community:trends of prevelence, detection tretment, and control of hypertension in the MONICA Project, Augsburg 1984-1995. J of Human Hypertension. 2001;15:27-36.
[44] Brownson R.C, Baker E.A, Leet T.L, Gillespie K.N. Evidence-based public health. Oxford University Press 2003.
[45] Merzel C, D'Affilitti J. Reconsidering community based health promotion:promise, performance and potential. Am J Public Health. 2003;93:557-574
[46] The Protocol for the WHO Study on the Effectiveness of Community-Based Programmes for the NCD Prevention and Control (COMPASS).WHO 2003.
[47] Bradley E.H, Tashonna W.R, Baker D, Schlesinger M. et all. Translating research into practice:Speeding the adoption of innovative health care programs. The Commonwealth Fund. July 2004.
[48] Israel B.A, Schulz A.J, Parker E.A, Becker A.B. Review of community-based research:Assesing partnership approaches to improve public health. Ann. Rev. Public Health. 1998;19:173-202.
[49] MacMahon B,Pugh T.F. Epidemiology.Principles and methods.Boston, 1970.
[50] Lilienfeld A.M, Lilienfeld D.E.Foundations of epidemiology.Oxford University Press 1980.
[51] Raljević E, Dilić M, Čerkez F. Prevencija kardiovaskularnih bolesti.Sarajevo 2003.
[52] Whelton P.K,Jiang H,Lawrence A.J. et all. Primary prevention of hypertension:Clinical and public health advisory from the National high blood pressure education program. JAMA. 2002;288(15):1882-1888.
[53] Kannel W.B, Garrison R.J, Dannenberg A.L et all. Secular blood pressure trends in normotensive persons:The Framingham study.Am Heart Journal.1993;125:1154-1158.
[54] Fields L.E,Burt V.L, Cutler J.A, Hughes J. Et all. The burden of adult hypertension in the United States 1999 to 2000. A Rising Tide. Hypertension.2004;44:389-404.
[55] Kastarinen MJ, Saloma VV, Vartiainen EA et al. Trend in blood pressure levels and control of hypertension in Finland from 1982-1997. J Hypertension 1998;16:1379-1387.

[56] Prevention and Treatment – Both work, says WHO Study on heart disease, Press Release WHO/10, February 2000.

[57] Milchak J.L, Carter B.L, James P.A, Ardery G. Measuring adherence to practice guidelines for the management of hypertension:An evaluation of the literature. Hypertension. 2004;44:602-608.

[58] Elder J.P, Ayala G.X, Harris S: Theories and Intervention approaches to health behaviour change in primary care.American Journal of Preventive medicine 1999;17(4):275-284

[59] Montgomery A.A, Fahey T, Peters T.J. et all. Evaluation of computer based clinical decision support sytem and risk chart for management of hypertension in primary care:randomised controlled trial.BMJ.2000;320:686-690.

[60] Kuulasmaa K, Tunstall-Pedoe H, Dobson A et all. For the WHO MONICA Project Estimation of contribution of changes in classic risk factors to trends in coronary-event rate across the WHO MONICA Project population. The Lancet 2000; 3555:675-687.

[61] Fuster V, Gotto A.M. Risk reduction.Circulation.2000;102:IV-94-IV-102.

[62] Carvalho JJM, Baruzzi RG, Howard P. Et all. Blood pressure in four remote populations in the INTERSALT study. Hypertension 1989;14:238-246.

[63] PREMIER Collaborative Research Group. Effects of comprehensive lifestyle modification on blood pressure control:Main results of the PREMIER Clinical Trial. JAMA. 2003;289(16):2083-2093.

[64] Geleijnse J.M,Kok F.J,Grobbee D.E. Impact of dietary and lifestyle factors on the prevalence of hypertension in Western population.European Journal of Public Health 2004;14:235-239.

[65] Kannel W.B. Risk stratification in hypertension:new insights from the Framingham study.Hypertension. 2000;13:3S-10S.

[66] Persson M, Carlberg B, Weinehall L, Nilsson L. Et all. Risk stratification by guidelines compared with risk assessment by risk equations applied to a MONICA sample. Journal of Hypertension. 2003;21:1089-1095.

[67] Conroy R.M, Pyorala K, Fitzgerald A.P, Sans S, Menotti A, De Backer G, De Bacquer D, Ducimetiere P, Jousilahti P, Keil U, Njřlstad I, Oganov R.G, Thomsen T, Tunstall-Pedoe H, Tverdal A, Wedel H, Whincup P, Wilhelmsen L, Graham I.M. on behalf of the SCORE project group. Estimation of ten-year risk of fatal cardiovasculardisease in Europe: the SCORE project. European Heart Journal 2003;24:987–1003

[68] Žarković G., Hrabač B., Nakaš B. Zdravstvena politika i upravljanje nacionalnim sistemima zaštite zdravlja:sa posebnim osvrtom na probleme bivših socijalističkih zemalja.ANU BIH. Sarajevo 1999.

[69] Egan B.M. hypertension in the 21st Century: The tide is rising; Our Daze Must End. Hypertension. 2004;44:389.

[70] Pilav A. Algorithm for the Control of Hypertension at Community Level. European Federation for Medical Informatics - Special Topic Conference 2007. Brioni, Croatia, May 30 – June 1, 2007

[71] Pilav A. Zdravstveni indikatori i značaj njihove primjene u svakodnevnom radu. Med. Arhiv. 1999;53 (4,supl. 3): 51-53

[72] Rychetnik L, Frommer M, Hawe P. Et all. Criteria for evaluating evidence on public health interventions.Journal of Epidemilogy and Community Health 56:119-127.2002.

4

The Use of Reynolds Risk Score in Cardiovascular Risk Assessment in Apparently Healthy Bosnian Men and Women: Cross-Sectional Study

Asija Začiragić

Department of Physiology, School of Medicine, University of Sarajevo,
Bosnia and Herzegovina

1. Introduction

Cardiovascular diseases (CVD) remain a major burden for public health worldwide. Pivotal concern of primary prevention is identification of individuals that are at risk for developing cardiovascular disease. The use of different algorithms for an assessment of cardiovascular risk allows physicians to identify and treat in a simple and cost-effective manner individuals that may be at high long-term cardiovascular risk.

A cardiovascular risk factor represents a condition that is related to increased risk for the development of cardiovascular disease. This relation is used in statistical terms. If certain individual has particular risk factor he/she has increased probability for the development of CVD. However, not all individual with cardiovascular risk will develop CVD and sometimes coronary events may occur in the absence of major risk factors (Ridker et al, JAMA 2007). Identification of individuals at cardiovascular risk results in a cost-effective prevention. Significant efforts are made to ensure most reliable tools in cardiovascular risk assessment. For a risk factor to be useful in routine clinical diagnostics, following criteria must be fulfilled: its analysis must be easy and available, there must be pathophysiological evidence that confirms causal link of risk factor with the disease, and also there must be certain knowledge on treatment options for patients with established high values of a certain risk factor (Thomas et al, 2009).

Cardiovascular risk factors are divided into three main categories: non-modifiable (age, gender, heredity); modifiable (increased blood pressure, dyslipidemia, fibrinogen, obesity, glucose intolerance, diabetes, left ventricular hypertrophy, cocaine, behavioral factors); and protective factors (HDL-cholesterol, exercise, estrogen, moderate alcohol intake). It is important to emphasize that treatment of certain modifiable cardiovascular risk factor will not result in total elimination of probability in CVD development, but the possibility of CVD development will be reduced.

As for non-modifiable cardiovascular risk factors, many epidemiological studies have reported age as one of the strongest predictors of CVD. Furthermore, investigations have shown that men are more prone to CVD development then women for reason yet not completely understood. In most societies, development of cardiovascular risk factors begins in younger age, and manifests itself in middle age. Almost 85% of all deaths due to CVD occur in people 65 years of age or older. It has been reported that mortality rate for men before the age of 50 with no pre-existing myocardial infarction or stroke was 20%, which increased up to 80 % in those older then 70 years of age (Wannamethee et al, 1995).

Inherited likelihood for the development of CVD has been well documented. In some cases, such as familial hypercholesterolemia ways of inheritance are well defined. However, for other cardiovascular risk factors pattern of inheritance is still unknown. According to current assumptions, role of heredity in the development of CVD is multifactorial with genetic, environmental, and behavioral component (Phillips et al, 1988). Studies have shown that risk of developing premature CVD was increased more then threefold when any first-degree relative was affected and about sixfold when at least two first-degree relatives had a history of CVD (Eaton et al, 1996).

Of all the modifiable cardiovascular risk factors, hypertension is best investigated. Both systolic and diastolic blood pressures are important in the assessment of individual's risk. However, majority of complications of hypertension are attributed to systolic blood pressure. Studies have indicated that the risk of a cardiac event increases by 1.6 in men and 2.5 in women when blood pressure rises from an optimal (<120/80 mmHg) to high normal (130-139/85-89 mmHg) level (Vasan et al, 2000). Although hypertension is an independent cardiovascular risk factor, data have shown its strong relations with other risk factors, such as age, sex, race and hypercholesterolemia.

Increased levels of serum lipids are another common modifiable cardiovascular risk factor. According to current guidelines fasting lipoprotein profile (total cholesterol, triglycerides, LDL-cholesterol and HDL- cholesterol) should be preformed every five years in all adults age 20 years and older. Level of total cholesterol is strong predictor of CVD and to a lesser degree of stroke. Close linear relationship exists between cholesterol level and the mortality rate. Studies have shown that low-density cholesterol (LDL-C) and high-density cholesterol (HDL-C) and their relationship may have even more significant prognostic value in the prediction of CVD then total cholesterol. Men aged 45 to 65 years with total serum cholesterol level < 240 mg/dL and/or LDL-cholesterol > 160 mg/dL are considered to be at an increased risk for CVD (Wilson et al, 1998). Reduction of increased levels of total cholesterol and LDL-cholesterol is accompanied with the decline of cardiovascular risk. Earlier studies failed to demonstrate predictive value of triglycerides, but results of novel studies point to possible importance of triglycerides in the prediction of cardiovascular risk, especially in women and patients with diabetes. HDL-cholesterol attenuates atherogenicity of LDL-cholesterol. High levels of HDL-cholesterol have protective properties, while its low levels represent a major risk for CVD (P.W. Wilson, 1990; Schafer et al, 1994).

Recent data report on possible role of fibrinogen as cardiovascular risk factors. Even though mechanisms by which fibrinogen fulfills this role are still not completely known, it is believed that individuals with raised fibrinogen are more susceptible to the development of clots in arteries, and thereby have increased risk of heart attack or stroke. Evidences have shown that fibrinogen levels have tendency to rise with advancing age and in that sense fibrinogen does not represent modifiable cardiovascular risk factor. However, it has been

The Use of Reynolds Risk Score in Cardiovascular Risk Assessment in Apparently Healthy
Bosnian Men and Women: Cross-Sectional Study

59

proven that smoking cessation reduces fibrinogen levels which make fibrinogen a cardiovascular risk factor that can be controlled. In a 13-year longitudinal CARDIA study (D. Green et al, 2010) higher levels of fibrinogen during young adulthood were positively associated with incidence of subclinical atherosclerosis and coronary artery calcification in middle-age. However, study has shown that this association declines with advancing age.

A major contributor to CVD is cigarette smoking. It is estimated that out of approximately 500.000 deaths from coronary heart disease, 30-40% can be attributed to smoking. Studies have shown that risk of sudden death increases more then tenfold in men and almost fivefold in women who smoke. Smoking is associated with accelerated atherosclerosis and inflammatory processes. Smoking cessation and reduced tobacco exposure result in decrease of inflammatory component of CVD and this decrease is reversible (Bakhru & Erlinger, 2005; Tracy et al, 1997; Dobson et al, 1991).

Obese individuals (more then 30% over ideal body weight) are more likely to develop CVD, even in absence of other cardiovascular risk factors. A strong association has been found between overweight that begins in childhood and the development of other risk factors over time, such as hypertension and diabetes. The cause of overweight and obesity in majority of cases is excessive food intake and sedentary lifestyle. A study among middle-aged men has shown that risk of developing fatal and non-fatal CVD increased up to 72% if their body mass index (BMI) increased from less then 23 to the range of 25-29 (Rimm et al, 1995). For all of these reasons obese individuals tend to be at high risk for CVD, and weight management is extremely important lifestyle intervention that can lead to significant reduction of cardiovascular risk.

Individuals with glucose intolerance and diabetes mellitus have increased risk for CVD. These two conditions are often accompanied with raised levels of insulin that in this setting increases blood pressure and aids in plaque deposition. As a result of these insulin actions, atherosclerosis and its complications will develop. Data have reported that there is a liner association between glucose levels and CVD mortality (Balkaue et al, 1999). It is of note that influence of diabetes mellitus on the development of CVD differs among ethnic groups. A prospective study in individuals of African-American origin has shown that 27% of women and 8% of men had CVD that could be attributed to diabetes mellitus. In individuals of Caucasian origin, 15% of men and 12% of women had CVD that could also be attributed to diabetes mellitus (Folsom et al, 1997)

Even though certain authors disagree, many others find behavioral risk factors such as type A personality and stress as important risk factors for CVD. Type A or coronary-prone personality is an individual that is always in hurry, under pressure by time, becomes upset often with no objective reason, has chronic impatience and sometimes overwhelming hostility. Results from GAZEL French prospective study have demonstrated that neurotic hostility, coronary-prone personality and antisocial personality are all predictive of mortality outcomes (Nabi et al, 2008).

Left ventricular hypertrophy (LVHT) is a major independent risk factor for cardiovascular mortality. Studies have shown that individuals with LVHT are more susceptible to arrhythmias, heart failure and sudden death and this condition is often accompanied with hypertension. Appropriate treatment of these conditions reduces cardiovascular risk. Novel findings suggest that there are racial and ethnic differences in cardiovascular mortality related to LVHT. It has been demonstrated that LVHT contributes more to the risk of cardiovascular mortality in African American then it does in White individuals (Havranek et al, 2008).

Cocaine is a sympathomimetic agent that can cause hypertension, arrhythmias, angina and sudden death. Cocaine is also a risk for congenital heart disease. Main mechanism of cocaine action is that it constricts coronary blood vessels and reduces oxygen supply to the heart. It has been reported that concomitant use of cigarettes exacerbates the deleterious effects of cocaine on myocardial oxygen supply and demand (Lange et al, 2004).

Alongside with non-modifiable and modifiable cardiovascular risk factors, there are also some proven protective factors that in fact protect from the development of CVD. Sedentary life-style is associated with the development of obesity, metabolic risk factors, insulin resistance, and early onset of diabetes mellitus type 2. Regular exercise is one of those protective factors that helps in weight management, increases HDL-cholesterol concentration, enhances utility of insulin in organism, reduces stress and decreases blood pressure. There are convincing data that it also reduces chances for having a myocardial infarction. Significant changes in classical cardiovascular risk factors are preceded by reductions of vascular functions. Important guidelines for primary and secondary prevention settings should be based on the encouragement of regular physical activity that has been shown to have many beneficial effects on the vascular wall (D.J. Green et al, 2008). Studies have found that increased physical activity leads to the decline of CVD mortality (Blair et al, 1995). Results of a meta-analysis reported that physical activity was inversely associated to the development of CVD, with a relative increased risk of 1.9 in people with sedentary lifestyle compared to physically active individuals (Berlin et al, 1990).

Another protective factor against CVD is estrogen. It reduces likelihood of heart attack by increase in HDL-cholesterol levels. However, once women reach an age of menopause this protective action of estrogen diminishes, and women are at same cardiovascular risk as men. According to recent findings, estrogen decreases production of reactive oxygen species in mitochondria. Studies have shown that estrogen promotes angiogenesis, enhances endothelial vasodilator function and modulates autonomic function (Miller et al, 2008).

Moderate alcohol consumption is proven to have protective effects against atherosclerosis and coronary heart disease. Mechanisms by which these effects are achieved are still not completely understood, but it seems that consumption of one or two drinks a day increases levels of HDL-cholesterol. A systematic review of literature and meta-analysis on association between alcohol consumption and overall mortality from CVD, incidence of and mortality from coronary heart disease, and incidence of and mortality from stroke has observed that light to moderate alcohol consumption is associated with reduced risk of multiple cardiovascular outcomes (Ronksley et al, 2011). However, consumption of alcohol in larger amounts increases blood pressure and risk of CVD.

Prevalence of cardiovascular risk factors differs around the globe. Data from USA indicate that nearly 70% of adult Americans are overweight or obese. Less than 15% of adults or children exercise sufficiently, and over 60% do not engage in vigorous activity. Among adult population, 11%–13% have diabetes, 34% have hypertension, 36% have prehypertension, 36% have prediabetes, and 12% have both prediabetes and prehypertension, At least one cardiovascular risk factor is present in 50% of adults. Furthermore, almost 65% of patients do not have their traditional cardiovascular risk biomarkers under control (Kones, 2011).

Another study in US population (Danaei et al, 2009) aimed to assess the number of disease-specific deaths attributable to all non-optimal levels of risk factors exposure, by age and sex. Results have shown that in year 2005, cigarette smoking was responsible for an estimated 467.000 deaths and high blood pressure for 395.000 deaths in US adults. Overweight-obesity, physical inactivity, and high blood glucose caused 8%-9% of all deaths in same population. Other dietary risk factors also caused significant number of deaths in the US.

A comprehensive, population-based study compared cardiovascular risk profiles among individuals of white, South Asian, Chinese and black ethnic groups living in Canada (Chiu et al, 2010). Results have shown that there is a considerable variation in the prevalence of smoking, hypertension, obesity, and diabetes mellitus among four ethnic groups included in the study. Authors concluded that these results may lead to the development of CVD prevention programs for specific ethnic groups.

Prediction of risk for future cardiovascular events or stratification of healthy individuals into risk categories by different algorithms has been widely used in clinical practice. Important issue is critical appraisal of implemented prediction models. Even though validity of models can be evaluated by different means, calibration and discrimination represent two most important measures of accurate models assessment. Calibration is a measure of how well predicted probabilities agree with actual observed risk, whereas calibration is a measure of how well the model can separate those who do and do not have the disease of interest. A measure of discrimination that is broadly used is c statistics, also known as the area under the Receiver Operating Characteristic (ROC) curve, or c index. Results of a Women Health Study have shown that use of c statistics can be advocated because of its specificity and sensitivity in differentiating between those who do and those who do not have a certain disease. Also, its use may contribute to more exact reclassification of large proportion of patients into higher- risk or lower-risk categories. However, it seems unlikely that it can be used in the evaluation of algorithms that predicts future risk or stratify individuals into risk categories. Another conclusion of this study was that use of c statistics as the only measure of the possible usefulness of traditional or novel risk factors could not be advised (Cook N, 2007). Finally, decision on inclusion of novel risk marker in prediction algorithms should be based on the knowledge whether measurement of potential risk marker will result in different treatment options, and whether it has perspectives in disease prevention.

Etiology of CVD is multifactorial. In order to better assess cardiovascular risk, new biomarkers have been introduced as part of global cardiovascular risk assessment. Novel findings suggest that important role in atherosclerosis has inflammation. These conclusions led to the measurement of numerous markers of inflammatory processes to better identify individuals that are at the increased risk. C-reactive protein (CRP) is currently most studies and best validated biomarker of inflammatory processes. It is an acute phase protein, which is primarily synthesized in the liver and it represents a marker of systemic, non-specific, inflammation. CRP production is stimulated by cytokines (in particular interleukin-6, interleukin-1, and tumor necrosis factor-alpha) in response to systemic or local infection or inflammation by variety of cells, including adipocytes (Pepys & Hirschfield, 2003).

The Centers for Disease Control and Prevention and the American Heart Association published a statement in 2003 in which measurement of CRP is given at the discretion of physicians to be used in clinical practice as part of global risk assessment in adults (Pearson et al, 2003). According to existing guidelines, individuals with CRP values < 1 mg/L are considered to be in low, those with CRP values 1-3 mg/L in moderate and those with CRP values > 3 mg/L in high cardiovascular risk (Packard et al, 2008).

Current main goal in CRP testing is to identify individuals that can benefit from lipid-lowering treatment in order to prevent first cardiovascular event, especially for those individuals that have CRP > 3mg/L, and are in intermediate risk (10-20% 10-year predicted risk). However, it is of critical importance in any interpretation of CRP values to differentiate modest increase of CRP baseline values from its major rise that occurs in conditions such as tissue necrosis, sepsis and acute trauma. Furthermore, because of its completely unspecific nature, it is not possible or clinically appropriate to interpret CRP values without full medical information of individual, including history, physical examination, and results of all investigations (Casas et al, 2008). Although more sophisticated inflammatory biomarkers (such as interleukin-6, intercellular adhesion molecule-1, macrophage inhibitory cytokine-1, and CD40 ligand) have been shown to be predictive of cardiovascular disease, their use in routine clinical evaluation is highly unlikely because of short half-lives of these proteins (Katrinchak &Fritz, 2007).

Findings of many clinical, experimental, prospective epidemiological and cohort studies have demonstrated that CRP may play role in atherogenesis, since it was found in endothelial atherosclerotic lesions, and raise in CRP concentrations is linked with the increased prevalence of myocardial infarction, peripheral vascular disease, and stroke. Furthermore, CRP provides additional information for the prevention of cardiovascular disease, has a prognostic value of incident cardiovascular events in those with and without preexisting CVD, the increased risk associated with high CRP is independent of other established risk factors, and CRP is biologically stable over time and assays for its measurements are standardized (de Ferranti et al, 2007). For all of the stated properties, certain authors believe that CRP represents not only a marker but as well a mediator of cardiovascular disease (Ridker et al, 2004). Conversely, there are studies that reported that CRP is only a relatively modest predictor of coronary heart disease, and suggest that its use in the prediction of coronary heart disease development should be revised (Danesh et al, 2004).

Data have shown that conventional cardiovascular risk factors fail to predict development of coronary heart disease in 25-50% of cases. Certain authors believe that possible explanation of observed discrepancy may be endothelial dysfunction that may be a missing link between atherosclerotic disease and cardiac risk factors (Reriani et al, 2010). According to relatively recent hypothesis endothelial dysfunction has significant impact on the development and progression of atherosclerosis and atherothrombosis. One of the currently mostly used markers of endothelial dysfunction is asymmetric dimethylarginine (ADMA). ADMA is a endogenous inhibitor of all three isoforms of the enzyme nitric oxide synthase (NOS) and causes endothelial dysfunction by inhibiting production of nitric oxide (one of the major endothelium-derived vasoactive mediators). Prospective clinical studies have shown that elevated levels of ADMA are related to increased incidence of cardiovascular events, as well as with overall mortality (Anderssohn et al, 2010). Large multicentric CARDIAC study has found that elevated ADMA concentration significantly increases the risk of coronary heart disease (Landim et al, 2009). These findings point to the important role of functional vascular status in cardiovascular prognosis. However, it remains unclear whether increased values of ADMA represent only a marker of endothelial dysfunction that may be used in cardiovascular risk assessment or elevated ADMA concentration itself predispose the development of CVD.

Alongside with conventional biomarkers for the prediction of incident cardiovascular events, there are also some other novel biomarkers that are tested for their possible usefulness in cardiovascular risk assessment. Recent Swedish study assessed a panel of contemporary biomarkers, such as mid-regional-pro-atrial natriuretic peptide, N-terminal pro-B-type natriuretic peptide (N-BNP), mid-regional-pro-adrenomedullin (MRproADM), lipoprotein-associated phospholipase-2, and cystatin C in prediction of future cardiovascular events. Results have shown that 10-year incidence of coronary events was 4.4%. Another important finding of the study was that selected biomarkers may be used in the prediction of future cardiovascular events, but benefits over traditional risk factors are minimal. Furthermore, their use did not reclassify a substantial proportion of individuals to higher or lower risk categories (Melander et al, 2009).

A study in Hispanic population used standard risk assessment tools and the B-type natriuretic peptide biomarker to assess coronary heart disease risk (Macabasco-O'Connell et al, 2011). Based on their findings, authors concluded that the inclusion of B-type natriuretic peptide to the traditional risk scores may be helpful in cardiovascular risk prediction.

One of the most frequently used cardiac risk prediction model in clinical practice is Framingham Risk Score. Its use started in the 1980s and based on its implementation in cardiovascular risk assessment, individuals can be divided in those at low (less then 5%), intermediated (6-20%) and high (>20%) cardiovascular risk (Ridker et al, 2004). However, over time, Framingham Risk Score showed certain limitations. Evidences have shown that cardiovascular events occur in every fifth individual in whom classical risk factors have not been recognized. Furthermore, there is a limitation in specificity of conventional risk factors and it has been shown that overall cardiovascular risk differs across populations. It has also been concluded that intermediate risk category is broad and that there is a necessity for better risk stratification of that risk category. For all of the above reasons, there was a need for new and more comprehensive cardiovascular risk prediction tools.

So far, several other risk prediction models have been proposed to be used in every-day clinical practice for cardiovascular risk assessment, such as: Adult Treatment Panel III, ASSIGN (Assessing Cardiovascular Risk to Scottish Intercollegiate Guidelines Network), QRISK (QRESEARCH Cardiovascular Risk Algorithm), and SCORE (Systematic Coronary Risk Evaluation) project (Berger et al, 2010).

Majority of the studies so far evaluated risk of CVD in a 10-year or shorter time period. Contrary to these studies, there is a study in which individuals, free of conditions at baseline, were followed-up for 30-years and in that period incidence of CVD and death was ascertained. Results of this study demonstrated that standard risk factors remain highly predictive of cardiovascular risk over 30-years follow-up period and their impact is significant even if levels are not updated (Pencina et al, 2009).

A global vascular risk score was recently designed and validated that combines conventional risk factors with behavioral (alcohol consumption and physical activity) and anthropometric risk factors in African-American and Hispanic individuals at risk for vascular disease (Sacco et al, 2009). The use of this risk prediction model demonstrated an improvement in the prediction of global vascular risk.

Reynolds Risk Score (RRS) represents risk prediction algorithm that was designed, validated and used in the prediction of 10-year cardiovascular risk in initially healthy men and women. It is based on two separate large prospective studies that included more then 20.000 women, 45 years of age and older, with median follow-up period of 10.2 years and more the 10.000 men, 50 years of age and older, that were followed up over a median period of 10.8 years for incident myocardial infarction, stroke, coronary revascularization, or cardiovascular death (Ridker 2007, 2008). The main aim of these two studies was to compare predictive value of traditional risk prediction model based on age, blood pressure, smoking status, total cholesterol and high-density lipoprotein cholesterol and RRS in which alongside with traditional risk markers, hsCRP and parental history of cardiovascular diseases are included. Results have confirmed significant predictive value of traditional risk factors as well as of hsCRP and parental history. Furthermore, both of the studies have shown that RRS had better predictive value in the prediction of incident cardiovascular events in women and in men compared to traditional cardiovascular risk prediction model. Study in initially healthy female subjects have also demonstrated that use of RRS improved risk stratification in a sense that 40-50% of women that were previously categorized to be at intermediate risk could be reclassified into higher or lower risk categories. Study in initially healthy male subjects showed that up to 20% of men previously categorized to be at intermediate risk could be reclassified into higher or lower risk categories. Conclusion derived from both of the studies was that use of RRS can serve in primary prevention settings to better targeting of treatments in order to increase benefits and reduce toxicity. RRS comprises of four 10-year risk categories: 0% to less then 5% - low risk category, 5% to less then 10% - low to medium risk category, 10% to less then 20% - medium to high risk category, and > 20% – high risk category (Ridker et al, 2004; Cook et al, 2006).

To date, no data exist on use of RRS in cardiovascular risk assessment among apparently healthy Bosnian men and women. To address this issue, we used Reynolds Risk Score calculator (http://www.reynoldsriskscore.org) to ascertain 10-year cardiovascular risk with the use of traditional factors such as age, smoking status, systolic blood pressure, blood levels of total cholesterol, HDL-cholesterol, as well as hcCRP and parental history of myocardial infarction and stroke before the age 60 in our study sample.

2. Methods

2.1 Subjects

Between February and March 2011, 230 of men and 270 women visited Family Medicine Out-Patient Clinic "Visnjik", Sarajevo, Bosnia and Herzegovina, for general health screening. Among them, 200 of men and 250 women signed informed consent. Excluding subjects with history of cardiovascular disease, malignancy, liver disease, alcohol abuse, use of antidiabetic, antihypertensive, or lipid-lowering drugs, or CRP values > 10 mg/L, and those aged < 45 years, the resulting 76 men and 120 women comprised the subjects in the present study. The study was approved by the Ethics Committee of the Medical Faculty University of Sarajevo. Written informed consent was obtained from all subjects included in the study. Participants

The Use of Reynolds Risk Score in Cardiovascular Risk Assessment in Apparently Healthy
Bosnian Men and Women: Cross-Sectional Study

65

underwent a medical history, physical examination and laboratory assessment. Investigations were carried out in accordance with the Declaration of Helsinki as revised in 2000.

2.2 Blood sampling

Blood was collected in the morning after an overnight fast and after a 30-minutes rest in a semi-recumbent position. Sampling was done without stasis, using the vacutainer technique.

2.3 Blood chemistry analysis

High sensitivity CRP was determined by means of particle enhanced immunonephelometry (BN Systems, Dade Behring, Marburg, Germany). The lower limit of detection of this assay was 0.18 mg/L. Levels of hs-CRP >10mg/L were excluded from the analysis, as they are likely related to infections or other acute inflammatory processes. Total cholesterol, HDL - cholesterol, triglycerides were measured by direct colorimetric reflectance spectrophotometry using Dimension clinical chemistry system (Dade Behring, Marburg, Germany). LDL - cholesterol was calculated by means of Friedwald formula.

2.4 Blood pressure measurements

Three supine blood pressure recordings were made after a 5-minutes rest using an Omron 705c oscillometric device. The mean of the second and third readings was used. Hypertension was defined as systolic blood pressure ≥140 mmHg, diastolic pressure ≥90 mmHg, or self-reported high blood pressure with use of anti-hypertensive medications. Prehypertension was defined as systolic blood pressure of 120–140 mmHg or diastolic blood pressure of 80–90 mmHg.

None of the included subjects was pregnant or had a history of intercurrent diseases. Parental history of myocardial infarction or stroke before the age 60 (genetic factor) was defined as family history of heart disease or stroke. Smoking status and genetic factor were assessed by self-administrated questioner.

Statistical analysis. The Kolmogorov-Smirnov test of normality was used to test the distribution of variables. Normally distributed data are presented as mean ± SEM and skewed variables as median and interquartile ranges. An unpaired Student t-test or Mann-Whitney U-test was used to compare the difference between two groups, as appropriate. Frequencies were tested by Chi-square test. In order to determine the factors associated with absolute 10 year Reynolds Risk Score, multiple regression analysis was performed. A p value of less then 0.05 was considered statistically significant. The software used was SPSS for Windows (version 17.0; SPSS, Chicago, IL, USA).

3. Results

Variables	Men (n=76)	Women (n=120)	p<
Age (yrs)	58.64±2.12	57.06±1.67	NS
Smoking (yes/no)	(29/47)	(36/84)	NS
SBP (mmHg)	136.43±2.13	130.92±1.71	0.05

Variables	Men (n=76)	Women (n=120)	p<
TC (mmol/L)	5.48±0.13	6.01±0.12	0.001
HDL (mmol/L)	1.22±0.04	1.39±0.03	0.001
hsCRP (mg/L)	1.33(0.78-3.92)	1.71(0.80-3.92)	NS
GF (yes/no)	(17/59)	(11/109)	0.05
Absolute RRS (%)	19.37±1.67	9.76±1.03	0.0001

Data are presented as mean ± SEM, median and inter-quartile range, or in total count. SBP: systolic blood pressure; TC: total cholesterol; HDL-cholesterol: high density lipoprotein – cholesterol; hsCRP: high sensitivity C-reactive protein; GF: genetic factor; Absolute RRS: absolute Reynolds Risk Score, n: number of subject.

Table 1. The values of Reynolds Risk Score factors in apparently healthy male and female subjects. Subjects did not differ in age, smoking status and CRP values. Statistically significant difference was observed in systolic blood pressure, total cholesterol, HDL-cholesterol, genetic factor presence and in absolute Reynolds risk score values between men and women.

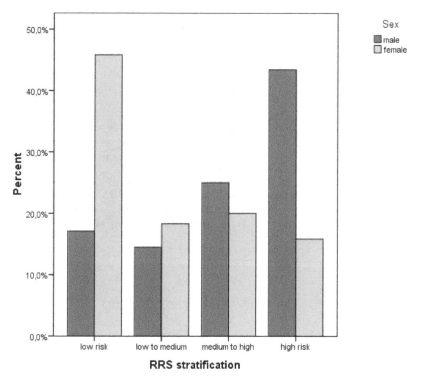

Fig. 1. Frequency of Reynolds Risk Score categories by gender. Results have shown that 6.63% of men and 28.6% of women were in low risk category, 5.6% of men and 11.2% of women in low to medium risk category, 9.7% of men and 12.2% of women in medium to high risk category, and 16.8% of men and 9.7% of women in high risk category.

Independent Variables	ß coefficient	t value	p<
Age (yrs)	0.553	7.753	0.0001
Smoking (yes/no)	0.023	0.359	NS
SBP (mmHg)	0.420	5.905	0.0001
TC (mmol/L)	0.095	1.422	NS
HDL (mmol/L)	-0.016	-0.244	NS
hsCRP (mg/L)	-0.005	-0.073	NS
GF (yes/no)	-0.143	-2.244	0.05

Table 2. Results of multiple regression analysis for absolute 10-year Reynolds Risk Score as dependent variable in men. Multiple regression analysis revealed that in male subjects most predictive value in cardiovascular risk assessment had age followed by systolic blood pressure and genetic factor, respectively.

Independent Variables	ß coefficient	t value	p<
Age (yrs)	0.287	4.394	0.0001
Smoking (yes/no)	-0.230	-4.265	0.0001
SBP (mmHg)	0.561	8.647	0.0001
TC (mmol/L)	0.093	1.701	0.092
HDL (mmol/L)	0.012	0.222	0.825
hsCRP (mg/L)	0.075	1.367	0.174
GF (yes/no)	-0.044	-0.804	0.423

Table 3. Results of multiple regression analysis for absolute 10-year Reynolds Risk Score as dependent variable in women. In female subjects most predictive value in cardiovascular risk assessment had systolic blood pressure, followed by age and smoking, respectively.

4. Discussion

CVD is one of the leading causes of death worldwide. It is estimated that for individuals at age of 50 years, the lifetime risk of CVD is, on average, for men 52% and 39% for women (Berger et al, 2010).

To the best of our knowledge, we are the first to report high prevalence of cardiovascular risk factors in apparently healthy Bosnian men and women with the use of Reynolds Risk Score calculator. Results have shown that in a total study sample, 34.7% of subjects were in low, 16.8% in low to medium, 21.9% in medium to high, and 26.5% of subjects were in high cardiovascular risk category. Our results are consistent with previous report (Cushman et al, 2009). Majority of women in both studies belonged to low and low to medium risk category group, and majority of men belonged to medium to high and high risk category group. The mean absolute 10-year cardiovascular risk determined with RRS calculator in men included in our study was 19.37%, and 9.97% in women. Our observations are not in accordance with the study among commercial pilots in UK that revealed that 9.7% of all male pilots were at high cardiovascular risk and that the mean 10-year cardiovascular risk for the entire pilot population was 8.41% (Houston et al, 2010).

Data on prevalence of cardiovascular risk factors in less developed countries are not abundant. In urban Tanzania, prevalence of cardiovascular risk factors was high, especially in women. The age-adjusted prevalence of obesity in men was 13%, and 35% in women. In men, BMI and waist circumference (WC) were significantly correlated with blood pressure, triglycerides, total cholesterol, LDL- cholesterol, and HDL-cholesterol (BMI only), and fasting glucose. Conversely, in women only blood pressure was positively associated with BMI and WC (Njelekela et al, 2009).

Study in urban Asian Indian subjects observed low prevalence of smoking, hypertension, dyslipidemia, metabolic syndrome and diabetes in adolescents, with rapid escalation of these risk factors by age of 30-39 years (Gupta et al, 2009).

Results of a first nationwide survey on cardiovascular risk factors in Grand-Duchy of Luxembourg have shown the most predominant cardiovascular risk factors was dyslipidemia (69.9%), followed with hypertension (34.5%), smoking (22.3%), and obesity (20.9%), while diabetes was present in 4.4% of study population. Furthermore, only 14.7% of men and 23.1% of women were free of any cardiovascular risk factor (Alkerwi et al, 2010).

Studies have demonstrated that incidence and prevalence of CVD increase with advancing age. However, the predictive value of classic risk factors diminishes with age. The mean value of age of male participants in our study was 58.64 years, and of female participants 57.06 years. There was no significant difference in age between these two groups. Population based observational cohort study in very old people (aged 85 years) with no history of CVD aimed to assess classic risk factors and some new biomarkers (homocysteine, folic acid, CRP, interleukin– 6) as predictors of cardiovascular mortality in this age group. Their results have shown that homocysteine alone accurately identified individuals at high cardiovascular risk, whereas classic risk factors included in the Framingham risk score did not (de Ruijter et al, 2008).

A study that investigated age relations of blood pressure, anthropometric indexes, serum lipids, and hemostatic variables in a population of Papua New Guinea (Lindberg et al., 1997) has found that diastolic blood pressure was not associated with age, while systolic blood pressure linearly increased after 50 years of age in both sexes. BMI decreased with age in both sexes. Serum total cholesterol, triglycerides, LDL-cholesterol increased in males between 20 and 50 years of age, whereas HDL-cholesterol decreased. Authors concluded that some of the relations of age with other cardiovascular risk factors represent effects of biological aging.

Results from EURIKA study (Guallar et al, 2011), which involved participants from 12 European countries with at least one cardiovascular risk, but without CVD reported that the average 10-year risk of CVD death in study participants was 8.2%. Hypertension was responsible for 32.7%, hyperlipidemia for 15.1%, smoking for 10.4%, and diabetes for 16.4% of CVD risk. The four risk factors accounted for 57.7% of CVD risk, representing a 10-year excess risk of CVD death of 5.66%. Study also demonstrated that lack of control of these cardiovascular risk factors was responsible for almost 30% of the risk of CVD death.

Besides age, hypertension, smoking, diabetes, and hyperlipidemia, risk factors for CVD also include obesity, physical inactivity and insulin resistance. A study conducted among adults seeking primary care in Germany reported high prevalence of overweight and obese individuals. Furthermore, a high waist to hip ratio (WHR) was associated with an increased prevalence of high triglycerides, a high blood pressure, an increased fasting glucose, and the presence of diabetes mellitus. On the other hand, a family history of myocardial infarction was not more frequent in patients with high WC compared to patients with normal WC. The prevalence of smoking was significantly lower in overweight men with an elevated and high WC, but not in women (Hauner et al, 2008).

According to Seventh Report of the Joint National Committee on Prevention, Detection, Evaluation, and Treatment of High Blood Pressure, systolic blood pressures of 120–139 mmHg and/or diastolic blood pressures of 80–89 mmHg are classified as prehypertension. Individuals with this condition are thought to be at increased risk of CVD. Results from a cross-sectional study in Jamaica have shown that the prevalence of prehypertension among Jamaicans was 30%. Prehypertension was found in 35% of male subjects, and 25 % of female subjects. Almost 46% of study participants were overweight; 19.7% were obese; 14.6% had hypercholesterolemia; 7.2% had diabetes mellituss, and 17.8% smoked cigarettes. With the exception of cigarette smoking and low physical activity, all the CVD risk factors had significantly higher prevalence in the prehypertensive and hypertensive groups compared to the normotensive group (Ferguson et al, 2008). Results of our study have shown that mean value of systolic blood pressure both in men and in women was bellow 140 mm/Hg. Men had significantly higher values of systolic blood pressure compared to women. Another observation of our study was that there was no significant difference in smoking status between men and women.

Diets high in fat, especially saturated fat, are frequently associated with hypercholesterolemia, hypertension and obesity. Resent findings have reported significant increase in the prevalence of obesity in all age groups, including children, adolescents and adults. A study conducted among physically active college students reported that 45% of participants were overweight or obese. Furthermore, positive association between grain consumption, alcohol intake and BMI was observed. Another finding of this study was that high percentage of subjects had high WHR, elevated systolic and diastolic blood pressure, blood glucose and total cholesterol levels (Sharma et al, 2008). The average value of total cholesterol level both in men and women in our study was above referent limits. On the contrary, average values of HDL-cholesterol in both groups were within normal range. However, since we did not conduct a survey on dietary habits of our participants, we are in no position to draw any conclusions whether there is an association between total cholesterol and HDL-cholesterol values and dietary habits of our study sample. Future studies should address this issue, among population of Bosnia and Herzegovina, since it has been well documented that caloric intake differs between ethnicities, age and socioeconomic groups.

The growing evidence supports the hypothesis that there is ethnic variation in CRP levels. Results of a large population-based study in Black and White men and women in the United States have shown that increased CRP values were more common among women than men, blacks than whites, and in the stroke belt compared to the rest of the U.S. Results of a same study also demonstrated that the use of RRS reclassified population to a different 10-year vascular risk level than the new Framingham Vascular Score (Cushman et al, 2009)). Our results did not show significant difference in CRP values between men and women included in our study. Thus, we were not able to confirm previous findings that gender influences CRP levels. However, this could be due to a limited size of our study sample.

Earlier results have demonstrated that inclusion of CRP in global risk prediction model improves risk classification in women (Cook et al, 2006). On the contrary, critical appraisal of literature on CRP measurement for the prediction of coronary heart disease event (Shah et al, 2009) have revealed that benefits of addition of CRP to models based on traditional risk factors are small and are only slightly resulting in better improvement in risk classification and reclassification.

It is of interest to note that in the present study CRP did not show significant predictive value in cardiovascular risk assessment both in men and in women. Thus, data on possible use of CRP in cardiovascular risk assessment remain conflicting and inconsistent. Possible explanation for the observed inconsistency may be a fact that normal functions of CRP as well as its possible roles in diseases are yet incompletely defined (Casas et al, 2008). The reason for this is that so far no deficiency or structural polymorphism of human CRP have been reported nor is any therapeutic intervention available which specifically inhibits CRP in vivo. Consequently, until today the effects of absence, lack of function or inhibition of human CRP have not been tested.

A large prospective study in Chinese male adults has demonstrated that hypertension and cigarette smoking were the leading predictive parameter for CVD (Ji et al, 2011). Our study had similar observations. We established that in male subjects most predictive value in cardiovascular risk assessment had age followed by systolic blood pressure and genetic factor, respectively. In female subjects, most predictive value in cardiovascular risk assessment had systolic blood pressure followed by age and smoking, respectively.

Limitations of our study merit careful considerations. Importantly, present study was cross-sectional and we did not include prediction of cardiovascular events. Subjects were not a general population but visitors to a Family Medicine Out-patient Clinic in capital city of an urban region in Bosnia and Herzegovina. Longitudinal studies and in larger populations are warranted to test present findings. Another limitation is that this study relied on self- reported smoking history and parental history of myocardial infarction which could bias the validity of findings. However, this potential limitation is extremely unlikely, because self-reported risk factors are commonly used in studies with reasonable accuracy (Sesso et al, 2001).

5. Conclusion

In conclusion, results of this cross-sectional study showed that significant proportion of our study sample belong to medium to high and high cardiovascular risk category. Significant reduction in cardiovascular risk can be achieved by scheduled cardiovascular risk assessment accompanied with appropriate interventions. One of the purposes of the present study was to inform physicians, especially in Bosnia and Herzegovina, about advantages of possible use of web-based RRS calculator in cardiovascular risk assessment of patients they treat in their everyday practice.

The advantage of RRS is that it includes traditional cardiovascular risks accompanied with blood-based biomarkers and parental history of cardiovascular disease that results in better risk assessment and is easily accessible and cost-effective in primary prevention. With the use of RRS, we were able to identify individuals who may require more comprehensive risk stratification. Moreover, findings of the present study suggest that use of RRS may serve in better targeting of treatments in primary prevention settings.

RRS calculator provides information not only on total cardiovascular risk but also how control of certain cardiovascular risk can lead to the reduction of absolute cardiovascular risk in percentages. The use of RRS in cardiovascular risk assessment may result in a better compliance of patients and physicians in their joint efforts to achieve better control of cardiovascular risks.

Based on the results of present study, physicians are strongly encouraged to promote and to intensify well established interventions such as blood pressure control, lipid reduction, smoking cessation, heart-healthy diet, physical activity and weight reduction. One can not foreseen that CVD will be eliminated in a near future, but education, screening, monitoring, and appropriate treatment will certainly lead to the decrease of the morbidity and mortality of these diseases.

6. References

Alkerwi, A., Sauvageot, N., Donneau, A-F., Lair, M-L., Couffignal, S., Beissel, J., Delagardelle, C., Wagener, Y., Albert, A., Guillaume, M. (2010) First nationwide survey on cardiovascular risk factors in Grand-Duchy of Luxembourg (ORISCAV-LUX). *BMC Public Health* 10:468.

Anderssohn, M., Schwedhelm, E., Lüneburg, N., Vasan, RS., Böger, RH. (2010) Asymmetric dimethylarginine as a mediator of vascular dysfunction and a marker of cardiovascular disease and mortality: an intriguing interaction with diabetes mellitus. *Diab Vasc Dis Res.* 7(2):105-18.

Bakhru, A., Erlinger, TP. (2005) Smoking Cessation and Cardiovascular Disease Risk Factors: Results from the Third National Health and Nutrition Examination Survey. *PLoS Med* 2(6): e160.

Balkau, B., Bertrais, S., Ducimetiere, P., Eschwege, E. (1999) Is there a glycemic threshold for mortality risk? *Diabetes Care* 22:696-699.

Berger, JS., Jordan, CO., Lloyd-Jones, D., Blumenthal, RS. (2010) Screening for cardiovascular risk in asymptomatic patients. *J Am Coll Cardiol.* 55(12):1169-77.

Berlin, JA., Colditz, GA. (1990) A meta-analysis of physical activity in the prevention of coronary heart disease. *Am J Epidemiol* 132:612-628.

Blair, SN., Kohl, HW III., Barlow, CE., Paffenbarger, RS Jr., Gibbons, LW., Macera, CA. (1995) Changes in physical fitness and all-cause mortality: a prospective study of healthy and unhealthy men. *JAMA* 273: 1093-1098.

Casas, JP., Shah, T., Hingorani, AD., Danesh, J., Pepys. MB. (2008) C-reactive protein and coronary heart disease: a critical review. *J Intern Med* 264:295-314.

Chiu, M., Austin, PC., Manuel, DG., Tu, JV. (2010) Comparison of cardiovascular risk profiles among ethnic groups using population health surveys between 1996 and 2007. *CMAJ* 182(8):301-310.

Cook, NR., Buring, JE., Ridker, PM. (2006) The effect of including C-reactive protein in cardiovascular risk prediction models for women. *Ann Intern Med.* 145(1):21-29.

Cook, NR. (2007) Use and Misuse of the Receiver Operating Characteristic Curve in Risk Prediction. *Circulation* 115;928-935.

Cushman, M., McClure, LA., Howard, VJ., Jenny, NS., Lakoski, SG., Howard G. (2009) Implications of Elevated C-reactive Protein for Cardiovascular Risk Stratification in Black and White Men and Women in the United States. *Clin Chem.* 55(9): 1627–1636.

Danaei, G., Ding, EL., Mozaffarian, D., Taylor, B., Rehm, J., Murray, CJL., Ezzati M. (2009) The Preventable Causes of Death in the United States: Comparative Risk Assessment of Dietary, Lifestyle, and Metabolic Risk Factors. *PLoS Med* 6(4): e1000058.

Danesh, J., Ch, B., Phil, D., Wheeler, JG., Hirschfield, GM., Eda, S., Eiriksdottir, G., Rumley, A., Lowe, GDO., Pepys, MB., Gudnason V. (2004) C-reactive protein and other circulating markers of inflammation in the prediction of coronary heart disease. *N Engl J Med* 350:1387-1397.

de Ferranti, SD., Rifai, N. (2007) C-reactive protein: a nontraditional serum marker of cardiovascular risk. *Cardiovasc Pathol.* 16:14-21.

de Ruijter, W., Westendorp, RGJ., Assendelft, WJJ., den Elzen, WPJ., de Craen, AJM., le Cessie, S., Gussekloo, J. (2008) Use of Framinghamrisk score andnewbiomarkers to predict cardiovascular mortality in older people: population based observational cohort study. *BMJ* 337:a3083.

Dobson, AJ., Alexander, HM., Heller, RF., Lloyd, DM. (1991) How soon after quitting smoking does risk of heart attack decline? *J Clin Epidemiol* 44:1247-1253.

Eaton, CB., Bostom, AG., Yanek, L. (1996) Family history and premature heart disease. *J Am Board Fam Pract* 9:312-318.

Ferguson, TS., Younger, NOM., Tulloch-Reid, MK., Wright, MBL., Ward, EM., Ashley, DE., Wilks, RJ. (2008) Prevalence of prehypertension and its relationship to risk factors for cardiovascular disease in Jamaica: Analysis from a cross-sectional survey. *BMC Cardiovascular Disorders* 8:20.

Folsom, AR., Szklo, M., Stevens, J., Liao, F., Smith, R., Eckfeldt, JH. (1997) A prospective study of coronary heart disease in relation to fasting insulin, glucose, and diabetes: the Atherosclerosis Risk in Communities (ARIC) Study. *Diabetes Care* 20:935-942.

Green, DJ., O'Driscoll, G., Joyner, MJ., Cable, NT. (2008) Exercise and cardiovascular risk reduction: Time to update the rationale for exercise? *J Appl Physiol.* 105(2):766-768.

Green, D., Chan, C., Kang, J., Lin, K., Schreiner, P., Jenny, N., Tracy, RP. (2010) Longitudinal assessment of fibrinogen in relation to subclinical cardiovascular diseases: the CARDIA study. *J Thromb Haemost* 8(3):489-495.

Guallar, E., Banegas, JR., Blasco-Colmenares, E., Jiménez, FJ., Dallongeville, J., Halcox, JP., Borghi, C., Massó-González, EL., Tafalla, M., Perk, J., Backer, GD., Steg, PG., Rodríguez-Artalejo, F. (2011) Excess risk attributable to traditional cardiovascular risk factors in clinical practice settings across Europe – The EURIKA Study. *BMC Public Health* 11:704.

Gupta, R., Misra, A., Vikram, NK., Kondal, D., Gupta, SS., Agrawal, A., Pandey, RM. (2009) Younger age of escalation of cardiovascular risk factors in Asian Indian subjects. *BMC Cardiovascular Disorders* 9:28.

Havranek, EP., Froshang, DB., Emserman, CDB., Hanratty, R., Krantz, MJ., Masoudi, FA., Dickinson, LM., Steiner, JF. (2008) Left ventricular hypertrophy and cardiovascular mortality by race and ethnicity. *Am J Med.* 121(10):870-875.

Hauner, H., Bramlage, P., Lösch, C., Steinhagen-Thiessen, E., Schunkert, H., Wasem, J., Jöckel, K-H., Moebus, S. (2008) Prevalence of obesity in primary care using different anthropometric measures – Results of the German Metabolic and Cardiovascular Risk Project (GEMCAS). *BMC Public Health* 8:282.

Houston, S., Mitchell, S., Evans, S. (2010) Application of a cardiovascular disease risk prediction model among commercial pilots. *Aviat Space Environ Med.* 81(8):768-73.

Ji, J., Pan, E., Li, J., Chen, J., Cao, J., Sun, D., Lu, X., Chen, S., Gu, D., Duan, X., Wu, X., Huang, J. (2011) Classical risk factors of cardiovascular disease among Chinese male steel workers: a prospective cohort study for 20 years. *BMC Public Health* 11:497.

Katrinchak, C., Fritz, K. (2007) Clinical implications of C-reactive protein as a predictor of vascular risk. *J Am Acad Nurse Pract.* 19:335-340.

Kones, R. (2011) Primary prevention of coronary heart disease: integration of new data, evolving views, revised goals, and role of rosuvastatin in management. A comprehensive survey. *Drug Des, Devel Ther.* 5: 325–380.

Landim, MB., Casella-Filho, A., Chagas, AC. (2009) Asymmetric dimethylarginine (ADMA) and endothelial dysfunction: implications for atherogenesis. *Clinics (Sao Paulo).* 64(5):471-478.

Lange, RA., Cigarroa, JE., Hillis, LD. (2004) Theodore e. Woodward award: cardiovascular complications of cocaine abuse. *Trans Am Clin Climatol Assoc.* 115:99-114.

Lindberg, S., Berntrop, E., Nilsson-Ehle, P., Terent, A., Vessby, B. (1997) Age relations of cardiovascular risk factors in traditional Melanesian society: the Kitava Study. *Am J Clin Nutr.* 66:845-852.

Macabasco-O'Connell, A., Danwalder, S., Sinha, K. (2011) Cardiac risk scores in high-risk Hispanics and the predictive value of BNP. *J Clin Nurs.* (epub ahead of print)

Melander, O., Newton-Cheh, C., Almgren, P., Hedblad, B., Berglund, G., Engström, G., Persson, M., Smith, JG., Magnusson, M., Christensson, A., Struck, J., Morgenthaler, NG., Bergmann, A., Pencina, M., Wang, TJ. (2009) Novel and conventional biomarkers for the prediction of incident cardiovascular events in the community. *JAMA* 302(1):49–57.

Miller, VM., Duckles, SP. (2008) Vascular actions of estrogens: functional implications. *Pharmacol Rev.* 60(2): 210-241.

Nebi, H., Kivimaki, M., Zins, M., Elovainiio, M., Conseli, SM., Cordier, S., Ducimetiere, P., Goldberg, M., Singf-Manoux, A. (2008) Does personality predict mortality? *Int J Epidemiol.* 37(2):386-396.

Njelekela, MA., Mpembeni, R., Muhihi, A., Mligiliche, NL., Spiegelman, D., Hertzmark, E., Liu, E., Finkelstein, JL., Fawzi, WW., Willett, WC., Mtabaji, J. (2009) Gender-related differences in the prevalence of cardiovascular disease risk factors and their correlates in urban Tanzania. *BMC Cardiovascular Disorders* 9:30.

Packard, RRS., Libby, P. (2008) Inflammation in atherosclerosis: from vascular biology to biomarker discovery and risk prediction. *Clin Chem.* 54(1):24-38.

Pearson, TA., Mensah, GA., Alexander, RW., Anderson, JL., Cannon, RO., Criqui, M. (2003) Markers of inflammation and cardiovascular disease: application to clinical and public health practice: A statement for healthcare professionals from the Centers for Disease Control and Prevention and the American Heart Association. *Circulation* 107:499–511.

Pencina, MJ., D'Agostino, Sr. RB., Larson, MG., Massaro, JM., Vasan, RS. (2009) Predicting the Thirty-year Risk of Cardiovascular Disease: The Framingham Heart Study. *Circulation* 119(24): 3078–3084.

Pepys, M., Hirschfield, G. (2003) C-reactive protein: a critical update. *J Clin.Invest.* 111:1805-1812.

Phillips, AN., Shaper, AG., Pocock, SJ., Walker, M. (1988) Parental death from heart disease and risk of heart attack. *Eur Heart J* 9:243-251.

Reriani, MK., Lerman, LO., Lerman, A. (2010) Endothelial function as a functional expression of cardiovascular risk factors. *Biomark Med.* 4(3):351–360.

Ridker, PM., Wilson, PWF., Grundy, SM. (2004) Should C-reactive protein be added to metabolic syndrome and to assessment of global cardiovascular risk? *Circulation* 109(23):2818-2825.

Ridker, PM., Buring, JE., Rifai, N., Cook, NR. (2007) Development and validation of improved algorithms for the assessment of global cardiovascular risk in women: The Reynolds Risk Score. *JAMA* 297(6):611-619.

Ridker, PM., Paynter, NP., Rifai, N., Gaziano, JM., Cook, NR. (2008) C-Reactive Protein and Parental History Improve Global Cardiovascular Risk Prediction: The Reynolds Risk Score for Men. *Circulation* 118;2243-2251.

Rimm, EB., Stampfer, MJ., Giovannuci, E. (1995) Body size and fat distribution as predictors of coronary heart disease among middle-age and older U.S. men. *Am J Epidemiol* 141:1117-1127.

Ronksley, PE., Brien, SE., Turner, BJ., Mukamai, KJ., Ghali, WA. (2011) Assocaition of alcohol consumption with selected cardiovascular diseases outcomes: a systematic review and meta-analysis. *BMJ* 342:d671.

Sacco, RL., Khatri, M., Rundek, T., Xu, O., Gardener, H., Boden-Albala, B., Di Tullio MR., Homma, S., Mitchell SVE., Paik, MC. (2009) Improving Global Vascular Risk Prediction with Behavioral and Anthropometric Factors: The Multi-ethnic Northern Manhattan Cohort Study. *J Am Coll Cardiol.* 54(24): 2303–2311.

Schaefer, EJ., Lamon-Fava, S., Ordovas, JM. (1994) Factors associated with low and elevated plasma high density lipoprotein cholesterol and apolipoprotein A-I levels in the Framingham offspring study. *J Lipid Res* 35:871-882.

Sesso, HD., Lee, IM., Gaziano, JM., Rexrode, KM., Glynn, RJ., Buring, JE. (2001) Maternal and paternal history of myocardial infarction and risk of cardiovascular disease in men and women. *Circulation* 104:393-398.

Shah, T., Casas, JP., Cooper, JA., Tzoulaki, I., Sofat, R., McCormack, V., Smeeth, L., Deanfield, JE., Lowe, GD., Rumley, A., Fowkes, GR., Humphries, SE., Hingorani, AD. (2009) Critical appraisal of CRP measurement for the prediction of coronary heart disease events: new data and systematic review of 31 prospective cohorts. *Int J Epidemiol.* 38:217–231.

Sharma, SV., Bush, JA., Lorino, AJ., Knoblauch, M., Abuamer, D., Blog,G., Bertman D. (2008) Diet and Cardiovascular Risk in University Marching Band, Dance Team and Cheer Squad Members: a cross-sectional study. J Int Soc Sports Nutr. 5:9.

Thomas, JC., Vohra, RS., Beer, S., Bhatti, K., Ponnambalam, S., Homer-Vanniasinkam, S. (2009) Biomarkers in peripheral arterial disease. *Trends Cardiovasc Med.* 19(5):147-151.

Tracy, RP., Psaty, BM., Macy, E., Bovill, EG., Cushman, M. (1997) Lifetime smoking exposure affects the association of C-reactive protein with cardiovascular disease risk factors and subclinical disease in healthy elderly subjects. *Arterioscler Thromb Vasc Biol* 17: 2167–2176.

Vasan, RS., Larson, MG., Kannel, WB., Levy, D. (2000) Evolution of hypertension from non-hypertensive blood pressure levels: rates of progression in the Framingham Heart Study (abstract 869-2). *J Am Coll Cardiol* 35:292A.

Wannamethee, G., Whincup, PH., Shaper, AG., Walker, M., MacFarlane, PW. (1995) Factors determining case fatality in myocardial infarction "who dies in a heart attack?" *Brit Heart J* 74:324-331.

Wilson, PF., D'Agostino, RB., Levy, D., Belanger, AM., Silbershatz, H., Kannel, WB. (1998) Prediction of coronary heart disease using risk factor categories. *Circulation* 97:1837-1847.

Wilson, PW. (1990) High-density lipoprotein, low-density lipoprotein, and coronary artery disease. *Am J Cardiol* 66:7A-10A.

5

Theoretical Identification of Behavioral Risk Factors Among Multiple Risk Factors Causing Morning Onset of Cardiac Events due to Circadian Variations

Fumiko Furukawa[1] and Tatsuya Morimoto[2]
[1]School of Nursing, University of Shizuoka
[2]School of Pharmaceutical Sciences, University of Shizuoka
Japan

1. Introduction

Circadian variations of cardiac events exist, although times of onset differ slightly between studies (Atkinson et al., 2010; Muller et al., 1989; Quyyumi, 1990; Scheer et al., 2010; Willich et al., 1987). However, several studies have confirmed the occurrence of more events in the morning than in the evening (Atkinson et al., 2010; Mulcahy et al., 1988; Scheer et al., 2010). Two peaks of onset of cardiac events were found: a high frequency of cardiac events in the hours after rising in the morning and in the evening hours (Atkinson et al., 2010; Hjalmarson et al., 1989; Mulcahy et al., 1988; Muller, 1987).

Because cardiac events occurred more frequently in the morning than at any other times of the day, the occurrences of these events are discussed relative to the time after awakening (Kiowski & Osswald, 1993). A specific single factor causing circadian variation in the morning has not been identified. It has been suggested that interactions between multiple factors during transition from the sleep state to the waking stage may occur simultaneously or as a self-sustaining reaction (Atkinson et al., 2010; Scheer et al., 2010).

Evidence regarding physiological risk factors for morning onset of cardiac events has been used when selecting the most appropriate time for taking antihypertensive or anti-arrhythmic medications (Athyros et al., 1998; Mulcahy, 1999; Redon, 2004). For example, Redon (2004) indicated that the angiotensin II blocker telmisartan with a long half-life given once daily is likely to confer benefit in terms of 24-hour blood pressure control and reduce early morning surge in blood pressure. Despite applications of this evidence to medical treatment, few studies examine use of behavioral risk factors related to morning onset of cardiac events. For example, final decisions based on evidence regarding the safest time to exercise during the day are still pending (Atkinson et al., 2006; Atkinson & Davenne, 2007; Murray et al.,1993; Shiotani et al., 2009; White, 2003).

Even though Ebrahim et al. (2006, 2011) indicated that intervention using educational method may be effective in reducing mortality in cardiac high risk population, few discussions have taken place regarding how to apply the current evidence regarding morning onset of cardiac events to patient education. In particular, knowledge about preventive strategies for self-care that minimize the chance of recurrent morning onset of cardiac events is lacking. Amazingly, most patient educational materials about cardiac disease do not contain information about risks of morning behaviors.

Although behavioral risk factors for cardiac events will not significantly influence daily life if they occur once in a while at an early age, human behaviors tend to be unconscious and habitual throughout life. By identifying behavioral risk factors among multiple risk factors that can trigger morning onset of cardiac events, patients with cardiac disease may be able to avoid life-threatening conditions and reconsider their daily lives, including the cycle of activity, rest, and sleep that is associated with quality of life (Baas, 2004; Condon & McCarthy, 2006; Kristofferzon et al., 2007; Noriss et al., 2004). By controlling behavioral risks among the multiple risk factors for cardiac events in the morning, it might be possible to reduce the frequency of early morning cardiac events.

Reviewing evidence regarding behavioral risk factors of morning onset of cardiac events may be helpful for health professionals including doctors and nurses in the cardiovascular community to educate the patients. Furthermore, interventions supported by research that ameliorate life-threatening conditions may improve the quality of patient education. Thus, the primary aim of this chapter is to identify behavioral risk factors among possible causes of morning onset of cardiac events. To develop interventions leading to evidence-based practice, the secondary aim is to suggest strategies for controlling behavioral risk factors that trigger morning onset of cardiac events.

2. Methods

Material reviewed in this chapter was based on journals reporting risk factors related to cardiac events. First, focus of the review was put on the physiological perspective in nature, and then behavioral risk factors were reviewed to suggest strategies for controlling such risk factors. Because physiological conditions are usually deteriorated by behavioral risk factors under the occurrence of cardiac events, it is importance to recognize how each physiological risk factor is progressed and interacted with each other (Deedwania, 1996). Recognition regarding physiological risk factors is also important to develop effective strategies for controlling behavioral risk factors (Baxendale, 1992).

The electronic databases of PubMed (1950 to 2011), CINAHL (1998 to 2011), and the COCHRANE Library (1998 to 2011) were searched for topics related to morning cardiac events and their mechanism. Key words were as follows: circadian variation, sleep, ischemic episodes, cardiac events, cardiac disease, autonomic nervous system activation, physical stress (abrupt upright posture), mental stress, endothelial response of the coronary blood vessels, morning surge of blood pressure, and blood components (Carnethon et al., 2002; Cooke-Ariel, 1998; Furukawa et al., 1998; Khoury et al., 1992; Scheer et al., 2010; Thrall et al., 2007; White, 2003). By searching the database for these key words, evidence regarding behavioral risks factors triggering morning cardiac events was identified, and preventive patient education strategies to decrease morning onset of cardiac events are proposed.

All journals used for this review were limited in only English language, and findings from the animal study were included to understand mechanism of the morning onset of cardiac events in patients with cardiac disease. Also the findings reported in the 1998 review

(Furukawa et al., 1998) were used in part in this review. Permission for utilization of the findings was obtained from the editor.

3. Results

Possible risk factors for cardiac events were as follows: 1) coronary artery blood flow dynamics during sleep; 2) physiology of sympathetic nervous system activation in the morning; 3) pathophysiology of sympathetic nervous system activation in the morning, including coronary blood flow, α- and β-adrenergic receptor responses of coronary artery endothelial cells to sympathetic nerves, platelet aggregation and atherosclerosis with sympathetic nervous activation, neurotransmitters and hormonal elements, and other risk factors for cardiac events, such as morning surge in blood pressure and seasonal variations; and 4) behavioral risk factors immediately after awakening, including abrupt changes of body position.

3.1 Coronary artery blood flow dynamics during sleep

Because of the sleeping state in relation to patterns of REM and non-REM sleep (Aserinsky & Kleitman, 1953; Jouvet, 1967; Steriade, 1992), the morning onset of cardiac events should be discussed from this point. One sleeping cycle is made up of one REM and one non-REM sleep period, and four to six cycles are repeated during the night in adults. Non-REM sleep has four sub-stages, from I to IV, during one cycle, and the depth of sleep increases progressively toward stage IV and then decreases in REM sleep. People wake up mostly at the end of the last rapid eye movement sleep (Willis, 1981).

During the night, arterial blood pressure falls progressively by 5% to 23% from the wakening state to stage IV of non-REM sleep (Martin, 1984). Giles (2005) indicated blood pressure in most people is from 10% to 20% lower than the mean daytime value (Giles, 2005). Cardiac output is minimized during the last rapid eye movement sleep period before arousal and is 25% lower than that during wakening (Martin, 1984). Changes in blood flow of the coronary artery vessels from the beginning of sleep to the time of awakening make insufficient blood flow in cardiac muscles at the time of restart of physical activity immediately upon awakening.

In healthy subjects, increased blood flow by sustained physical activity might lead to vasodilatation, which is induced by endothelial derived relaxing factor released from endothelial cells (Furchgott, 1983). This is a compensation mechanism to increase the blood supply to cardiac muscle. However, such mechanism may not work in patients with cardiac disease. The sudden rises in heart rate at each transition from non-REM sleep (deeper sleep) to REM sleep (lighter sleep), or increase in blood pressure at awakening may precipitate cardiac events (Viola et al., 2002).

3.2 Physiology of sympathetic nervous system activation in the morning

Coronary blood flow is determined by five factors (West, 1990): metabolic control (oxygen demand), coronary perfusion pressure, systolic compression, autonomic nervous system, and circulating catecholamine and other vasoactive substances. Determinants for coronary blood flow are conveyed by auto-regulatory mechanisms. Sympathetic nerve fibers stimulate α-adrenergic receptors of the endothelial cells to respond to vasoconstriction so as to increase coronary vascular resistance (Laxson et al., 1992; Baran et al., 1992; Quyyumi et al., 1992). Stimulation of β-adrenergic receptors of the endothelial cells is a response to coronary vasodilatation (Baran et al., 1992; Quyyumi et al., 1992).

Epinephrine, norepinephrine, and acetylcholine also act through adrenergic receptors of smooth muscle in the coronary arteries (Furchgott, 1983; Kuo et al., 1993). In the transition period from resting to activity in healthy person in the morning, coronary arteries of the human heart can receive signals normally from the sympathetic nervous system due to the increased physical and mental stress associated with awakening, and the compensatory mechanisms of the coronary artery function are well activated to meet oxygen demands.

3.3 Pathophysiology of sympathetic nervous system activation in the morning

In this section, 1) coronary blood flow, 2) α- and β-adrenergic receptor responses of coronary artery endothelial cells to the sympathetic nervous system, 3) platelet aggregation and atherosclerosis with sympathetic nervous activation, 4) neurotransmitters and hormonal elements under sympathetic nervous activation, and 5) other risk factors are reviewed.

3.3.1 Coronary blood flow

Ischemic episodes occur if the increase in coronary blood flow is inadequate for the myocardial oxygen demand. The frequency of ischemic episodes is maximized in the first 2 hours after awakening (Quyyumi, 1990; Rocco, 1990). Coronary spasms due to vasoconstriction are a trigger for ischemic episodes (Sugiishi & Takatsu, 1993). Coronary artery constriction is more severe in the early morning than in the late afternoon, and coronary blood flow at rest in the morning is lower than in the afternoon under comparable hemodynamic conditions (Fujita & Franklin, 1987).

Vascular resistance increases due to the decreased blood flow in patients with hypertrophy or elevated left ventricular diastolic pressure (Duncker et al., 1993). When coronary vascular resistance is increased in the morning, the ischemic threshold is lower than in the afternoon (Benhorin et al., 1993; Quyyumi et al., 1992). Also, the cardiac output during the last REM sleep period before arousal is lowest, and it is one fourth of that while wakening (Martin, 1984). These studies indicate that abrupt and vigorous physical stress becomes a risk factor for cardiac events.

3.3.2 α- and β-adrenergic receptor response of coronary artery endothelial cells to the sympathetic nervous system

The vascular endothelium modifies the contractile characteristics of vascular smooth muscle (Greenberg et al., 1990). When the vasodilator response to acetylcholine in endothelial dysfunction is eliminated, the coronary perfusion rate increases (Furchgott et al., 1980). Endothelial injury initiated by atherosclerotic change leads to plaque formation in a variety of conditions (Zemel & Sowers, 1990; Baxendale, 1992).

Similarly, injury to the endothelial wall triggers monocyte and platelet aggregation, which leads to release of growth factors into the smooth muscle of coronary arteries (Lucchesi,

1990). In particular, the injured endothelial vessel wall produces a paradoxical response that alters the normal response against α- and β-receptors on the vessel walls (Ludmer et al., 1986). The neural sympathetic tone, which increases in the morning, may cause an increased stimulation of α-adrenergic receptors, leading to coronary and peripheral vasoconstriction.

The presence of enough β-adrenergic receptors is necessary to adapt to the increased oxygen demand (Hammond et al., 1992; Figueras & Lindon, 1995). However, the number of β-adrenergic receptors decreases if there is volume overload–induced myocardial hypertrophy, or if the endothelial cells of the coronary artery are impaired (Figueras & Lidon, 1995; Hammond et al., 1992). Patients with unstable angina during bed rest and with significant coronary disease demonstrate a lower ischemic threshold early in the morning (Figueras & Lindon, 1995). Usually, plasma levels of norepinephrine are increased and myocardial levels of norepinephrine are decreased in patients with fewer β-adrenergic receptors (West, 1990; Hammond et al., 1992). The increased plasma norepinephrine over-stimulates sympathetic nervous activity and acts mostly on α-adrenergic receptors, causing vessel constriction (Hammond et al., 1992; Kuo et al., 1993; West, 1990).

3.3.3 Platelet aggregation and atherosclerosis with sympathetic nervous activation

Accelerated platelets aggragation is one of significant risk factors for the morning onset of ischemic episodes (Andrews et al., 1996; Quyyumi, 1990; Braunwald, 1995). The plasma levels of fibrin peptide (thrombin generator) in patients with variant angina are significantly higher from midnight to early morning than other times (Masuda et al., 1994). The plasma norepinephrine concentration (Brezinski et al., 1988), renin activity, and angiotensin II concentration (Oparil et al., 1970; Schachter, 2004) are all increased with change of platelet levels.

Activated platelets release potent vasoactive factors due to adherence of atherosclerotic plaque and cause vasoconstriction or vasospasms (Kaul et al., 1993; Vanhoutte & Huston, 1985). A plaque rupture associated with well-developed atherosclerotic conditions in the coronary artery is often occurred in the morning as sympathetic activity is upregulated, and this induced increase in blood pressure (Shimada et al., 2001; Stone, 1990). Fibrinogen is also involved in this process (Palmieri et al., 2003), and leads to increased blood viscosity (Jay et al., 1990; Lowe et al., 1980).

Plasma fibrinogen has further been found to stimulate red cell aggregation in familial hypercholesterolemia (Jay et al., 1990). The increased fibrinogen and red blood cells lead to increased blood viscosity (Yarnell et al., 1991). In addition, body fluid during sleep usually shifts from the vascular space to the interstitial space (Jacob et al., 1998). These conditions may lead to vasoconstriction and cause vessel occlusion in the presence of atherosclerosis and physical stress in the morning.

3.3.4 Neurotransmitters and hormonal elements

Neurotransmitters and hormonal elements such as epinephrine, norepinephrine, neuropeptide Y, and acetylcholine also participate in cardiac events through aggregation (Eisenhofer et al., 1992; Pernow et al., 1988; Svendsen et al., 1990; Yang & Levy, 1993) and interrelations with endothelial dysfunction (Ludmer et al., 1986), sympathetic nervous system activation (Drager et al., 2009), degrees of coronary blood flow (Fujita & Franklin, 1987; Kuo et al., 1993; Young & Vatner, 1986), level of co-existing atherosclerosis (Ludmer et al., 1986), sleep cycle during the morning transitional phase (Culebras, 1992; Steriade, 1992; Viola et al., 2002), and sleep duration (Cappuccio et al., 2011).

In particular, plasma epinephrine and norepinephrine levels were shown to increase rapidly while plasma volume induced by an abrupt upright posture fell by 13% over 14 minutes (Jacob et al., 1998). Epinephrine approached baseline values by 20 minutes of standing, but norepinephrine spillover increased by 80% and clearance decreased by 30% with 30 minutes of standing (Jacob et al., 1998). Inhibition of the morning surge in catecholamine levels may reduce the risk of thrombotic vascular events in atherosclerosis (Andwers et al., 1999).

3.3.5 Other risks factors

The morning increase in blood pressure, called the morning surge, is one of the risk factors for cardiac events (Giles, 2005; Ohkubo et al., 2008; White, 2001). In addition, morning onset of cardiac events might occur more easily in winter if the body is suddenly exposed to a cold environment (Peters et al., 1996). Mental stress also may cause stress-induced cardiac arrhythmic vulnerability associated with sudden cardiac death (Critchley et al., 2005).

3.4 Behavioral risk factors immediately after awakening

Physical activity, such as standing up immediately after awakening, affects the blood components. In healthy men, a significant change in platelet aggregation occurs as a result of a compensatory homeostatic mechanism against the immediate change to the upright position (Muller et al., 1989; Krantz et al., 1996). Adaption to the change of position after awakening causes persistent platelet aggregation for the next 90 minutes; this platelet aggregation is greater than walking up and down stairs. (Muller et al., 1989). If activities such as walking up and down stairs are performed immediately after waking, platelet aggregation becomes greater than just staying in the upright position (Muller et al., 1989). Because the abrupt upright position after awakening brings a significant change in platelet aggregation with persistent manner, patients with cardiac disease may experience an adverse effect of exercise in the morning (Hilberg et al., 2000).

Also, the upright posture from spine position made plasma volume fell by 13% over approximately 14 minutes in healthy subjects, after which time it remained relatively stable (Jacob et al., 1998). This occurs as a result of compensatory homeostatic mechanisms responding to the initial decrease in central blood and stroke volume from the heart induced by the physical stress (Ahmadizad et al., 2006; Thrall et al., 2007). The sudden rises in heart rate in this case may occur to compensate cardiac output based on the intense of activity. These changes in platelet aggregation and plasma volume occurred in healthy subjects may become severe triggers of cardiac events for patients with cardiac disease.

4. Discussion and conclusion

Cardiac events often occur in the morning after awakening. Many studies report similar findings in terms of the circadian variation of the cardiac events. The significant behavioral risk factor was an abrupt upright position at awakening and seriously acted on

Theoretical Identification of Behavioral Risk Factors Among Multiple Risk Factors Causing
Morning Onset of Cardiac Events due to Circadian Variations

81

physiological risk factors at the occurrence of the cardiac events. The most plausible underline cause of cardiac events in the morning in patients with progressed atherosclerosis was activation of the sympathetic nervous system due to activity immediately upon rising (Kiowski & Osswald, 1993; Stone, 1990; Umemura et al., 1987). Studies on physical stress for cardiac disease under variety of settings were available (Camici et al., 1992; Herd, 1991), but only a few studies of the relation between physical stress and morning onset of the cardiac events were found. The activation of the sympathetic nervous system by physical activity after rising (Umemura et al., 1987) should be considered in relation to levels of atherosclerosis and sleeping stages. The nature of sleep (Culebras, 1992; Steriade, 1992) plays an important role in the morning onset of cardiac events.

A shift change of domination in the autonomic nervous system occurs upon awakening, so that the sympathetic nervous system is activated to prepare for physical and mental activities in the morning. The morning surge of blood pressure can be explained by this shift change, because the sympathetic nervous system is activated by exogenous factors (Leary et al., 2002; van Eekelen et al., 2004a). It should be noted that domination of the sympathetic nervous system in the morning may play a major role on the occurrence of cardiac events (Atkinson et al., 2010; van Eekelen et al., 2004a, 2004b).

In particular, patients who have atherosclerosis may experience a paradoxical response in their vessels under sympathetic nervous system activation with abrupt physical activities undertaken after awakening in the morning (Ludmer et al., 1986). Atherosclerosis triggers cardiac events by creating a paradoxical response in the injured endothelial cells of coronary vessels, providing the greatest vulnerability to sympathetic nervous activity (Ludmer et al., 1986). Thus, normal daytime activity may become a powerful stimulus if it is undertaken in the morning by patients with coronary artery disease (Freed et al., 1989; Herd, 1991; Meller et al., 1979).

It can be assumed that we might experience cardiac events at the time of awakening in the morning because our lives repeat to follow a daily active-sleep cycle, and nobody can develop atherosclerosis with aging. The last REM sleep at the time of awakening is needed to create a smooth transition from parasympathetic to sympathetic nervous activation. As one study indicated, REM sleep works to increase pulse rate (Martin, 1984). The last REM sleep may bring a wake-up ready condition by increasing pulse rate through gradually stimulating the sympathetic nervous system (Martin, 1984) and decreasing parasympathetic nervous system activation (van Eekelen et al., 2004a). Using evidence on the nature of sleep is beneficial if strategies for controlling the morning onset of cardiac events are developed.

Waking-up at REM sleep, not at non-REM sleep may be important for decreasing cardiac events in the morning. REM sleep provide a waking-up ready condition to cardiovascular system. To facilitate waking-up at rapid eye movement sleep, it is better to avoid utilizing an alarm clock, and use non-artificial stimuli such as sunlight providing a natural wake-up call. People should sleep with the shades and curtains open so that they are woken up with natural sunlight that will lead us to wake up at REM sleep.

Similarly, it is important for patients with cardiac disease to not wake up in the morning during non-REM sleep. Because coronary blood flow is the lowest at the last non-REM sleep (Martin, 1984), cardiac output in patients with cardiac disease might not respond adequately to a sudden increase of coronary blood flow at the time of wakening (Kuo et al., 1993), so that supply and demand become unbalanced (Li, 2003). If patients with cardiac disease show non-movement of eyelids, smooth movement of the chest, and quiet breathing indicating non-REM sleep (Aserinski & Kleitman, 1953; Aserinski & Kleitman, 2003), it is better for them to be left until waking-up by themselves.

In addition to sensitivity to REM sleep and non-REM sleep, levels of catecholamine and coronary tone should be considered because they are lowest just before awakening (Linsell et al., 1985). During the transitional phase from sleep state to physical activity state in patients with atherosclerosis, insufficient oxygen supply to the heart occurs. The high levels of catecholamine at awakening may produce a severe paradoxical response to the coronary vessel wall in patients with progressing atherosclerosis, leading to vasospasm (Ludmer et al., 1986). Such vasospasms might trigger a cardiac event. Atherosclerosis of artery walls develops over a long period and progresses with a high-fat diet and a sedentary lifestyle. The cardiovascular system should be maintained in a healthy condition by an adequate caloric intake and an active lifestyle (Ebrahim et al., 2011). From the viewpoint of human evolution, modern life with excess caloric intake and sedentary lifestyles may contribute to the increased number of cardiac events that occur in the morning.

Although atherosclerotic changes are significantly associated with aging, platelet aggregation may not be. Platelet aggregation has shown to be triggered in healthy young people who assume an abrupt upright position in the morning (Muller et al., 1989; Tofler et al., 1987) and works with fibrinogen levels to significantly contribute to morning onset of cardiac events (Braunwald, 1995). Abruptly assuming an upright position immediately after awakening is now a known risk factor for cardiac events, and may create a life-threatening condition in patients with the major cardiac risk factors. However, such behavior seems to be recognized as a small factor that can be modified, and the effects of this change have not been studied.

Abrupt changes in blood pressure and heart rate due to adoption of an upright position after awaking in the morning may trigger platelet aggregation, enhancing the degree of occlusion of the coronary artery with aging (Storm et al., 1989). Once platelet aggregation occurs, it lasts for hours (Muller et al., 1989). Activated platelets release potent vasoactive factors due to adherence of atherosclerotic plaque, and cause vasoconstriction or vasospasms (Kaul et al., 1993; Vanhoutte & Huston, 1985). This phenomenon may create a morning peak in cardiac events. Patients with cardiac disease should take their time getting up in the morning, engaging only in slow activities until platelet aggregation subsides. Furthermore, they should maintain ideal fibrinogen levels by taking part in regular exercise (Furukawa et al., 2008).

Cold temperatures with seasonal variations at the transitional phase in the morning are also a risk factor triggering cardiac events (Peters et al., 1996). These temperatures may increase blood pressure by constricting peripheral vessels. Increased blood pressure might create rupture of the vessel's wall and release clots, leading to ischemic events (Shimada et al., 2001). Here again, rupture of the vessel wall leads to an increase in platelets (Shimada et al., 2001). Abruptly assuming an upright posture, which causes platelet aggregation, will precipitate ischemic events during a few hours after awakening in the morning. Therefore, before patients rise from bed, they should lay quietly in bed for a few minutes.

In general, four strategies are recommended to reduced cardiac events in the early morning, especially for people with any cardiac disease: waking up at the end of rapid eye movement sleep, laying in bed for a few minutes after awakening, slowly raising the body from bed, and staying relaxed at least 30 minutes after awakening. Staying relaxed in 30 minutes is suggested because the once increased norepinephrine spillover by standing mostly decreased after 30 minutes (Jacob et al., 1998). Relaxation therapy is also recommended in the morning to control sympathetic nervous activation in patients with cardiac disease (Benson et al., 1974; Guzzetta, 1989; Hoffman et al., 1982; Melville, 1987).

From a preventive perspective for self-care, health professionals might intervene in awakening behavior to control one of the risk factors that triggers cardiac events in the morning. Based on findings of this review, an experimental study should be conducted to identify the effects of interventions associated with the four wakening behaviors identified.

In conclusion, evidence indicates that activation of the sympathetic nervous system due to physical stress in the morning is a significant factor causing morning cardiac events in relation to the pattern of REM and non-REM sleep stages in patients with atherosclerosis. In addition to controlling the major cardiac risk factors causing cardiac events, four strategies for controlling the abrupt upright position at wakening should be included in patient education to reduce cardiac events for patients with cardiac disease. These strategies include waking up at the end of REM sleep, laying in bed for a few minutes after awakening, slowly raising the body from bed, and staying relaxed at least 30 minutes after awakening. Health professionals play vital roles on identifying novel behavioral risk factors that trigger morning cardiac events. Because it is important to maintain continuity of the activity, rest, sleep cycle of daily life in patients with cardiac disease, strategies for patient education should focus on preventive behaviors that control triggers of cardiac events.

5. Clinical implications for managing behavioral risk factors for morning cardiac events

Health professionals should develop educational strategies to reduce the frequency of cardiac events by modifying the patient behaviors such as abruptly assuming an upright position upon awakening in the morning. When patients wake up, they should stay in bed for few minutes and slowly sit up, then stand and walk in relaxed manner. In addition, running up and down stairs, smoking, mental stress, and other behaviors immediately after awakening should be avoided.

6. References

Ahmadizad, S., El-Sayed, M.S., & Maclaren, D.P. (2006). Responses of Platelet Activation and Function to a Single Bout of Resistance Exercise and Recovery. *Clinical Hemorheology and Microcirculation*, Vo.35, No.1-2, pp159-168, ISSN 1386-0291

Andrews, N.P., Goldstein, D.S., & Quyyumi, A.A. (1999). Effect of Systemic Alpha-2 Adrenagic Blockade on the Morning Increase in Platelet Aggragation in Normal Subjects. *American Journal of Cardiology*, Vol.84, No.3, pp. 316-320, ISSN 0002-9149

Andrews, N.P.,Gralnick, H.R., & Merryman, P., et al. (1996). Mechanisms Underlying the Morning Increase in Platelet Aggregation: a Flow Cytometry Study. *American Journal of Cardiology*, Vol.28, No.7, pp.1789-1795,ISSN 0002-9149

Aserinsky, E., & Kieitman, N.(1953). Regularly Occurring Periods of Eye Motility and Concomitant Phenomena during Sleep. *Science,* Vol.118, No.3062, pp. 273-274, ISSN 0036-8075

Aserinsky, E. & Kleitman, N. (2003). Regularly Occurring Periods of Eye Motility and Concomitant Phenomena during Sleep. 1953. *Journal of Neuropsychiatry Clinical Neuroscience,* Vol.15, No.4, pp. 454-455, ISSN 0895-0172

Athyros, V.G., Didangelos, T. P., & Karamitsos, D. T., et al. (1998).Long-term Effect of Converting Enzyme Inhibition on Circadian Sympathetic and Parasympathetic Modulation in Patients with Diabetic Autonomic Neuropathy. *Acta Cardiologica,* Vol.53, No.4, pp.201-109, ISSN 0001-5385

Atkinson, G. & Davenne, D. (2007). Relationship between Sleep, Physical Activity and Human Health. *Physiology & Behavior,* Vol.90, No.2-3, pp. 229-235, ISSN 0031-9384

Atkinson, G., Jones, H. & Ainslie, P.N. (2010). Circadian Variation in the Circulatory Responses to Exercise: Relevance to the Morning Peaks in Strokes and Cardiac Events. *European Journal of Applied Physiology,* Vol.108, No.1, pp. 15-29, ISSN 1439-6319.

Atkinson, G., Drust, B., & George, K. (2006). Chronobiological Considerations for Exercise and Heart Disease. *Sports Medicine,* Vol.36, No.6, pp. 487-500, ISSN 0112-1642

Baran, K.W., Bache, R.J., & Dai, X.Z., et al. (1992).Effect of α- adrenergic Blocked with Prazosin on Large Coronary Diameter during Exercise. *Circulation,* Vol.85, No. 3, pp. 1139-1145, ISSN 0009-7322

Baas, L.S. (2004). Self-care Resources and Activity as Predictors of Quality of Life in Persons after Myocardial Infarction. *Dimensions of Critical Care Nursing,* Vol.23, No.3, pp. 131-138, ISSN 0730-4625

Baxendale, L.M. (1992). Pathophysiology of Coronary Artery Disease. *Nursing Clinic of North America,*Vol.27, No.1, pp143-152, ISSN 0029-6465

Benhorin, J., Banai, S., & Moriel, M., et al. (1993). Circadian Variations in Ischemic Threshold and Their Relation to the Occurrence of Ischemic Episodes. *Circulation,* Vol.87, No.3, pp. 808-814, ISSN 0009-7322

Benson, H., Rosner, B.A., & Marzetta, B.R., et al (1974). Decreased Blood Pressure in Pharmacologically Treated Hypertensive Patients Who Regularly Elicited the Relaxation Response. *Lancet,* Vol.1, No.7852, pp. 289-291, ISSN 0140-6736

Braunwald, E. (1995). Morning Resistance to Thrombolytic Therapy. *Circulation,* Vol.91, No.5, pp. 1604-1606, ISSN 0009-7322

Brezinski, D.A., Tofler, G.H., & Muller, J.E., et al.(1988). Morning Increase in Platelet Aggragability. Association with Assumption of the Upright Posture. *Circulation,* Vol.78, No. 1, pp. 35-40, ISSN 0009-7322

Camici, P.G., Gistri,R., & Lorenzoni, R., et al. (1992). Coronary Reserve and Exercise ECG in Patients with Chest Pain and Normal Coronary Angiograms. *Circulation,* Vol.86, No.1, pp179-186, ISSN 0009-7322

Cappuccio, F.P., Cooper, D., & D'Elia, L., et al. (2011). Sleep Duration Predicts Cardiovascular Outcomes: a Systematic Review and Meta-analysis of Prospective Studies. *European Heart Journal,* Vol.32, No.12, pp.1484-1492, ISSN 0195-668X

Carnethon, M.R., Liao, D., & Evans, G.W., et al. (2002). Does the Cardiac Autonomic Response to Postural Change Predict Incident Coronary Heart Disease and

Mortality? The Atherosclerosis Risk in Communities Study. *American Journal of Epidemiology*, Vol.155, No.1, pp. 48-56, ISSN 0002-9262

Condon, C. & McCarthy, G. (2006). Lifestyle Changes Following Acute Myocardial Infarction: Patients Perspectives. *European Journal of Cardiovascular Nursing*, Vol.5, No.1, pp. 37-44, ISSN 1479-5151

Cooke-Ariel, H. (1998). Circadian Variation in Cardiovascular Function and their Relation to the Occurrence and Timing of Cardiac Events. *American Journal of Health-System Pharmacy*, Vol. 55, Suppl.3, pp.S5-S11, ISSN 1079-2082

Critchley, H.D., Taggart, P., & Sutton, P.M., et al. (2005). Mental Stress and Sudden Cardiac Death: Asymmetric Midbrain Activity as a Linking Mechanism. *Brain*, Vol.128, (Pt 1), pp. 75-85, ISSN 0006-8950

Culebras, A. (1992). The Neurology of Sleep: Introduction. *Neurology*, Vol. 42, (7 Supple 6), pp. 6-8, ISSN 0028-3878

Deedwania, P.C. (1996). Hemodynamic Changes as Triggers of Cardiovascular Events. *Cardiology Clinics*, Vol.14, No.2, pp. 229-238, ISSN 0733-8651

Drager, L.F., Ueno, L.M., & Lessa, P.S., et al. (2009). Sleep-related Changes in Hemodynamic and Autonomic Regulation in Human Hypertension. *Journal of Hypertension*, Vol.27, No.8, pp. 1655-1663, ISSN 0263-6352

Duncker, D.J., Zhang, J., & Bache, R, J. (1993). Coronary Pressure-flow Relation in Left Ventricular Hypertrophy. Importance of Changes in Back Pressure versus Changes in Minimum Resistance. *Circulation Research*, Vol.72, No. 3, pp579-587, ISSN 0009-7330

Ebrahim, S., Beswick, A., & Burke, M. et al. (2006). Multiple Risk Factor Interventions for Primary Prevention of Coronary Heart Disease. *Cochrane Database System Reviews (Online)*, (4), CD001561. ISSN 1469-493X

Ebrahim, S., Taylor, F.,& Ward, K., et al. (2011). Multiple Risk Factor Interventions for Primary Prevention of Coronary Heart Disease. *Cochrane Database System Reviews (Online)*, (1), CD001561. ISSN 1469-493X

Eisenhofer, G., Esler, M.D., & Meredith, I.T., et al. (1992). Sympathetic Nervous Function in Human Heart as Assessed by Cardiac Spillovers of Dihydroxyphenylglycol and Norepinephrine. *Circulation*, Vol.85, No.5, pp. 1775-1785, ISSN 0009-7322

Figueras, J., & Lidon, R.M. (1995). Early Morning Reduction in Ischemic Threshold in Patients with Unstable Angina and Significant Coronary Disease. *Circulation*, Vol. 92, No.7, pp. 1737-1742, ISSN 0009-7322

Freed, C.D., Thomas, S A , & Lynch, J.J., et al. (1989). Blood Pressure, Heart Rate, and Heart Rhythm Changes in Patients with Heart Disease during Talking. *Heart & Lung*, Vol.18, No.1, pp. 17-22, ISSN 0147-9563

Fujita, M. & Franklin, D. (1987). Diurnal Changes in Coronary Blood Flow in Conscious Dogs. *Circulation*, Vol.76, No.2, pp. 488-491, ISSN 0009-7322

Furchgott, R.F., & Zawadzki,J.V. (1980).The Obligatory Role of Endothelial Cells in the Relaxation of Arterial Smooth Muscle by Acethlcholine. *Nature*, Vol.288 , No.5789, pp.373-376, ISSN 0028-0836

Furchgott, R.F. (1983). Role of Endothelium in Responses of Vascular Smooth Muscle. *Circulation Research*, Vol.53, No.5, pp. 557-573, ISSN 0009-7330

Furukawa, F., Kazuma, K., & Kojima, M., et al. (2008). Effects of an Off-site Walking Program of Fibrinogen and Exercise Energy Expenditure in Women. *Asian Nursing Research*, Vol.2, No.1, pp. 35-45, ISSN 1976-1317

Furukawa, F., Nagano, M., & Ueda, E., et al. (1998). Mechanisms of Ischemic Morning Episodes of Coronary Artery Disease Following Awakening: a Review. *Tenri Medical Bulletin*, Vol.1, No.1, pp. 126-138, ISSN 1433-1817

Giles, T. (2005). Relevance of Blood Pressure Variation in the Circadian Onset of Cardiovascular Events. *Journal of Hypertension Supplement*, Vol.23, Suppl 1, pp. S35-S39, ISSN 0952-1178

Greenberg, S.S., Diecke, F.P., & Peevy, K., et al.(1990). Release of Norepinephrine from Adrenagic Nerve Endings of Blood Vessels is Modulated by Endothelium-derived Relaxing Factor. *American Journal of Hypertension*,Vol.3, No.3, pp. 211-218, ISSN 0895-7061

Guzzetta, C.E. (1989). Effects of Relaxation and Music Therapy on Patients in a Coronary Care Unit with Presumptive Acute Myocardial Infarction. *Heart & Lung*, Vol.18, No.6, pp. 609-619, ISSN 0147-9563

Hammond, H.K., Roth, D.A., & Insel, P.A., et al. (1992). Myocardial Beta-adrenergic Receptor Expression and Signal Transduction after Chronic Volume-overload Hypertrophy and Circulatory Congestion.*Circulation*,Vol.85, No.1, pp. 269-280, ISSN 0009-7322.

Herd, J.A. (1991). Cardiovascular Response to Stress. *Physiological Reviews*, Vol.71, No.1, pp. 305-330, ISSN 0031-9333

Hilberg, T., Nowacki, P.E., & Muller-Berghaus, G., et al. (2000). Changes in Blood Coagulation and Fibrinolysis Associated with Maximal Exercise and Physical Conditioning in Women Taking Low Dose Oral Contraceptives. *Journal of Science and Medicine in Sport*, Vol.3, No.4, pp.383-390, ISSN 1440-2440

Hjalmarson, A., Gilpin, E.A., & Nicod, P., et al.(1989). Differing Circadian Patterns of Symptom Onset in Subgroups of Patients with Acute Myocardial Infarction. *Circulation*, Vol.80, No.2, pp. 267-275, ISSN 0009-7322

Hoffman, J.W., Benson, H., & Arns,P.A., et al. (1982). Reduced Sympathetic Nervous System Responsivity Associated with the Relaxation Response. *Science*, Vol.215, No.4529, pp. 190-192, ISSN 0036-8075

Jacob, G., Ertl, A.C., & Shannon, J.R., et al. (1998). Effect of Standing on Neurohumoral Responses and Plasma Volume in Healthy Subjects. *Journal of Applied Physiology*, Vol.84, No.3, pp. 914-921, ISSN 8750-7587

Jouvet, M. (1967).Neurophysiology of the States of Sleep. *Physiological Reviews*, Vol.47, No.2, pp.117-177, ISSN 0031-9333

Jay, R.H., Rampling, M.W., & Betteridge, D.J. (1990). Abnormalities of Blood Rheology in Familial Hypercholesterolaema: Effects of Treatment. *Atherosclerosis*, Vol.85, No,2-3, pp. 249-256, ISSN 0021-9150

Kaul, S., Waack, B.J., & Padgett, R.C., et al. (1993).Altered Vascular Responses to Platelets from Hypercholesterolemic humans, .*Circulation Research*, Vol.72, No.4, pp. 737-743, ISSN 0009-7330.

Khoury, A.F., Sunderajan, P., & Kaplan, N.M. (1992). The Early Morning Rise in Blood Pressure is Related Mainly to Ambulation. *American Journal of Hypertension*, Vol. 5, No.(6 Pt 1), pp. 339-344, ISSN 0895-7061

Theoretical Identification of Behavioral Risk Factors Among Multiple Risk Factors Causing
Morning Onset of Cardiac Events due to Circadian Variations

87

Kiowski, W., & Osswald, S. (1993).Circadian Variation of Ischemic Cardiac Events. *Journal of Cardiovascular Pharmacology*, Vol.21, Suppl 2, ppS45-S48, ISSN 0160-2446

Krantz, D.S., Kop,W.J., & Gabbay, F.H., et al.(1996). Circadian Variation of Ambulatory Myocardial Ischermia: Triggering by Daily Activities and Evidence for an Endogenous Circadian Component. *Circulation*, Vol.93, No.7, pp. 1364-1371, ISSN 0009-7322

Kristofferzon, M.L., Lofmark, R., & Carlsson, M. (2007). Striving for Balance in DailyLlife: Experiences of Swedish Women and Men Shortly after a Myocardial Infarction, *Journal of Clinical Nursing,*Vol.16, No.2, pp. 391-401, ISSN 0962-1067.

Kuo, L.,Arko, F., & Chilian, W.M., et al. (1993). Coronary Vascular Responses to Flow and Pressure, *Circulation Research*, Vol.72, No.3, pp. 607-615, ISSN 0009-7330

Laxson, D.D., Dai, X.Z., & Homan, D.C., et al. (1992). Coronary Vasodilator Reserve in Ischemic Myocardium of the Exercising Dog.*Circulation,*Vol.85, No.1, pp. 313-322, ISSN 0009-7322

Leary, A.C., Struthers, A.D., & Donnan, P.T., et al. (2002). The Morning Surge in Blood Pressure and Heart Rate is Dependent on Levels of Physical Activity after Waking. *Journal of Hypertension*, Vol.20, No.5, pp. 865-870, ISSN 0263-6352

Linsell, CR., Lightman, S.L., & Mullen, P.E., et al.(1985). Circulation Rhythms of Epinephrine and Norepinephrine in Man. *Journal of Clinical Endocrinology & Metabolism.* Vol. 60, No.6, pp.1210-1215, ISSN 0021-972X

Lowe, G.D., Drummond, M.M., & Lorimer, A,R., et al. (1980). Relation between Extent of Coronary Artery Disease and Blood Viscosity. *British Medical Journal*, Vol.280, No.6215, pp. 673-674, ISSN 0959-8138

Li, J.J. (2003). Circadian Variation in Myocardial Ischemia: the Possible Mechanisms Involving in this Phenomenon. *Medical Hypotheses*, Vol.61, No.2, pp. 240-243, ISSN 0306-9877

Lucchesi, B. (1990). Myocardial Ischemia, Reperfusion, and Free Radical Injury. *American Journal of Cardiology*, Vol.65, No.19, pp.141-231, ISSN 0002-9149

Ludmer, P.L., Selwyn, A.P., & Shook, T.L., et al.(1986). Paradoxical Vasoconstriction Induced by Acetylcholine in Atherosclerotic Coronary Arteries. *The New England Journal of Medicine*, Vol. 315, No.17, pp. 1046-1051, ISSN 0028-4793

Martin, R.J. (1984). Cardiorespiratory Disorders during Sleep. 2nd. Future Pub Co., ISBN 978-0-87993-208-4, New York, USA

Masuda, T., Ogawa, H., & Miyao, Y. (1994). Circadian Variation in Fibrinolytic Activity in Patients with Variant Angina. *British Heart Journal*, Vol.71, No.2, pp.156-161, ISSN 0007-0769

Meller, J., Goldsmith, S. J., & Rudin, A. (1979). Spectrum of Exercise Thallium-201 Myocardial Perfusion Imaging in Pateints with Chest Pain and Normal Coronary Angiograms. *American Journal of Cardiology*, Vol.43, No.4, pp. 717-723, ISSN 0002-9149

Melvile, S.B. (1987). Relaxation Techniques in Acute Myocardial Infarction: the Theoretic Rationale. *Focus on Critical Care*, Vol.14, No.1, pp. 9-11, ISSN 0736-3605

Mulcahy, D.(1999). "Circadian" Variation in Cardiovascular Events and Implications for Therapy? *Journal of Cardiovascular Phamacology*, Vol.34, Suppl 2, pp. S3-S8, Disscussion, S29-S31, ISSN 0160-2446

Mulcahy, D., Keegan, J., & Cunningham, D., et al. (1998). Circadian Variation of Total Ischemic Burden and Its Alteration with Anti-anginal Agents. *Lancet*, Vol.2, No.8614, pp. 755-759, ISSN 0140-6736

Muller, J.E., Ludmer, P.L., & Willich, S.N., et al. (1987). Circadian Variation in the Frequency of Sudden Cardiac Death. *Circulation*, Vol.75, No. 1, pp. 131-138, ISSN 0009-7322

Muller, J.E., Tofler, G.H., & Stone, P.H. (1989). Circadian Variation and Triggers of Onset of Acute Cardiovascular Disease. *Circulation*, Vol. 79, No.4, pp. 733-743, ISSN 0009-7322

Murray, P.M., Herrington, D.M., & Pettus, C.W., et al. (1993).Should Patients with Heart Disease Exercise in the Morning or Afternoon. *Archives of Internal Medicine*, Vol.153, No.7, pp. 833-836, ISSN 0003-9926

Norris, C.M., Ghali, W.A., & Galbraith, P.D., et al. (2004). Women with Coronary Artery Disease Report Worse Health-related Quality of Life Outcomes Compared to Men. Health and Quality of Life Outcomes, Vo.2, No. 21, pp.1-11 (page number not for citation prupoes), Published online 2005 May 5 doi:10. ISSN 1186/1477-7525-2-21.

Ohkubo, T., Metoki, H., & Imai, Y. (2008). Prognostic Significance of Morning Surge in Blood Pressure: Which Definition, Which Outcome? *Blood Pressure Monitoring*, Vol.13, No,3, pp.161-162, ISSN 1359-5237

Oparil, S., Vassaux, C., & Sanders, C.A., et al. (1970).Role of Renin in Acute Postural Hemostasis.*Circulation*,Vol.41, No.1, pp. 89-95, ISSN 0009-7322.

Palmieri, V., Celentano, A., & Roman, M.J., et al. (2003). Relation of Fibrinogen to Cardiovascular Events is Independent of Preclinical Cardiovascular Disease: the Strong Heart Study. *American Heart Journal*, Vol.145, No.3, pp. 467-474, ISSN 0002-8703

Pernow, J., Lundberg, J.M., & Kaijser, L. (1988). Alph-adrenoceptor Influence on Plasma Level of Neuropeptide Y-like Immunoreactivity and Catecholamines during Rest and Sympathoadrenal Activation in Humans. *Journal of Cardiovascular Phamacology*,Vol.12, No.5, pp. 593-599, ISSN 0160-2446

Peters R.W., Brooks, M.M., & Zoble, R.G., et al. (1996). Chronobiology of Acute Myocardial Infarction: Cardiac Arrhythmia Suppression Trial (CAST) Experience. *The American Journal of Cardiology*, Vol.78, No.11, pp.1198-1201, ISSN 0002-9149

Quyyumi, A.A. (1990).Circadian Rhythms in Cardiovascular Disease. *American Heart Journal*.Vol.120, No.3, pp.726-733, ISSN 0002-8703

Quyyumi, A.A., Panza, J.A., & Diodati,J.G., et al. (1992). Circadian Variation in Ischemic Threshold: A Mechanimic Underlying the Circadian Variation in Ischemic Events. *Circulation*, Vol.86, No.1, pp. 22-28, ISSN 0009-7322

Redon, J. (2004). The Normal Circadian Pattern of Blood Pressure: Implications for Treatment. *International Journal of Clinical Practice*,Vol.58, Supplement 145, pp. 3-8 ISSN 1368-504X

Rocco, M.B. (1990). Timing and Triggers of Transient Myocardial Ischemia. *American Journal of Cardiology*.Vol.66, No.16, pp. 18G-21G, ISSN 0002-9149

Schachter, M. (2004).Diurnal Rhythms, the Rennin-angiotensin System and Antihypertensive Therapy. *British Journal of Cardiology*, Vol.11, No. 4, pp. 287-290, ISSN 0969-6113

Scheer, F.A., Hu, K., & Evoniuk, H., et al. (2010). Impact of the Human Circadian System, Exercise, and Their Interaction on Cardiovascular Function. *Proceeding of National*

Theoretical Identification of Behavioral Risk Factors Among Multiple Risk Factors Causing
Morning Onset of Cardiac Events due to Circadian Variations

89

Academy of Science of the United States of America, Vol. 107, No.47, pp20541-20546, ISSN 0027-8424

Shimada, K., Kario, K., & Umeda, Y., et al. (2001). Early Morning Surge in Blood Pressure. *Blood Pressure Monitoring,* Vol.6, No.6, pp. 349-353, ISSN 1359-5237

Shiotani, H., Umegaki, Y., & Tanaka, M.., et al. (2009).Effects of Aerobic Exercise on the Circadian Rhythm of Heart Rate and Blood Pressure. *Chronobiology International,* Vol.26, No.8, pp. 1636-1646, ISSN 0742-0528

Steriade, M. (1992). Basic Mechanisms of Sleep Generation. *Neurology,* Vol.42, 7Supple 6, pp. 9-17, ISSN 0028-3878

Stone, P.H. (1990). Triggers of Transient Myocardial Ischemia: Circadian Variation and Relation to Plaque Rupture and Coronary Thrombosis in Stable Coronary Artery Disease. *American Journal of Cardiology.*Vol.66, No.16, pp. 32G-36G, ISSN 0002-9149

Storm, D.S., Metzger, B.L., & Therrien, B. (1989). Effects of Age on Autonomic Cardiovascular Responsiveness in Healthy Men and Women. *Nursing Research,* Vol.38, No.6, pp. 326-300, ISSN 0029-6562

Sugiishi, M., & Takatsu, F. (1993). Cigarette Smoking is a Major Risk Factor for Coronary Spasms. *Circulation,* Vol. 87, No.1, pp. 76-79, ISSN 0009-7322

Svendsen, J.H., Sheikh, S.P., & Jorgensen, J., et al. (1990). Effect of Neuropeptide Y on Regulation of Blood Flow Rate in Canine Myocardium. *American Journal of Physiology,* Vol.259, No.6, pt 2, pp.H1709-H1717, ISSN 0363-6135

Thrall, G., Lane, D., & Carroll, D., et al. (2007). A Systematic Review of the Prothrimbotic Effects of an Acute Change in Posture: a Possible Mechanism Underlying the Morning Excess in Cardiovascular Events? *Chest,* Vol.132, No.4, pp. 1337-1347, ISSN 0012-3692

Tofler, G.H., Brezinski, D., & Schafter, A.I., et al. (1987). Concurrent Morning Increase in Platelet Aggregability and the Risk of Myocardial Infarction and Sudden Cardiac Death. *New England Journal of Medicine,* Vol.316, No.24, pp. 1514-1518, ISSN 0028-4793

Umemura, S., Tochikubo, O., & Noda, K. (1987). Changes in Blood Pressure and Plasma Norepinephrine during Sleep in Essential Hypertension. *Japanese Circulation Journal.* Vol. 51, No.11, pp1250-1256, ISSN 0047-1828

van Eekelen, A.P., Houtveen, J.H. & Kerkhof, G.A. (2004a). Circadian Variation in Cardiac Autonomic Activity: Rreactivity Measurements to Different Type of Stressors. *Chronobiology International,* Vol.21, No.1, pp107-129, ISSN 0742-0528

van Eekelen, A.P., Houtveen, J.H., & Kerkhof, G.A.(2004b).Circadian Variation in Base Rate Measures of Cardiac Autonomic Activity. *European Journal of Applied Physiology,* Vol.93, No.1-2. pp.39-46, ISSN 1439-6319

Vanhoutte, A.M., & Huston, D.S. (1985).Platelets, Endothelium and Vasospasm. *Circulation,* Vol.72, No.4, pp. 728-743, ISSN 0009-7322

Viola, A.U., Simon, C., & Ehrhart, J., et al. (2002). Sleep Processes Exert a Predominant Influence on the 24-h Profile of Heart Rate Variability. *Journal of Biological Rhythms,* Vol.17, No.6, pp. 539-547, ISSN 0748-7304

West, J.B. (1990). *Best and Taylor's Physiological Basis of Medical Practice.* 12[th]ed, Williams & Wilkins, ISBN 0-683-08947-1, Baltimore, USA

White, W.B. (2001). Cardiovascular Risk and Therapeutic Intervention for the Early Morning Surge in Blood Pressure and Heart Rate. *Blood Pressure Monitoring,* Vol.6, No.2, pp.63-72, ISSN 1359-5237

White, W.B. (2003). Relevance of Blood Pressure Variation in the Circadian Onset of Cardiovascular Events. *Journal of Hypertension, Supplement*, Vol. 21(S6), pp. S9-S15, ISSN 0952-1178

Willich, S.N., Levy, D., & Rocco, M.B., et al. (1987). Circadian Variation in the Incidence of Sudden Cardiac Death in the Framingham Heart Study Population. *American Journal of Cardiology*, Vol.60, No.10, pp.801-806, ISSN 0002-9149

Willis, W.D. & Grossman, R.G. (1981).*Medical Neurobiology*. 3rd CV Mosby Co, ISBN 978-0-8016-5582-1, St. Luis, USA

Yang, T., & Levy, M.N. (1993). Effects of Intense Antecedent Sympathetic Stimulation on Sympathetic Neurotransmission in the Heart. *Circulation Research,*Vol.72, No.1, pp. 137-144, ISSN 0009-7330

Yarnell, J.W., Baker, I.A., & Sweetnam, P.M., et al. (1991). Firbirnogen, Viscosity, and White Blood Cell Count are Major Risk Factors for Ischemic Heart Disease. The Caerphilly and Speedwell Collaborative Heart Disease Studies. *Circulation,* Vol.83, No.3, pp.836-844, ISSN 0009-7322

Young, M.A., &Vatner, S.F. (1986). Regulation of Large Coronary Arteries. *Circulation Research,* Vol.59, No.6, pp. 579-596, ISSN 0009-7330

Zemel, P.C. , & Sowers, J.R. (1990). Relation between Lipids and Atherosclerosis: Epidemiologic Evidence and Clinical Implications. *American Journal of Cardiology,* Vol.66, No. 21, pp.71-121, ISSN 0002-9149

6

Anger, Hostility and Other Forms of Negative Affect: Relation to Cardiovascular Disease

Marco A.A. Torquato Jr., Bruno P.F. de Souza,
Dan V. Iosifescu and Renerio Fraguas
University of São Paulo, Institute of Psychiatry,
Brazil

1. Introduction

The link between psychological factors and cardiovascular disease goes far beyond well-established psychiatric diagnoses such as major depressive disorder, generalized anxiety disorder or panic disorder. The literature describes several mental and behavioral concepts which are not captured in the current nomenclature as independent mental disorders but show some degree of association with cardiovascular disease. We will discuss them in this chapter under the larger category of "negative affect". The most common constructs we subsume in this category are Anger, Hostility, Aggressiveness, Negative Emotion, Negative Affectivity, Vital Exhaustion (VE), Type D Personality, and Type A Behavior Pattern (TABP). We chose the "negative affect" category as a mean to discuss together these different mood states having in common their potential negative impact on the cardiovascular system.

Some of these constructs have different definitions and are measured by diverse instruments. This variety of approaches reflects the complexity of the field and explains, at least in part, some disparity in results relating them to cardiovascular disease.

In this chapter, we review these constructs included in "negative affect" and the instruments that have been developed to assess them. Additionally, we will review the studies investigating their relationship with cardiac conditions, emphasizing the pathophysiological mechanisms that could mediate the relationship between negative affect and cardiac pathology . Finally, we will discuss potential treatments of negative affect and their eventual impact on cardiac conditions.

2. The mix of concepts: Hostility, anger, aggression and other negative affect

Over the past decades, a large number of studies have investigated the association between negative affect and coronary heart disease (CHD). Many were cross-sectional case-control studies, which have been criticized for the recall bias of the CHD diagnosis and for the memory distortion (Chida and Steptoe 2009). More recently, several prospective longitudinal studies with more rigorous methodology have also been developed. Notwithstanding, results from this studies are not homogeneous, with both positive and negative results. Although more rigorous in their methodology, the prospective studies use diverse and partially overlapping concepts to define negative affect associated with CHD (Table 1). Since each study analyzes only a single psychological construct at a time and since these concepts are only partially overlapping, it is not surprising to note the conflicting results in the literature. In addition, the single-factor approach ignores the clustering of psychosocial risk factors for physical disease, which may act synergistically (Suls and Bunde 2005). Another view, from a twin-designed study, is that some of this negative affect concepts may have a single common genetic factor and a nonshared environmental factor, i.e., enviroments uncorrelated between twins, such as accidents.(Raynor, Pogue-Geile et al. 2002).

Type A Behavior Pattern	Type D Personality	Vital exhaustion	Hostility	Anger	Aggression	Negative Affectivity	Negative emotions
An action-emotion complex induced by environmental factors, involving psychomotor mannerisms, vigorous voice, hard-driving, time envolvement-pressured job, competitiveness, impatience and easy triggering anger and hostility (Friedman and Rosenman 1959)	Negative affectivity, social inhibition and feeling of distress (Denollet 1998).	An unusual tiredness, increased irritability and feelings of demoralization (Appels, Hoppener et al. 1987).	A tendency to view the world in a negative, cynical fashion; a primarily cognitive construct involving negative attitude toward others, consisting of enmity, denigration, and ill will (Smith, Glazer et al. 2004).	An affective experience, ranging in intensity from mild annoyance to fury and outrage. Two subtypes "anger-out", a combination of anger and aggression and "anger-in", a tendency to feel anger and suppress it (Schulman and Stromberg 2007) .	A physical or verbal behavior including attacking destructive or hurtful actions, may be considered a personality trait.	Abroadband personality dimension caracterized by a general disposition to chronically experience anxiety, sadness, guilt, anger, irritability, and other negative emotions.	Depression, anger, anxiety and hostility are emotions that range from normal to pathological in a continuum (Kubzansky and Kawachi 2000; Kubzansky, Davidson et al. 2005; Kubzansky 2007).

Table 1. Concepts.

Some authors have proposed that anger, hostility and aggression should be considered a syndrome and other include anger and hostility in the concept of aggression. For others, hostility is characterized by interrelated elements of cynical beliefs and attributions, angry emotional states, and aggressive or antagonistic behaviors. Martin et al. advocate for the standardization of these concepts emphasizing that anger corresponds to *affect*, aggression to *behavior*, and hostility (or cynicism) to *cognition*. Together the three constructs form a three-factor "ABC" model of trait anger (Martin, Watson et al. 2000).

Aside from hostility, anger and aggression, VE and distressed personality are more complex concepts. Although they overlap partially, these constructs include specific patterns and aspects not captured by general scales for hostility, anger and aggression. Last but not least, the concept of negative affectivity posits that these symptoms represent markers of a trait characterized by hypersensitivity to negative stimuli (Watson and Clark 1984) and the concept of negative emotions postulate the existence of a continuum across these affective states.

3. Depression: The mix beyond the negative affects

Beyond negative affect, depression and, secondarily, anxiety have the strongest evidence for associations with CHD, even after controlling for traditional CHD risk factors, such as serum cholesterol, blood pressure, and smoking. Intriguingly, as it has been pointed out by Suls and Bunde, there is an appreciable construct and measurement overlap across anger, anxiety, and depression, which creates ambiguity both for theory testing and for interpretation of available evidence (Suls and Bunde 2005). Ravaja et al., have proposed that depression would be a moderator of the relationship between cardiovascular risk factors and anger (Ravaja, Kauppinen et al. 2000). They reported a negative association between hostility and cardiovascular risk factors in patients with high depressive tendencies. Patients with severe depression and lack of anger or hostility would represent the most severe form of exhaustion where the individual had "given-up"(Ravaja, Kauppinen et al. 2000).

Irritability has been considered a diagnostic feature of MDD in children and adolescents (American Psychiatric Association 1994). Actually, a hostile depressive subtype has been proposed in 1966 (Overall, Hollister et al. 1966). However, unfortunately, most standard rating scales of depressive symptom severity do not specifically measure irritability (Hamilton 1960; Montgomery and Asberg 1979). A particular form of irritable depression marked by recurrent anger attacks, spontaneous episodes characterized by feelings of rage and symptoms of physiologic arousal similar to panic attacks and accompanied by chronic irritability, has been reported to occur in 20-60% of patients with unipolar depression and nearly two-thirds of patients with bipolar depression (Perlis, Smoller et al. 2004) (Baker, Dorzab et al. 1971; Overall, Goldstein et al. 1971; Snaith and Taylor 1985) (Gould, Ball et al. 1996; Fava, Uebelacker et al. 1997; Morand, Thomas et al. 1998; Mischoulon, Dougherty et al. 2002; Posternak and Zimmerman 2002; Dougherty, Rauch et al. 2004). Data have suggested that depression with anger may be associated with distinct abnormalities of subcortical white matter structure (Iosifescu, Renshaw et al. 2007) and brain metabolism (Dougherty, Rauch et al. 2004), and possibly with increased serotonergic dysfunction (Fava, Vuolo et al. 2000). It is possible that anger may be a marker of a depressive variant with increased cardiovascular risk (Fava, Abraham et al. 1996; Painuly, Sharan et al. 2005; Fraguas, Iosifescu et al. 2007). Anger attacks in MDD patients were independently associated with smoking (for periods >11 years) and with total serum levels of cholesterol ≥ 200mg/dL, after adjusting for age, gender, BMI, and baseline severity of depression (Fraguas, Iosifescu et al. 2007).

Major depression is a mental disorder and has reliable operational diagnostic criteria. However, the limit between major depressive disorder and subsyndromal depressive symptoms and the relevance of irritability/anger/hostility in depressed patients involve multiple non answered questions. For example, little is known about the distinction between irritable depression and depression with comorbid personality disorders or other psychiatric diagnoses associated with high rates of irritability. The interaction between temperament, personality is a complex phenomenon (Clark, Watson et al. 1994). The nature of depressive symptoms may be influenced by personality traits; in this model, irritability may be one manifestation of sensitivity to negative stimuli (Watson and Clark 1984), or interpersonal sensitivity(Bagby, Kennedy et al. 1997). Also, increased anxiety levels may define a specific subtype of MDD (Fava, Alpert et al. 2004) and irritability is often manifested in the presence of increased anxiety (as an inadequate response of individuals overwhelmed by stress and anxiety); in a factor analysis, this continuum of symptoms in depression appears to be best captured by a common anxiety/irritability factor (Gullion and Rush 1998).

4. Instruments

The variety of instruments (Table 2) used to evaluate negative affect makes standardization or even comparison between studies difficult (Davidson 2008). We describe the instruments when addressing each "negative affect" construct separately (Item 6). However, some general limitations should be discussed. For example, some instruments are composed of multidimensional items mixing several concepts and including definitional caveats. For example, the Potential for Hostility subcomponent of the Structured Inverview for the TABP

Type A Behavior Pattern	Type D Personality	Vital exhaustion	Hostility	Anger	Agresssion
Among the self-report instruments there is the Jenkins Activity Scale (JAS) (Jenkins, Rosenman et al. 1967) and the Framingham Type A scale (FTAS) (Levenkron, Cohen et al. 1983). Among the instruments used by an interviewer there is the Rosenman and Friedman structured interview (MacDougall, Dembroski et al. 1979).	The Type D Scale-14 (DS14) evaluate the two components of Type D, the negative affectivity and social inhibition (Denollet 2005).	The 21-item Maastricht Questionnaire evaluates VE including factors such as depressive symptoms, sleep problems and lack of concentration (Appels, Hoppener et al. 1987).	The Cook and Medley Hostility scale (CMHS, or Ho scale) includes 50 items, true or false, evaluates cynicism and distrust (Smith, Glazer et al. 2004); the Buss-Durkee Hostility Inventory (Buss and Durkee 1957) assesses expressive hostility or antagonism (physical and verbal aggression) and neurotic or experiential hostility; the Interpersonal Hostility Assessment Technique (IHAT) is a structured interview that classifies the hostile behavior in four styles (Brummett, Maynard et al. 2000).	The Anger Expression scales (Spielberger et al., 1985), and Framingham Anger Reaction or Expression Scales (Haynes, Feinleib et al. 1980; Eaker, Pinsky et al. 1992); the Spielberger State-Trait Anger Expression Inventory is a self-report Inventory and assess anger expression ("anger-in" and "anger out"); the Anger Attacks Questionnaire evaluates the presence of anger attacks, spells of anger that are inappropriate to the situation and have physical features resembling panic attacks(Fava, Rosenbaum et al. 1991).	The Aggressio n Questionn aire (AQ), developed by Buss and Perry (1992) contains subscales to measure anger, hostility and verbal and physical aggression (Buss and Perry 1992).

Table 2. Instruments

has elements of hostile cynicism and anger affect , although it primarily assesses antagonistic expression (Dembroski, MacDougall et al. 1989). In addition, the same questionnaires identified as measures of anger and hostility by some authors are described as measures of aggression by others (Felsten and Hill 1999).

Raynor et al., using twin analyses, found that covariation among the Beck Depression Inventory, the Interpersonal Support Evaluation List and the Cook-Medley Hostility Scale could be explained by a single common genetic factor and a common nonshared environmental factor. They challenged the conventional approach of examining these psychosocial variables as independent risk factors for cardiovascular disease and argued for the importance of investigating specific causes for their covariation(Raynor, Pogue-Geile et al. 2002).

Devidson et. al. (Davidson 2008) performed a comparative analysis between the association of different instruments for measuring anger and hostility and CHD. The Minnesota Multiphasic Personality Inventory (MMPI) and the Cook-Medley Hostility Scale (CMHS) were positively associated with CHD in populations with and without psychiatric pathology. The Spielberger Trait Anger Scale (TAS) tended to show higher association with CHD compared with the overall effect in disease studies, while the Spielberger anger expression scale showed no association with CHD.

5. Neurophysiological bases for the relationship between negative affect and the cardiovascular system

Many authors attribute the possible influence of psychological traits on CHD to the impact of these affect states on promoting cardiovascular high-risk behaviors such as smoking, poor eating habits, low physical activity, poor sleep quality and low adherence to drug treatment (Scherwitz, Perkins et al. 1992). However, physiological pathways have been studied, suggesting that these affective constructs may be associated with autonomic, inflammatory and neuroendocrine changes that increase the risk for CHD (Table 3). Aspects of the proposed mechanisms of impact on the cardiovascular system are also discussed in the each of the negative affect categories in section 6.

The *reactivity hypothesis* offers a comprehensive model to understand the mechanisms connecting negative affect and increased cardiovascular morbidity. This hypothesis states that exaggerated physical or psychological responses can identify individuals at increased risk of cardiovascular disease. Based on this model, psychological traits and states would lead to increased risk through cardiovascular and neuroendocrine responses to environmental stressors. Lovallo and Gerin (2003)(Lovallo and Gerin 2003), divided the physiological mechanisms responsible for cardiovascular reactivity in three levels: 1) exaggerated cognitive-emotional responses; 2) increased brain stem and hypothalamus responsiveness; 3) Abnormalities in peripheral tissue modifications. In this paper, we discuss the first level, since it concerns the influence of personality traits on physiological responses of the organism.

Neurophysiologically, Lovallo and Gerin (2003)(Lovallo and Gerin 2003), outline two brain circuits through which the frontal lobe modulates and controls emotions. The first one includes the premotor region of the frontal cortex, connected to the anterior cingulate cortex, responsible for the selection of motor responses due to a motivated behavior. The second involves the orbital prefrontal cortex, which regulates the activity of the brain stem and hypothalamus secondary to the conscious evaluation of external events. It is worth mentioning the important connection of the orbital prefrontal cortex to the ventromedial prefrontal cortex, which has extensive dopaminergic and serotonergic areas, and is activated by signals ascending from the amygdala, the bed nuclei of the stria terminalis and septal regions. Thus, this second circuit would provide "emotional color" to the experiences.

After the cognitive and emotional evaluation, such areas send signals to the hypothalamus and brain stem, originating a wide range of physiological, endocrine, visceral and motor changes. Thus, specific cognitive and affective dispositions would lead to specific (and possibly persistent) changes in these systems (Lovallo and Gerin 2003).

This model is supported by several studies (Everson, McKey et al. 1995; Drevets 1999; Schaefer, Abercrombie et al. 2000; Pizzagalli, Pascual-Marqui et al. 2001) which indicate the importance of the quality of the stressor event (and not just its intensity) in the increased reactivity in susceptible individuals.

5.1 Proposed mechanisms: Chronic versus acute risk

The impact of negative affect on the cardiovascular system may be chronic or acute. For instance, hostility may be a personality trait with considerable stability across years and can be considered a character trait. In this situation the negative affect may chronically contribute to the morbidity of the cardiovascular system such as an association with increased levels of cholesterol (Table 3) (Dujovne and Houston 1991). On the other hand, anger attacks occurring episodically may acutely damage the cardiovascular system, such as an anger attack causing a heart attack (Mittleman, Maclure et al. 1995).

Regarding emotional states precipitating acute cardiac events, the evidence is very robust. Epidemiological studies have shown a significant increase of sudden cardiac death in populations submitted to disasters such as wars or earthquakes. In records of patients with implantable cardioverter-defibrillator (ICD), it was noticed that individual intense emotions such as anger or anxiety could trigger arrhythmias in susceptible patients. Lampert R et al, 2002, (Lampert, Joska et al. 2002) conducted a controlled prospective study, where ICD patients were requested to record in a diary the intensity of their emotions in the 15 minutes before shocks and, also, during the two hours to 15 minutes before the shock. As a control, the study assessed the diaries of the same patients during the same periods, one week after the shocks registration. Patients identified anger significantly more in the 15 minutes before the shock than during the control period. The association between the shocks and acute anger showed to be higher than the association with other measured emotions such as joy, sadness, worry and anxiety. The same group had previously reported that induced arrhythmias in patients undergoing mental stress (eg, performing arithmetic calculation or remembering stressful events) were faster in onset and more difficult to be extinguished than in those without such exposure.

Regarding psychological precipitants for acute myocardial infarction (MI), Culic V., et al, 2005 (Culic, Eterovic et al. 2005), performed a meta-analysis which found that emotional stress could immediately precedes MI in 7% of all cases of MI.

The relevance of considering both patterns is that affective traits may increase the frequency of acute subtle cardiovascular episodes.

Type A Behavior Pattern	Type D Personality	Vital exhaustion	Hostility	Anger
-Short-term responses to stress in physiological variables that are controlled by sympathetic nervous system(Oishi, Kamimura et al. 1999); - Increased cardiovascular risk factors as atherogenic lipid profile(Niaura, Stoney et al. 1992), -Increased thickness of the carotid intima-media (Keltikangas-Jarvinen, Hintsa et al. 2007).	-Overstated cardiovascular activity in daily life, mediated by an enhanced sympathetic drive and decreased vagal control of the heart including endothelial function, platelet function, altered lipid profile, altered activity of the hypothalamus-pituitary-adrenal cortex (HPA) axis and enhanced inflammatory activity of the immune system; -Increased negative behavioral factors; enhanced cortisol reactivity to stress and heightened blood pressure reactivity (Habra, Linden et al. 2003).	-Decreased ACTH and cortisol activation of inflammation; decreased slow wave sleep; reactivated cytomegaloviru s fosters growth of atherosclerosis; -Increased production of cytokines and decreased negative feedback from the HPA-axis upon the sympathic adrenomedular system.	-Increased blood pressure, heart rate, and levels of norepinephrine, cortisol and testosterone after stress (Suarez, Kuhn et al. 1998); -Decreased adaptation of blood pressure and heart rate to different stressors (mainly those related to interpersonal activities).(Everso n, McKey et al. 1995).	-Increased levels of catecholamines and decreased vagal stimulation; increased risk of cardiac arrhythmias (Verrier, Calvert et al. 1975; Stopper, Joska et al. 2007; Ziegelstein 2007; Yu-Wai-Man, Griffiths et al. 2010); -Increased hypertension (Ohira 2010).

Table 3. Proposed Mechanisms

6. The negative affects

6.1 Type A Behavior Pattern (TABP)

The TABP was described by Meyer Friedman and Ray Rosenman, two American cardiologists in the decade of 1950. The TABP is an action-emotion complex induced by environmental factors, involving psychomotor mannerisms, vigorous voice, hard-driving, time envolement-pressured job, competitiveness, impatience and easy triggering anger and hostility (Friedman and Rosenman 1959) (Table 1). During the decades of 1960 and 1970 various studies demonstrated a significant association between high levels of TABP measures and the development of cardiovascular disease (Jenkins, Rosenman et al. 1974; Rosenman, Brand et al. 1976). However, subsequent studies found did not confirm the relevance of the TABP as a predictor of CHD (Ragland and Brand 1988; Ragland and Brand 1988; Schulman and Stromberg 2007). Therefore, many researchers changed the focus of their research to assess whether some aspects of the TABP, particularly anger and hostility, would be more closely linked with the development of heart disease.

Both self-report and investigator-administered instruments have been developed to recognize TABP. Among the self-report instruments are the Jenkins Activity Scale (JAS) (Jenkins, Rosenman et al. 1967) and the Framingham the Type A scale (FTAS) (Levenkron, Cohen et al. 1983). A reliable investigator-administered instrument is the Rosenman and Friedman structured interview (MacDougall, Dembroski et al. 1979). Use of this structured interview may result in different association with CHD than the self report evaluation (Dembroski, MacDougall et al. 1985; Schulman and Stromberg 2007), raising questions on the reliability of the self-report instruments.

6.2 Hostility

Various studies combine under the single label of hostility a variety of manifestations of anger and aggression. Nevertheless, those represent distinct cognitive, emotional and behavioral characteristics. Essentially, hostility generally reflects a person's tendency to view the world in a negative, cynical fashion. Smith et al (Smith, Glazer et al. 2004) define hostility as a primarily cognitive construct involving "negative attitude toward others, consisting of enmity, denigration, and ill will". The author describes its components: the cynicism (i.e., a belief that others are motivated primarily by selfish concerns); the mistrust (an expectation that people will tend to be hurtful); and denigration (i.e., a devaluation of other people's motivation and goals). Other authors define hostility as "antagonistic interpersonal attitude" including cognitions (cynicism and hostile attributions), affect (hostile emotions) and behaviors (aggressive responses) (Barefoot JC LI. The assessment of anger and hostility. In: Siegman AW, Smith TW, eds Anger, Hostility, and the Heart Hillsdale, NJ: Lawrence Erlbaum 1994:43– 66.

It is clear that these definitions, as well as the personality traits they originate from, are highly correlated and overlapping. Smith and Glazer (Smith, Glazer et al. 2004) point out the correlation among these phenomena, emphasizing that anger, hostility and aggression are not just different names for the same construct. Consequently, one could not presume that they have similar associations with cardiovascular pathology. Suarez et al (Suarez, Kuhn et al. 1998) conducted a randomized study in which men, stratified by high or low scores on the Ho scale, underwent an anagram-solving task while experiencing alternatively harassing and not harassing comments from the researcher. It was observed that, compared to men with low levels of hostility, those with higher scores on Ho scale showed greater increase in blood pressure, heart rate, and levels of norepinephrine, cortisol and testosterone. Interestingly, such increase occurred only during (and shortly after) the aversive comments. In a similar study Everson et al (Everson, McKey et al. 1995) evaluated men with high and low levels of hostility. They found that men with low levels of hostility experienced rapid adaption of heart rate and blood pressure elevations to task repetition, while men with high hostility experienced even larger increases in their rates of heart rate and blood pressure after repetitions of aversive tasks. From these two studies it can be concluded that personality traits influence physiological responses to different stressors, particularly those related to interpersonal activities. Smith and Glazer (Smith, Glazer et al. 2004) point out other social stressors also related to high reactivity among hostile individuals, such as recalling and discussing past anger-inducing events, discussions, watching anger-inducing movies and self-disclosure of personal problems. Some authors have emphasized the relevance of higher cynical hostility (Chaput, Adams et al. 2002). Various studies and meta-analyses have supported the role of hostility in increasing the risk of CHD and even cardiac death (Booth-Kewley and Friedman 1987; Friedman and Booth-Kewley 1987; Miller, Smith et al. 1996).

A variety of instruments have been used to evaluate hostility and the differences among them indicate the distinction among the subjacent concepts.

The Cook and Medley Hostility scale (CMHS, or Ho scale) consists of 50 items taken from the Minnesota Multiphasic Personality Inventory to be answered true or false. CMHS can be interpreted as a measure of cynicism and distrust (Smith, Glazer et al. 2004). This is a comprehensive scale that has been correlated with other features outside of the concept of hostility, such as neuroticism, depression and anxiety (Barefoot, Dodge et al. 1989; Steinberg and Jorgensen 1996). Although frequently used, its internal reliability is low and some authors advise to analyze its subscales separately(Barefoot, Dodge et al. 1989).

The Buss-Durkee Hostility Inventory (Buss and Durkee 1957) assesses mainly two interconnected dimensions: the expressive hostility or antagonism (physical and verbal aggression) and the neurotic or experiential hostility, which involves subjective experiences like resentment, suspicion, mistrust and irritation.

The Interpersonal Hostility Assessment Technique (IHAT) developed by Barefoot and colleagues (Brummett, Maynard et al. 2000) is a structured interview that classifies hostile behaviors in four types, based on the style (rather than content) of the responses to interviewer: direct challenges to the interviewer, indirectly or more subtle challenges, hostile withholding of information or evasion of the question, and irritation (Brummett, Maynard et al. 2000).

Although consistently associated with increased cardiovascular morbidity, the effect size of hostility has been considered low and its clinical relevance has been questioned by some authors (Myrtek 2001).

6.3 Anger

The concept of anger usually refers to an unpleasant emotion ranging in intensity from irritation or annoyance to fury or rage. Feelings of anger are elicited in situation of being treated unjustly and is accompanied by subjective arousal. As a personality trait it can be defined as the characteristic to experience frequent and pronounced episodes of this emotion.

Another relevant aspect of anger is its expression. In this context, two subtypes have been defined: "anger-out", a personality trait derived from a combination of anger and aggression (i.e, the expression of aggressive behavior when angry) and "anger- in", a tendency to feel anger and suppress it (Schulman and Stromberg 2007) . Anger is viewed by other authors (Norlander and Eckhardt 2005) as a multidimensional construct, involving physiological, behavioral, cognitive and phenomenological components. Scales have been developed to evaluate various aspects of anger. The Anger-Out scale of the Spielberger et al. (1985) Anger-Expression Questionnaire evaluates tendencies to express aggression outwardly using a self-report questionnaire format, whereas the Anger-In scale purportedly measures tendencies to suppress or withhold anger.

Evaluated as a trait, anger significantly predicted occurrence of another MI (Denollet and Brutsaert 1998). More recently, Ohira (Ohira 2010), 2010, in the Circulatory Risk in

Communities Study (CIRCS), evaluated the association of depressive symptoms, tension and anger expression with the incidence of cardiovascular disease in Japanese population. It was a pioneering study, since all previous relevant data are mostly limited to Western populations. As an instrument for measuring tension and anger expression, Ohira and colleagues used the Spielberger anger expression scale and the Framingham Tension Scale to evaluate 6292 men and women. In a cross-sectional examination, "anger-out" was inversely associated with hypertension in men. In longitudinal observation, anger-in score was positively associated with hypertension in men, even after further adjustment for BMI, alcohol intake and systolic blood pressure levels at baseline.

Besides working chronically as a personality trait, episodes of anger may acutely cause negative impact on the cardiovascular system. Anger attacks have been associated with sudden cardiac death, MI and ventricular arrhythmias.

Among the pathophysiological mechanisms linking anger attacks and acute cardiovascular changes, two are most studied: modifications in autonomic regulation and electrophysiological changes. The autonomic dysregulation caused by anger and other emotions is well described. Experimental studies show that intense emotional factors increase the level of catecholamines and decrease vagal stimulation. Other findings suggest that cardiac sympathetic activation (and the decrease of vagal stimulation) is arrhythmogenic (Lampert 2010). Of note, Verrier et al (Verrier, Calvert et al. 1975) reported the stimulation of the posterior hypothalamus (which increases sympathetic cardiac stimulation) produced a 40% reduction of the threshold for induction of ventricular fibrillation in dogs. Regarding arrhythmogenic electrophysiological changes induced by stress, interesting results were obtained by analyzing the T-wave alternation. This measure is considered a marker of the heterogeneity of repolarization and therefore to have a major role in arrhythmogenesis. T-wave alternation was enhanced during mental stress (Kovach, Nearing et al. 2001). In a previous study, increased T-wave alternation among patients experiencing emotional stressors correlated to a higher incidence of shocks of implantable cardioverter-defibrillator (ICD) which were in turn induced by acute ventricular arrhythmias (Stopper, Joska et al. 2007). Moreover, it is noteworthy that recent evidence obtained from neuroimaging studies using positron emission tomography suggest that the laterality of brain activity during stress is related to an increased susceptibility to ventricular arrhythmias (Ziegelstein 2007).

Psychological interventions may be used to improve the management of anger, and anger attacks may also decrease significantly with antidepressant treatment, particularly in those with depression (Fava, Rosenbaum et al. 1991; Fava, Alpert et al. 1996).

6.4 Type D

Type D personality, also known as *distressed* personality, is a construct that has also been associated with cardiovascular disorders. The core symptoms of this construct are *negative affectivity* and *social inhibition* (Denollet 1998). The *negative affectivity* refers to a tendency to experience distress over time and in various situations (Watson and Pennebaker 1989), while *social inhibition* refers to the tendency of consciously inhibit the expression of these negative emotions in social situations. A high score on both traits denotes those with a Type D personality (Pedersen and Denollet 2003). Therefore, the base of this construct is not just experiencing negative emotions, but the combination of negative emotion and suppressed emotional expression. Consequently, those with this personality experience distress which is not easily shared with others. Type D personality may be identified with the DS14, an instrument developed specifically to obtain standard assessment of negative affectivity and social inhibition (Denollet 2005).

Several studies established Type D personality as an independent predictor of cardiac mortality in patients with CHD (Denollet, Sys et al. 1995; Denollet, Vaes et al. 2000). It has also been reported that Type D personality increases the risk of sudden cardiac arrest (Appels, Golombeck et al. 2000) and is an independent predictor of mortality in patients with decreased left ventricular ejection fraction after MI (Denollet and Brutsaert 1998).

Direct mechanisms proposed for the impact of Type D personality in the cardiovascular system include cardiovascular autonomic nervous system activity, endothelial function, platelet function and altered lipid profile. Type D personality has been associated with greater cortisol reactivity to stress, heightened blood pressure reactivity (Habra, Linden et al. 2003) and increased circulating levels of the pro-inflammatory cytokine tumor necrosis factor (TNF-α) and TNF-α soluble receptors 1 and 2 (Denollet, Conraads et al. 2003).

6.5 Vital exhaustion

The most common definition of VE characterizes this condition by an unusual fatigue, increased irritability and feelings of demoralization. The assessment of VE can be made with the 21-item Maastricht Questionnaire (Appels, Hoppener et al. 1987) and, although there is an overlap between VE and depressive symptoms, there is evidence these are distinct conditions (Kopp, Falger et al. 1998).

Various studies have associated VE with CHD and chronic heart failure (Appels, Kop et al. 1995; Pedersen and Middel 2001; Smith, Gidron et al. 2009). VE has been associated with a twofold to threefold increased risk of mortality and morbidity in patients with CHD (Kop, Appels et al. 1994; Appels, Kop et al. 1995). It has also been associated with sudden cardiac arrest and adverse cardiac events in patients that underwent successful angioplasty(Kop, Appels et al. 1994; Appels, Golombeck et al. 2000). A recent study showed that four distinct VE trajectories may be found in cardiac patients: low VE, decreasing VE, increasing VE and severe VE; the last two (increasing VE and severe VE) trajectories were predictors of poor cardiovascular prognosis (Smith, Kupper et al. 2010).

Several possible biological pathways may link VE with cardiovascular disease. VE has been associated with increased lipid metabolism (van Doornen and van Blokland 1989), reduced fibrinolytic capacity (Kop, Hamulyak et al. 1998; van Diest, Hamulyak et al. 2002), parasympathetic withdrawal (Watanabe, Sugiyama et al. 2002), reduced heart rate recovery after exercise (von Kanel, Barth et al. 2009), increased levels of cytokines (van der Ven, van Diest et al. 2003; Janszky, Lekander et al. 2005), decreased slow wave sleep, reactivated cytomegalovirus fosters growth of atherosclerosis, decreased negative feedback from the HPA-axis onto the sympathetic-adrenomedular system (Appels 2004) and hypocortisolemia (Keltikangas-Jarvinen, Raikkonen et al. 1996; Nicolson and van Diest 2000).

Treatment of VE aims to reduce stressors causing exhaustion and to support recovery by promoting rest and by making rest more efficient. Group discussions may be used to identify stressors in the family and work domain, and to help patients to cope with these stressors. The process includes an evaluation of the optimum length of resting time, teaching relaxation exercises designed to make rest more efficient, stimulation of physical exercise and homework assignments(Appels 2004).

6.6 Aggression

Aggression refers to a physical or verbal behavior, typically defined as attacking, destructive, or hurtful actions. Aggressive behavior may be precipitated by anger, but it may be motivated by many other factors as well. Aggression may be considered a personality trait in those who tend to frequently exhibit such behavior. The Aggression Questionnaire (AQ), developed by Buss and Perry (1992) (Buss and Perry 1992), contains subscales to measure anger, hostility and verbal and physical aggression.

6.7 Negative affectivity and negative emotion

Watson & Clark (1984) have proposed the existence of a broadband personality dimension referred to as negative affectivity(Watson and Clark 1984). This construct includes all negative emotions and is characterized by a general disposition to chronically experience anxiety, sadness, guilt, anger, irritability, and other negative emotions.

These individuals tend to be internally focused and attuned to somatic sensations. This tendency leads them to experience body sensations as symptoms of physical illness.

Some data have offered a support for increased risk of CHD in individuals with increased levels of negative affectivity (Frasure-Smith and Lesperance 2003).

Besides negative affectivity, some studies have referred to depression, anger, anxiety and hostility as negative emotions. According to Kubzansky et al. anger, anxiety and depression are the three negative emotions with the largest evidence linking them etiologically to the development of CHD (Kubzansky and Kawachi 2000; Kubzansky, Davidson et al. 2005; Kubzansky 2007). According to these authors emotions occur in a continuum ranging from normal to pathological and there is evidence of a dose response between negative emotions and CHD risk (Kubzansky and Kawachi 2000; Everson-Rose and Lewis 2005; Rozanski, Blumenthal et al. 2005). Possibly all these negative emotions work as a general stressor of the cardiovascular system (Todaro, Shen et al. 2003). In the INTERHEART, a case-control study, the authors performed an analysis using a score integrating psychosocial factors including depression, locus of control, perceived stress and life events. They found that psychosocial factors had a greater relative risk of MI than well-established risk factors such as hypertension, abdominal obesity and diabetes (Yusuf, Hawken et al. 2004).

7. Treatment

Various strategies have been developed to treat negative affect (Table 4). Most of them focused in reducing TABP, including education about CHD and TABP; Relaxation Training (Relaxation excercises of the "deep-muscle" or "acobsonian"); Cognitive Therapy including restructuring techniques such as the identification and modification of TABP cognitions (e.g.,

"I have to get there faster" is changed to "I'm going fast enough"). Specific techniques are the *Imaging* strategy that includes imagining rousing situations such as a traffic jam or confrontation with a boss and the training to apply specific coping skills such as relaxation training or cognitive restructuring; the *Behavior Modification* that includes rehearsing of Type B coping skills through role playing or behavioral prescriptions that are given to be carried out between sessions; the *Emotional Support* that includes the encouragement to ventilate the painful affects and experiences in an empathic atmosphere. There is also the *Psychodynamic Interpretation* that includes the use of psychodynamic interpretations of the unconscious motives and conflicts underlying TABP (Nunes, Frank et al. 1987). A meta-analysis of 18 controlled studies of psychological treatment of TABP revealed an effect size of 0.61±0.21 indicating a reduction approximately by half a standard deviation (Nunes, Frank et al. 1987).

Type A Behavior Pattern	Type D Personality	Vital exhaustion	Hostility	Anger	Aggression
-Education about CHD and TABP; -Relaxation Training: Relaxation excercises; -Cognitive Therapy including cognitive restructuring techniques and also psychodynamic interpretation (Nunes, Frank et al. 1987)	-Patients may benefit from psychological treatment to deal with threatening issues and lighten the symptoms.	-Reduction of the stressors that cause exhaustion, -Support recovery by promoting rest and by making rest more efficient; -Group discussions may be used to identify stressors in the family and work domain, and to help patient in coping with these stressors; -Stimulation of physical exercise (Appels 2004).	-Cognitive-behavior interventions may reduce measures of hostility (Sloan, Shapiro et al. 2010); -SSRIs may reduce hostile affect (Kamarck, Haskett et al. 2009).	-Cognitive-behavioral and skills-based approaches may reduce anger (Blake and Hamrin 2007). -Anger attacks may decrease with SSRIs particularly in depressed patients (Fava, Rosenbaum et al. 1991; Fava, Alpert et al. 1996)	-SSRIs may reduce, physical and verbal aggression in women (Kamarck, Haskett et al. 2009).

Table 4. Treatments

There is no well-established treatment for type D personality, but these patients may benefit from psychological treatment to deal with threatening issues and lighten the symptoms. Interventions for VE focus on reducing the stressors associated with the exhaustion and support recovery by promoting rest and by making rest more efficient. Group discussions may be used to identify stressors in the family and work domain, to help patients to cope with these stressors and to stimulate physical exercise (Appels 2004). Kamark et al (Kamarck, Haskett et al. 2009) studied people with high hostility scores and with no Axis I diagnosis medicated with citalopram or placebo. The citalopram group showed significant reductions in state anger, and hostile affect, while physical and verbal aggression was reduced among women.

Cognitive-behavior interventions have shown to be effective in reducing measures of hostility and improving cardiac autonomic modulation (Sloan, Shapiro et al. 2010). In addition, Cognitive-behavioral and skills-based approaches may be effective in reducing anger and aggression in youth (Blake and Hamrin 2007). Anger attacks (Fava, Rosenbaum et al. 1991; Fava, Alpert et al. 1996) decreased significantly with fluoxetine treatment in depressed patients.

8. Discussion

Several studies have linked negative affect with cardiovascular morbidity. However, due to discrepancies among results, there is still some controversy regarding the existence, nature and magnitude of their relationship. In this context, Schulman and Stromberg, 2007, (Schulman and Stromberg 2007) conducted a review of the meta-analyses and systematic reviews on this subject. As inclusion criteria, the authors used the Database of Abstracts of Reviews of Effects (DARE) criteria and they chose to include only those reviews and meta-analyses which had measured the magnitude of the effect of anger, hostility and TABP on the cardiovascular outcomes. The final analysis included five systematic reviews (Hemingway and Marmot 1999; Rozanski, Blumenthal et al. 1999; Kuper, Marmot et al. 2002; Suls and Bunde 2005). As a common result, they showed positive results between TABP, hostility, anger and CHD in healthy populations. For individuals with heart disease the review showed conflicting results. The authors concluded that TABP, hostility, anger and anger expression may not constitute a risk factor for worse prognosis in all patient samples, and their effects would be more significant in a previously healthy population. In such patients negative affect could harm the cardiovascular system directly or indirectly by increasing cardiovascular risk factors such as hypertension and atherosclerosis (Matthews, Owens et al. 1998; Pollitt, Daniel et al. 2005).

In a more recent review and meta-analysis, Chida and Steptoe (2009) (Chida and Steptoe 2009) selected only prospective cohort studies, exploring the causal association of measures of anger and hostility and heart disease. A total of 21 cohorts with healthy patients at baseline with 71 606 individuals, and 18 cohorts of patients with existing CHD with 8120 individuals were included. These studies were published between 1983 and 2006 and performed in a wide range of countries (Europe, America and Australia). This meta-analysis found that 28% of studies with healthy individuals and 26.3% of studies with CHD patients showed significant harmful effects. The overall combined hazard ratio (HR) was 1.19 (95% CI 1.05 to 1.35) for the healthy population and 1.23 (95% CI 1.08 to 1.42) for the disease population, indicating a positive association. In subgroup analysis, it was found that cohorts with longer follow-up periods showed higher HR than the overall effect both in studies with healthy and with CHD individuals. Also, in studies with CHD patients, the HR was sustained even after controlling for baseline disease status and treatment (1.20 95% CI 1.0 to 1.44). Focusing on mortality analyses, a positive association was also found between anger and hostility and cardiovascular mortality. Thus, this review emphasizes the increased risk of negative affect for those with established CHD, in contrast to the results of Schulman and Stromberg.

The development of a validated gold standard for the assessment of negative affect is necessary to allow the comparison between studies. Moreover, the concepts of anger and hostility do not include a clear cutoff for its morbidity and consequently data about their prevalence, course, comorbidity and treatment response are lacking. Besides this difference in instruments, there is also a disagreement concerning the results of clinical studies focused on the relationship between psychological traits and cardiovascular disease.

Undeniably, a consistent body of evidence links negative affect with heart disease. In addition, the efficacy of psychotherapeutic interventions in cardiac patients was recently demonstrated (Linden, Phillips et al. 2007). While the clinical use of screening instruments for anger and hostility is not yet a reality, in the future the multi-disciplinary approach involving psychological techniques, possibly specifically focused on these traits, might become an important strategy in the management of patients with CHD. Moreover, recent advances in our understanding of pathophysiology involving physical and emotional changes will potentially allow specific case definitions and possible targeted drug therapies for certain forms of negative affect.

9. References

American Psychiatric Association (1994). Diagnostic and Statistical Manual of Mental Disorders. Washington, DC, American Psychiatric Association.

Appels, A. (2004). "Exhaustion and coronary heart disease: the history of a scientific quest." Patient Educ Couns 55(2): 223-229.

Appels, A., B. Golombeck, et al. (2000). "Behavioral risk factors of sudden cardiac arrest." J Psychosom Res 48(4-5): 463-469.

Appels, A., P. Hoppener, et al. (1987). "A questionnaire to assess premonitory symptoms of myocardial infarction." Int J Cardiol 17(1): 15-24.

Appels, A., W. Kop, et al. (1995). "Vital exhaustion, extent of atherosclerosis, and the clinical course after successful percutaneous transluminal coronary angioplasty." Eur Heart J 16(12): 1880-1885.

Bagby, R. M., S. H. Kennedy, et al. (1997). "Personality and symptom profiles of the angry hostile depressed patient." J Affect Disord 45(3): 155-160.

Baker, M., J. Dorzah, et al. (1971). "Depressive disease. classification and clinical characteristics." Compr Psychiatry 12(4): 354-365.

Barefoot, J. C., K. A. Dodge, et al. (1989). "The Cook-Medley hostility scale: item content and ability to predict survival." Psychosom Med 51(1): 46-57.

Blake, C. S. and V. Hamrin (2007). "Current approaches to the assessment and management of anger and aggression in youth: a review." Journal of child and adolescent psychiatric nursing : official publication of the Association of Child and Adolescent Psychiatric Nurses, Inc 20(4): 209-221.

Booth-Kewley, S. and H. S. Friedman (1987). "Psychological predictors of heart disease: a quantitative review." Psychol Bull 101(3): 343-362.

Brummett, B. H., K. E. Maynard, et al. (2000). "Reliability of interview-assessed hostility ratings across mode of assessment and time." J Pers Assess 75(2): 225-236.

Buss, A. H. and A. Durkee (1957). "An inventory for assessing different kinds of hostility." J Consult Psychol 21(4): 343-349.

Buss, A. H. and M. Perry (1992). "The aggression questionnaire." J Pers Soc Psychol 63(3): 452-459.

Chaput, L. A., S. H. Adams, et al. (2002). "Hostility predicts recurrent events among postmenopausal women with coronary heart disease." Am J Epidemiol 156(12): 1092-1099.

Chida, Y. and A. Steptoe (2009). "The association of anger and hostility with future coronary heart disease: a meta-analytic review of prospective evidence." J Am Coll Cardiol 53(11): 936-946.

Clark, L. A., D. Watson, et al. (1994). "Temperament, personality, and the mood and anxiety disorders." J Abnorm Psychol 103(1): 103-116.

Culic, V., D. Eterovic, et al. (2005). "Meta-analysis of possible external triggers of acute myocardial infarction." Int J Cardiol 99(1): 1-8.

Davidson, K. W. (2008). "Emotional predictors and behavioral triggers of acute coronary syndrome." Cleve Clin J Med 75 Suppl 2: S15-19.

Dembroski, T. M., J. M. MacDougall, et al. (1989). "Components of hostility as predictors of sudden death and myocardial infarction in the Multiple Risk Factor Intervention Trial." Psychosom Med 51(5): 514-522.

Dembroski, T. M., J. M. MacDougall, et al. (1985). "Components of Type A, hostility, and anger-in: relationship to angiographic findings." Psychosom Med 47(3): 219-233.

Denollet, J. (1998). "Personality and coronary heart disease: the type-D scale-16 (DS16)." Ann Behav Med 20(3): 209-215.

Denollet, J. (2005). "DS14: standard assessment of negative affectivity, social inhibition, and Type D personality." Psychosom Med 67(1): 89-97.

Denollet, J. and D. L. Brutsaert (1998). "Personality, disease severity, and the risk of long-term cardiac events in patients with a decreased ejection fraction after myocardial infarction." Circulation 97(2): 167-173.

Denollet, J., V. M. Conraads, et al. (2003). "Cytokines and immune activation in systolic heart failure: the role of Type D personality." Brain Behav Immun 17(4): 304-309.

Denollet, J., S. U. Sys, et al. (1995). "Personality and mortality after myocardial infarction." Psychosom Med 57(6): 582-591.

Denollet, J., J. Vaes, et al. (2000). "Inadequate response to treatment in coronary heart disease : adverse effects of type D personality and younger age on 5-year prognosis and quality of life." Circulation 102(6): 630-635.

Dougherty, D. D., S. L. Rauch, et al. (2004). "Ventromedial prefrontal cortex and amygdala dysfunction during an anger induction positron emission tomography study in patients with major depressive disorder with anger attacks." Archives of General Psychiatry 61(8): 795-804.

Drevets, W. C. (1999). "Prefrontal cortical-amygdalar metabolism in major depression." Annals of the New York Academy of Sciences 877: 614-637.

Dujovne, V. F. and B. K. Houston (1991). "Hostility-related variables and plasma lipid levels." Journal of behavioral medicine 14(6): 555-565.

Eaker, E. D., J. Pinsky, et al. (1992). "Myocardial infarction and coronary death among women: psychosocial predictors from a 20-year follow-up of women in the Framingham Study." Am J Epidemiol 135(8): 854-864.

Everson, S. A., B. S. McKey, et al. (1995). "Effect of trait hostility on cardiovascular responses to harassment in young men." International journal of behavioral medicine 2(2): 172-191.

Everson-Rose, S. A. and T. T. Lewis (2005). "Psychosocial factors and cardiovascular diseases." Annu Rev Public Health 26: 469-500.

Fava, M., M. Abraham, et al. (1996). "Cardiovascular risk factors in depression. The role of anxiety and anger." Psychosomatics 37(1): 31-37.

Fava, M., J. Alpert, et al. (1996). "Fluoxetine treatment of anger attacks: a replication study." Ann Clin Psychiatry 8(1): 7-10.

Fava, M., J. E. Alpert, et al. (2004). "Clinical correlates and symptom patterns of anxious depression among patients with major depressive disorder in STAR*D." Psychol Med 34(7): 1299-1308.

Fava, M., J. F. Rosenbaum, et al. (1991). "Anger attacks in depressed outpatients and their response to fluoxetine." Psychopharmacology bulletin 27(3): 275-279.

Fava, M., L. A. Uebelacker, et al. (1997). "Major depressive subtypes and treatment response." Biol Psychiatry 42(7): 568-576.

Fava, M., R. D. Vuolo, et al. (2000). "Fenfluramine challenge in unipolar depression with and without anger attacks." Psychiatry Research 94(1): 9-18.

Felsten, G. and V. Hill (1999). "Aggression Questionnaire hostility scale predicts anger in response to mistreatment." Behaviour research and therapy 37(1): 87-97.

Fraguas, R., D. V. Iosifescu, et al. (2007). "Major depressive disorder with anger attacks and cardiovascular risk factors." Int J Psychiatry Med 37(1): 99-111.

Frasure-Smith, N. and F. Lesperance (2003). "Depression and other psychological risks following myocardial infarction." Arch Gen Psychiatry 60(6): 627-636.

Friedman, H. S. and S. Booth-Kewley (1987). "The "disease-prone personality". A meta-analytic view of the construct." Am Psychol 42(6): 539-555.

Friedman, M. and R. H. Rosenman (1959). "Association of specific overt behavior pattern with blood and cardiovascular findings; blood cholesterol level, blood clotting time, incidence of arcus senilis, and clinical coronary artery disease." J Am Med Assoc 169(12): 1286-1296.

Gould, R. A., S. Ball, et al. (1996). "Prevalence and correlates of anger attacks: a two site study." J Affect Disord 39(1): 31-38.

Gullion, C. M. and A. J. Rush (1998). "Toward a generalizable model of symptoms in major depressive disorder." Biol Psychiatry 44(10): 959-972.

Habra, M. E., W. Linden, et al. (2003). "Type D personality is related to cardiovascular and neuroendocrine reactivity to acute stress." J Psychosom Res 55(3): 235-245.

Hamilton, M. (1960). "A rating scale for depression." J Neurol Neurosurg Psychiatry 23: 56-62.

Haynes, S. G., M. Feinleib, et al. (1980). "The relationship of psychosocial factors to coronary heart disease in the Framingham Study. III. Eight-year incidence of coronary heart disease." Am J Epidemiol 111(1): 37-58.

Hemingway, H. and M. Marmot (1999). "Evidence based cardiology: psychosocial factors in the aetiology and prognosis of coronary heart disease. Systematic review of prospective cohort studies." BMJ 318(7196): 1460-1467.

Iosifescu, D. V., P. F. Renshaw, et al. (2007). "Major depressive disorder with anger attacks and subcortical MRI white matter hyperintensities." J Nerv Ment Dis 195(2): 175-178.

Janszky, I., M. Lekander, et al. (2005). "Self-rated health and vital exhaustion, but not depression, is related to inflammation in women with coronary heart disease." Brain Behav Immun 19(6): 555-563.

Jenkins, C. D., R. H. Rosenman, et al. (1967). "Development of an objective psychological test for the determination of the coronary-prone behavior pattern in employed men." J Chronic Dis 20(6): 371-379.

Jenkins, C. D., R. H. Rosenman, et al. (1974). "Prediction of clinical coronary heart disease by a test for the coronary-prone behavior pattern." N Engl J Med 290(23): 1271-1275.

Kamarck, T. W., R. F. Haskett, et al. (2009). "Citalopram intervention for hostility: results of a randomized clinical trial." Journal of consulting and clinical psychology 77(1): 174-188.

Keltikangas-Jarvinen, L., T. Hintsa, et al. (2007). "Type A eagerness-energy across developmental periods predicts adulthood carotid intima-media thickness: the Cardiovascular Risk in Young Finns Study." Arteriosclerosis, thrombosis, and vascular biology 27(7): 1638-1644.

Keltikangas-Jarvinen, L., K. Raikkonen, et al. (1996). "Vital exhaustion, anger expression, and pituitary and adrenocortical hormones. Implications for the insulin resistance syndrome." Arterioscler Thromb Vasc Biol 16(2): 275-280.

Kop, W. J., A. P. Appels, et al. (1994). "Vital exhaustion predicts new cardiac events after successful coronary angioplasty." Psychosom Med 56(4): 281-287.

Kop, W. J., K. Hamulyak, et al. (1998). "Relationship of blood coagulation and fibrinolysis to vital exhaustion." Psychosom Med 60(3): 352-358.

Kopp, M. S., P. R. Falger, et al. (1998). "Depressive symptomatology and vital exhaustion are differentially related to behavioral risk factors for coronary artery disease." Psychosom Med 60(6): 752-758.

Kovach, J. A., B. D. Nearing, et al. (2001). "Angerlike behavioral state potentiates myocardial ischemia-induced T-wave alternans in canines." Journal of the American College of Cardiology 37(6): 1719-1725.

Kubzansky, L. D. (2007). "Sick at heart: the pathophysiology of negative emotions." Cleve Clin J Med 74 Suppl 1: S67-72.

Kubzansky, L. D., K. W. Davidson, et al. (2005). "The clinical impact of negative psychological states: expanding the spectrum of risk for coronary artery disease." Psychosom Med 67 Suppl 1: S10-14.

Kubzansky, L. D. and I. Kawachi (2000). "Going to the heart of the matter: do negative emotions cause coronary heart disease?" J Psychosom Res 48(4-5): 323-337.

Kuper, H., M. Marmot, et al. (2002). "Systematic review of prospective cohort studies of psychosocial factors in the etiology and prognosis of coronary heart disease." Semin Vasc Med 2(3): 267-314.

Lampert, R. (2010). "Anger and ventricular arrhythmias." Curr Opin Cardiol 25(1): 46-52.

Lampert, R., T. Joska, et al. (2002). "Emotional and physical precipitants of ventricular arrhythmia." Circulation 106(14): 1800-1805.

Levenkron, J. C., J. D. Cohen, et al. (1983). "Modifying the Type A coronary-prone behavior pattern." J Consult Clin Psychol 51(2): 192-204.

Linden, W., M. J. Phillips, et al. (2007). "Psychological treatment of cardiac patients: a meta-analysis." Eur Heart J 28(24): 2972-2984.

Lovallo, W. R. and W. Gerin (2003). "Psychophysiological reactivity: mechanisms and pathways to cardiovascular disease." Psychosom Med 65(1): 36-45.

MacDougall, J. M., T. M. Dembroski, et al. (1979). "The structured interview and questionnaire methods of assessing coronary-prone behavior in male and female college students." J Behav Med 2(1): 71-83.

Martin, R., D. Watson, et al. (2000). "A three-factor model of trait anger: dimensions of affect, behavior, and cognition." J Pers 68(5): 869-897.

Matthews, K. A., J. F. Owens, et al. (1998). "Are hostility and anxiety associated with carotid atherosclerosis in healthy postmenopausal women?" Psychosom Med 60(5): 633-638.

Miller, T. Q., T. W. Smith, et al. (1996). "A meta-analytic review of research on hostility and physical health." Psychol Bull 119(2): 322-348.

Mischoulon, D., D. D. Dougherty, et al. (2002). "An open pilot study of nefazodone in depression with anger attacks: relationship between clinical response and receptor binding." Psychiatry Res 116(3): 151-161.

Mittleman, M. A., M. Maclure, et al. (1995). "Triggering of acute myocardial infarction onset by episodes of anger. Determinants of Myocardial Infarction Onset Study Investigators." Circulation 92(7): 1720-1725.

Montgomery, S. A. and M. Asberg (1979). "A new depression scale designed to be sensitive to change." Br J Psychiatry 134: 382-389.

Morand, P., G. Thomas, et al. (1998). "Fava's Anger Attacks Questionnaire: evaluation of the French version in depressed patients." Eur Psychiatry 13(1): 41-45.

Myrtek, M. (2001). "Meta-analyses of prospective studies on coronary heart disease, type A personality, and hostility." Int J Cardiol 79(2-3): 245-251.

Niaura, R., C. M. Stoney, et al. (1992). "Lipids in psychological research: the last decade." Biological psychology 34(1): 1-43.

Nicolson, N. A. and R. van Diest (2000). "Salivary cortisol patterns in vital exhaustion." J Psychosom Res 49(5): 335-342.

Norlander, B. and C. Eckhardt (2005). "Anger, hostility, and male perpetrators of intimate partner violence: a meta-analytic review." Clin Psychol Rev 25(2): 119-152.

Nunes, E. V., K. A. Frank, et al. (1987). "Psychologic treatment for the type A behavior pattern and for coronary heart disease: a meta-analysis of the literature." Psychosom Med 49(2): 159-173.

Ohira, T. (2010). "Psychological distress and cardiovascular disease: the Circulatory Risk in Communities Study (CIRCS)." J Epidemiol 20(3): 185-191.

Oishi, K., M. Kamimura, et al. (1999). "Individual differences in physiological responses and type A behavior pattern." Applied human science : journal of physiological anthropology 18(3): 101-108.

Overall, J. E., B. J. Goldstein, et al. (1971). "Symptomatic volunteers in psychiatric research." J Psychiatr Res 9(1): 31-43.

Overall, J. E., L. E. Hollister, et al. (1966). "Nosology of depression and differential response to drugs." JAMA 195(11): 946-948.

Painuly, N., P. Sharan, et al. (2005). "Relationship of anger and anger attacks with depression: a brief review." Eur Arch Psychiatry Clin Neurosci 255(4): 215-222.

Pedersen, S. S. and J. Denollet (2003). "Type D personality, cardiac events, and impaired quality of life: a review." Eur J Cardiovasc Prev Rehabil 10(4): 241-248.

Pedersen, S. S. and B. Middel (2001). "Increased vital exhaustion among type-D patients with ischemic heart disease." J Psychosom Res 51(2): 443-449.

Perlis, R. H., J. W. Smoller, et al. (2004). "The prevalence and clinical correlates of anger attacks during depressive episodes in bipolar disorder." J Affect Disord 79(1-3): 291-295.

Pizzagalli, D., R. D. Pascual-Marqui, et al. (2001). "Anterior cingulate activity as a predictor of degree of treatment response in major depression: evidence from brain electrical tomography analysis." The American journal of psychiatry 158(3): 405-415.

Pollitt, R. A., M. Daniel, et al. (2005). "Mediation and modification of the association between hopelessness, hostility, and progression of carotid atherosclerosis." J Behav Med 28(1): 53-64.

Posternak, M. A. and M. Zimmerman (2002). "Anger and aggression in psychiatric outpatients." J Clin Psychiatry 63(8): 665-672.

Ragland, D. R. and R. J. Brand (1988). "Coronary heart disease mortality in the Western Collaborative Group Study. Follow-up experience of 22 years." Am J Epidemiol 127(3): 462-475.

Ragland, D. R. and R. J. Brand (1988). "Type A behavior and mortality from coronary heart disease." N Engl J Med 318(2): 65-69.

Ravaja, N., T. Kauppinen, et al. (2000). "Relationships between hostility and physiological coronary heart disease risk factors in young adults: the moderating influence of depressive tendencies." Psychological Medicine 30(2): 381-393.

Raynor, D. A., M. F. Pogue-Geile, et al. (2002). "Covariation of psychosocial characteristics associated with cardiovascular disease: genetic and environmental influences." Psychosom Med 64(2): 191-203; discussion 204-195.

Rosenman, R. H., R. J. Brand, et al. (1976). "Multivariate prediction of coronary heart disease during 8.5 year follow-up in the Western Collaborative Group Study." Am J Cardiol 37(6): 903-910.

Rozanski, A., J. A. Blumenthal, et al. (2005). "The epidemiology, pathophysiology, and management of psychosocial risk factors in cardiac practice: the emerging field of behavioral cardiology." J Am Coll Cardiol 45(5): 637-651.

Rozanski, A., J. A. Blumenthal, et al. (1999). "Impact of psychological factors on the pathogenesis of cardiovascular disease and implications for therapy." Circulation 99(16): 2192-2217.

Schaefer, S. M., H. C. Abercrombie, et al. (2000). "Six-month test-retest reliability of MRI-defined PET measures of regional cerebral glucose metabolic rate in selected subcortical structures." Human brain mapping 10(1): 1-9.

Scherwitz, L. W., L. L. Perkins, et al. (1992). "Hostility and health behaviors in young adults: the CARDIA Study. Coronary Artery Risk Development in Young Adults Study." Am J Epidemiol 136(2): 136-145.

Schulman, J. K. and S. Stromberg (2007). "On the value of doing nothing: anger and cardiovascular disease in clinical practice." Cardiol Rev 15(3): 123-132.

Sloan, R. P., P. A. Shapiro, et al. (2010). "Cardiac autonomic control and treatment of hostility: a randomized controlled trial." Psychosomatic medicine 72(1): 1-8.

Smith, O. R., Y. Gidron, et al. (2009). "Vital exhaustion in chronic heart failure: symptom profiles and clinical outcome." J Psychosom Res 66(3): 195-201.

Smith, O. R., N. Kupper, et al. (2010). "Vital exhaustion and cardiovascular prognosis in myocardial infarction and heart failure: predictive power of different trajectories." Psychol Med: 1-8.

Smith, T. W., K. Glazer, et al. (2004). "Hostility, anger, aggressiveness, and coronary heart disease: an interpersonal perspective on personality, emotion, and health." J Pers 72(6): 1217-1270.

Snaith, R. P. and C. M. Taylor (1985). "Irritability: definition, assessment and associated factors." Br J Psychiatry 147: 127-136.

Steinberg, L. and R. S. Jorgensen (1996). "Assessing the MMPI-based Cook-Medley Hostility Scale: the implications of dimensionality." J Pers Soc Psychol 70(6): 1281-1287.

Stopper, M., T. Joska, et al. (2007). "Electrophysiologic characteristics of anger-triggered arrhythmias." Heart rhythm : the official journal of the Heart Rhythm Society 4(3): 268-273.

Stopper, M., T. Joska, et al. (2007). "Electrophysiologic characteristics of anger-triggered arrhythmias." Heart Rhythm 4(3): 268-273.

Suarez, E. C., C. M. Kuhn, et al. (1998). "Neuroendocrine, cardiovascular, and emotional responses of hostile men: the role of interpersonal challenge." Psychosom Med 60(1): 78-88.

Suls, J. and J. Bunde (2005). "Anger, anxiety, and depression as risk factors for cardiovascular disease: the problems and implications of overlapping affective dispositions." Psychol Bull 131(2): 260-300.

Todaro, J. F., B. J. Shen, et al. (2003). "Effect of negative emotions on frequency of coronary heart disease (The Normative Aging Study)." Am J Cardiol 92(8): 901-906.

van der Ven, A., R. van Diest, et al. (2003). "Herpes viruses, cytokines, and altered hemostasis in vital exhaustion." Psychosom Med 65(2): 194-200.

van Diest, R., K. Hamulyak, et al. (2002). "Diurnal variations in coagulation and fibrinolysis in vital exhaustion." Psychosom Med 64(5): 787-792.

van Doornen, L. J. and R. W. van Blokland (1989). "The relation of type A behavior and vital exhaustion with physiological reactions to real life stress." J Psychosom Res 33(6): 715-725.

Verrier, R. L., A. Calvert, et al. (1975). "Effect of posterior hypothalamic stimulation on ventricular fibrillation threshold." The American journal of physiology 228(3): 923-927.

von Kanel, R., J. Barth, et al. (2009) "Heart rate recovery after exercise in chronic heart failure: Role of vital exhaustion and type D personality." J Cardiol 53(2): 248-256.

Watanabe, T., Y. Sugiyama, et al. (2002). "Effects of vital exhaustion on cardiac autononomic nervous functions assessed by heart rate variability at rest in middle-aged male workers." Int J Behav Med 9(1): 68-75.

Watson, D. and L. A. Clark (1984). "Negative affectivity: the disposition to experience aversive emotional states." Psychol Bull 96(3): 465-490.

Watson, D. and J. W. Pennebaker (1989). "Health complaints, stress, and distress: exploring the central role of negative affectivity." Psychol Rev 96(2): 234-254.

Yu-Wai-Man, P., P. G. Griffiths, et al. (2010). "Multi-system neurological disease is common in patients with OPA1 mutations." Brain : a journal of neurology 133(Pt 3): 771-786.

Yusuf, S., S. Hawken, et al. (2004). "Effect of potentially modifiable risk factors associated with myocardial infarction in 52 countries (the INTERHEART study): case-control study." Lancet 364(9438): 937-952.

Ziegelstein, R. C. (2007). "Acute emotional stress and cardiac arrhythmias." JAMA 298(3): 324-329.

7

Health Related Quality of Life in Coronary Patients

María Dueñas, Alejandro Salazar, Begoña Ojeda and Inmaculada Failde
Preventive Medicine and Public Health Department, University of Cádiz,
Spain

1. Introduction

The increase observed in the survival of patients with ischemic cardiopathy, together with the effect of the disease on the social, professional, and family life of those suffering from it, have led researchers to consider that the traditional ways of measuring morbidity and mortality are not adequate for assessing the potential benefits of health care interventions. For this reason, there is common agreement on the need to use an indicator of subjective assessment of health, and of health related quality of life (HRQL), as a complementary criterion for monitoring the results of medical interventions in these patients.

The term "quality of life" (QoL) or health related quality of life (HRQL) came into use during the 1970s as a multidimensional concept reflecting the overall subjective condition of the physical and mental welfare of the individual, which is a consequence not only of the disease but also of the family and social conditions forming the patient's environment.

The assessment of these patients' HRQL has been tackled by several authors using both disease-specific and generic instruments such as the Nottingham Health Profile, the Sickness Impact Profile, the SF-36 or the SF-12 health questionnaire. Both types of instrument have advantages and disadvantages, and they may provide additional information since they quantify the patient's overall health.

Using different multidimensional measures, poorer HRQL has been observed in patients with Acute Myocardial Infarction (AMI) and angina pectoris than in other populations, and these differences have been related to low social class, female sex, the presence of mental disorders and the severity of the clinical condition.

Measuring changes in the HRQL of coronary patients is also important as a way of assessing interventions and predicting needs for social care, because it has been shown that the focus of attention in the immediate period following a cardiac attack is generally the physical functioning, but following discharge from hospital and in the longer term, general health, vitality, social and emotional functions could be at least as important.

In this chapter, we aim to provide an overview of the concept of HRQL and the usefulness of this measure from the perspective of a coronary patient. Likewise, we intend to review the main instruments used to assess HRQL and we analyse the factors that have been seen to affect the quality of life of these patients.

2. Quality of Life and heart disease

2.1 The concept of Quality of Life and Health-Related Quality of Life

Quality of Life has generated interest for many years, and as early as 384-322 BC Aristotle noted "the good life" or "doing well" to be the same as "being happy". However, the advent of this concept as it is known today, and concern for its systematic and scientific assessment, is relatively recent. In the field of health sciences, one of the most important advances in recent decades has been to recognise that patients' perspective of their illness is just as legitimate and valid as that of healthcare professionals. This has led to the need to define the concept of Health Related Quality of Life (HRQL) and to its assessment as a way of subjectively measuring its effect on a disease. In addition, its treatment is considered with growing frequency as an indicator of the advances and innovations in healthcare services (Casas Anguita et al., 2001).

The most widely accepted definition of Quality of Life at the present time was proposed in 1994 by the World Health Organization (WHO); it is considered as an individual's perception of their position in life in the context of the culture and value systems in which they live and in relation to their goals, expectations, standards and concerns (Group, World Health Organization Quality of Life (WHOQOL), 1993). The term Health-Related Quality of Life (HRQL) emerged later to distinguish between QoL in its more general sense and the requirements of clinical medicine and clinical trials, and thus remove ambiguity. Shumaker et al. defined it as people´s subjective evaluations of the influences of their current health status, health care, and health promoting activities on their ability to achieve and maintain a level of overall functioning that allows them to pursue valued life goals and that is reflected in their general well-being. Although there is disagreement about which dimensions should be included in HRQL assessments, these authors have specified that the domains of functioning that are critical to HRQL include: social, physical and cognitive functioning; mobility and self-care; and emotional well-being (Shumaker & Berzon, 1995).

HRQL acts as a point of reference for measuring the effect of a disease on the individual, and is described and characterized by the patients themselves as the result of their appraisal of their health care (Urzúa M, 2010). One unifying and non-controversial theme throughout all the approaches is that this concept can only be assessed by subjective measures. It is precisely their subjective and multidisciplinary nature that has led to them being more widely used to complement the traditional physiological and biological measures of health status. However, their assessment requires instruments with suitable psychometric properties, something which must be taken into consideration before their implementation.

2.2 Assessing Quality of Life in coronary patients

One area of health care that has taken particular interest in the concept and measurement of Health-Related Quality of Life involves patients with coronary heart disease. This disease, besides being the main cause of death worldwide, has significant physical, emotional and social consequences for sufferers, so assessing their quality of life is not only necessary for assessing the success of a treatment or operation, but also for highlighting certain problems which are not assessed by traditional methods and that may be of use for modifying or improving the treatment given, or for providing alternatives that improve patients' clinical course (Fayers & Machin, 2007). Considering that the management of coronary artery disease mainly involves leading a healthy life style, instruments for measuring HRQL are one of the best ways of providing an assessment of the experience of the patients themselves with regard to their health problems in areas such a physical, emotional or social functioning, role accomplishment, pain and fatigue (Asadi-Lari et al., 2003).

Despite the accepted interest in the assessment of HRQL in coronary patients, one of the main problems posed in clinical practice is the choice of the right instrument. When choosing a tool to assess HRQL, researchers or clinicians must first consider whether the chosen instrument has really been developed and validated in a population with similar characteristics, and if it covers all the aspects that it is important to assess in coronary patients.

To be used with confidence, the tools must have a series of characteristics such as: validity, or the degree to which it measures what it aims to measure; reliability, or the degree to which a measure provides similar values for people with the same quality of life; and sensitivity to change, or the degree to which a measure manages to detect significant changes appropriate to clinical changes (Cepeda-Valery et al., 2011). Furthermore, these tools must be complete; that is, they must include all the aspects that may be affected by the disease and they should be easy to score and interpret. This last aspect is of utmost importance in clinical settings as being quick and easy to use are necessary qualities under these circumstances (McDowell & Newell, 1996).

The most widely-used tools for measuring the HRQL of coronary patients can be grouped in two types: generic and specific (Table 1). Both kinds have pros and cons, and deciding which to use depends on the type of intervention to be assessed and the aims to be reached. In general, generic tools are able to detect the effects on the health of a broad range of patients and diseases and so comparisons can be established between the effect of heart disease and that of other chronic diseases such as diabetes or COPD on HRQL. However, generic measures are less sensitive at detecting the effect that the specific symptoms of heart disease have on a patient's life.

		Dimensions	Items
Generic	SF-36	8	36
	SF-12		12
	EroQol (EQ-5D)	5	16
Specific	Seattle Angina Questionnaire (SAQ)	5	19
	The Angina Pectoris Quality of Life Questionnaire (APQLQ)	4	22
	Myocardial Infarction Dimensional Assessment Scale (MIDAS)	7	35
	The MacNew Heart Disease Health-related Quality of Life instrument (MacNew)	3	27
	Cardiovascular Limitations and Symptoms Profile (CLASP)	9	37

Table 1. Health Related Quality of Life Instruments for Coronary Disease

The IQOLA project (International Quality of Life Assessment) (Alonso et al., 2004; Gandek et al., 1998), which studied the general population in eight countries, is one of the few projects to examine the impact of a series of chronic diseases, including coronary disease, on HRQL. In this project, which used the SF-36 health questionnaire to assess HRQL, it is interesting to note how quality of life is affected in different ways depending on the chronic disease analysed. At the present time, the Medical Outcomes Study 36-item Short-Form Health Survey (SF-36) used in this project is the most valid instrument for measuring the quality of life of patients with coronary disease and its use has been proven in the clinical forms of both angina and myocardial infarction (Failde & Ramos, 2000). Likewise, it is an appropriate tool for use in patients who undergo heart surgery and as an evaluative measure in intervention programmes (Brown et al., 1999; Dougherty et al., 1998; Hawkes & Mortensen, 2006; Yu et al., 2003).

There are two versions of the SF-36 health questionnaire. Version 1, developed by Ware et al in the USA in 1992 (Ware et al., 1993) and version 2, revised and published by Ware himself (Ware, 2000). The latter, an improved version of the original, is made up of 36 items grouped into 8 dimensions: Physical Functioning (10 items), Social Functioning (2 items), Role-Physical (4 items) , Role-Emotional (3 items), Mental Health (5 items), Vitality (4 items), Bodily Pain (2 items), and General Health (6 items). For each of the 8 dimensions, the items are coded, aggregated and transformed to a scale ranging from 0 (the worst state of health for that dimension) to 100 (the best state of health). The instrument was not designed to produce of global index. However, it is possible to calculate two summary scores by combining the scores of each dimension: the physical and mental summary measures (PCS and MCS).

One of the short forms of this questionnaire, the SF-12, has also been shown to possess suitable psychometric properties for use in this field of medicine, and has been shown to have the advantage of being quicker to carry out while achieving the same results as the SF-36 (Failde et al., 2009). However, some studies carried out on patients after an acute myocardial infarction have found that the results of the SF-12 may not detect significant differences between the domains of QL affected by the disease, although this has been improved in version 2 of the questionnaire, in which it is possible to assess the same 8 dimensions included in the SF-36, and the summary dimensions (physical and mental). In patients with a recent myocardial infarction, the SF-36 has also been shown to be more sensitive at detecting improvements in HRQL after active intervention (Thompson & Yu, 2003).

Another of the most widely-used instruments for assessing HRQL is the EuroQol (EQ-5D). Like the SF-36, this questionnaire can be applied to a wide range of diseases. It provides a simple descriptive profile and a single index value for health status. The EQ-5D has three parts. The first enables the respondent to define their health status in accordance with the EQ-5D multi-attribute scale and is composed of 5 dimensions (mobility, self-care, usual activities, pain/discomfort, and anxiety/depression). Each of these has 3 levels of severity, where a higher score corresponds with a worse health status. The second part is a visual analogical scale ranging from 0 (worst health status imaginable) to 100 (best health status imaginable). The third part gathers other anonymous data to provide a demographic characterization of the group studied (Williams, 1990). This questionnaire has been validated among populations with heart disease and has been shown to possess good psychometric characteristics when compared with other previously-validated generic tools used with these populations (Ellis et al., 2005; Nowels et al., 2005).

In a recently published review it was revealed that the Stratification of EQ-5D index scores by disease severity decreased from a mean of 0.78 (SD 0.18) to 0.51 (SD 0.21) for mild to severe disease in heart failure patients and from 0.80 (SD 0.05) to 0.45 (SD 0.22) for mild to severe disease in angina patients (Dyer et al., 2010).

Unlike the generic tools mentioned previously, specific instruments which have been developed for one particular disease assess the effect that the disease, in this case coronary artery disease, has on the different dimensions of HRQL. This improves their sensitivity at detecting the clinical changes in the symptoms that most frequently affect individuals. They are also less likely to have a floor or ceiling effect, with high percentages of patients with minimum or maximum scores in the survey not being observed. On the other hand, a drawback with regard to generic tools is that they do not allow for comparisons between groups of patients with different diseases (Thompson & Yu, 2003).

In the field of cardiology, several scales have been developed that are specifically designed to assess the HRQL of patients with angina, myocardial infarction or heart failure. Among the specific tools for assessing the HRQL of patients with angina, one of the most widely used is the Seattle Angina Questionnaire (SAQ) (Spertus et al., 1995). This questionnaire comprises 19 items that quantify 5 relevant clinical domains for coronary disease: physical limitations of the patient due to angina; angina frequency (assessing the frequency of symptoms and the use of medication); angina stability (measuring recent changes in symptoms); treatment satisfaction (assessing general satisfaction, and satisfaction with the treatment and the doctor's explanations); and disease perception (measures the effect of angina on quality of life). All the items use 5 or 6 point descriptive scales. The global score is calculated by adding the score of the items within each dimension and transforming them to a scale of 0 to 100, where the highest scores show better functioning (less physical limitations, less angina, and better quality of life). Regarding its psychometric properties, it appears to have good validity characteristics (Dougherty et al., 1998) and each domain and dimension of the SAQ has been independently validated, proving to be both reliable and sensitive to clinical changes. Furthermore, several studies show that the questionnaire correlates well with variables that influence the disease such as age and gender (Cepeda-Valery et al., 2011).

The Angina Pectoris Quality of Life Questionnaire (APQLQ) (Marquis et al., 1995a) developed in France is another specific instrument for use with coronary patients. It comprises 22 items grouped into 4 domains: physical activity, somatic symptoms, emotional distress, and life satisfaction. The correlations with the SF-36 dimensions were consistent with what was expected. Its reliability, concurrent and clinical validity allowed its use in clinical trials. The distribution of the scores of the APQLQ according to the clinical severity of Angina Pectoris (AP) was as hypothesized: the more severe the AP, the more impaired the Quality of Life (Marquis et al., 1995b).

As with patients with Angina Pectoris, it is important to assess the HRQL of patients who have suffered a myocardial infarction as it provides a holistic examination of the results of treatment and does not only focus on the physical component. A few years ago, a group from the UK developed and validated a specific instrument for this kind of patients (Thompson & Roebuck, 2001) which is commonly used nowadays. Known as the Myocardial Infarction Dimensional Assessment Scale (MIDAS), this tool comprises a 35-item self-administered questionnaire covering seven dimensions related to health status (physical activity, insecurity, emotional reaction, dependency, diet, concerns over medications and side effects). The MIDAS showed excellent content validity, good criterion validity with good internal consistency, and sensitivity to change. Compared with other already validated questionnaires such as the SF-36, this tool showed a good correlation in most of the variables.

The MacNew Heart Disease Health-related Quality of Life instrument (MacNew) is a self-administered scale, a modified version of the original Quality of life after Myocardial Infarction Questionnaire (QLMI) (Oldridge et al., 1991). It is designed to assess the effect of coronary heart disease and its treatment (initially myocardial infarction, then extended to include angina pectoris) on everyday activities, and physical, emotional and social functioning. It comprises 27 items grouped into 3 dimensions: physical limitations, emotional functioning and social functioning. This new version of the instrument has good psychometric properties of validity, reliability and sensitivity to change, and is of proven use with patients after myocardial infarction. (Höfer et al., 2004).

Finally, it should be noted that it is sometimes difficult to establish an accurate diagnosis of coronary disease. It could begin with angina and proceed to a myocardial infarctus or heart failure. In these cases the Cardiovascular Limitations and Symptoms Profile (CLASP) can be extremely useful for assessing HRQL. The main advantage of this instrument is that it makes it possible to assess HRQL through different clinical situations, and is especially useful to check whether symptoms worsen or new ones develop. The CLASP, with 37 items grouped into 9 different dimensions (4 related to symptomatology and 5 with physical limations), can identify where there are difficulties for a patient, their importance, and the best treatment in each case. This instrument has been shown to be a reliable, valid and sensitive measure of health-related quality of life in patients with chronic stable angina (Lewin et al., 2002). However, further research is required before it can be recommended for routine use in clinical practice.

2.3 Factors related to Health Related Quality of Life in coronary patients

As mentioned above, quality of life measures have gained increasing attention as outcome variables in studies of cardiovascular disease in addition to the objective measures of cardiovascular status (Kaplan, 1988). Also, one main goal of coronary artery by-pass grafting (CABG) after a coronary event is to relieve angina and thereby to improve physical activity. This has consequences for work, leisure, mood, social, sexual activities, and also over quality of life (Duits et al., 1997).

Several studies carried out in coronary patients after CABG have shown some improvements in physical, social and sexual functioning (Stanton et al., 1984) as well as working status (Folks et al., 1986) 6 months after the intervention; and decreased anxiety, depression, fatigue, and sleep problems have been also reported at this time in this patients (Jenkins et al., 1983). On the other hand, some authors have found improvements in performance of everyday activities, mental state, and family life one year post-surgery (Mayou & Bryant, 1987) with general health status becoming very similar with those from a normal population (Caine et al., 1991).

Cross-sectional studies carried out in patients with angina and myocardial infarctus have shown that the SF-36 health questionnaire is a valid and reliable instrument for detecting differences between groups of coronary patients defined by age, gender, socio-economic status, and clinical condition (Hemingway et al., 1997a, 1997b), and that it is a useful tool in patients with stable angina (Charlier et al., 1997; Permanyer-Miralda et al., 1991). Likewise, it has been demonstrated using this tool that coronary patients have worse HRQL than general population (Figure 1) (Soto Torres et al., 2004); also being female, being older, not being married, having a history of the disease and having a mental illness are factors affecting the QoL of these patients. Moreover, patients with unstable angina have been found to have a worse QoL than those who suffered an AMI (Soto et al., 2005).

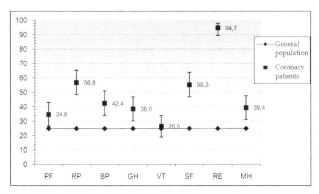

Fig. 1. Percentage of coronary patients below the 25th percentile of the general population, with the corresponding 95% confidence intervals. PF: Physical Functioning. RP: Role Physical . BP: Bodily Pain. GH: General Health. VT: Vitality. SF: Social Functioning. RE: Role Emotional. MH: Mental Health.

Despite this, and the fact that HRQL is a useful indicator of results in coronary patients who undergo revascularization, there are not many follow-up studies that analyse the evolution of HRQL and assess the effect of clinical and socio-demographic variables on the different clinical forms of the disease (angina vs myocardial infarction), even though it would be advisable to identify predictive factors to improve the development of interventions for subjects at risk (Bryant & Mayou, 1989).

Failde et al., in a study carried out in patients affected by both unstable angina and myocardial infarction (Failde & Soto, 2006), observed a significant decrease at 3 months of follow-up in the physical functioning, general health, and vitality dimensions, and the physical component summary (PCS) of the SF-36 health questionnaire. Also, the same authors have recently shown that HRQL is significantly impaired in coronary patients just after hospital discharge, with improvements being produced at 6 months, especially in the dimensions of the SF-36 related to bodily pain, general health, vitality, and the physical component summary (PCS) (Table 2) (data not yet published). In the same way, Höfer et al. (Höfer et al., 2006) also observed a significant positive change over time for the physical component summary dimension (PCS) of the SF-36, but not for the mental component summary dimension (MCS). However, other authors (Elliott et al., 2003; Mancuso et al., 2000; Wells et al., 1989) have shown that the SF-36 MCS is a good indicator of depression in general and diseased populations and Tavella et al. (Tavella et al., 2010) have even established a threshold score on the SF-36 MCS that would categorise a population with cardiac disease into depressed and non-depressed patients.

In the analysis of the factors affecting the change of HRQL in coronary patients Failde et al. observed that revascularization, age, and the interaction between a previous history of Coronary Heart Disease (CHD) and the presence of one or more risk factors affected negatively the physical component summary of the SF-36 at 3 months of follow-up (Failde & Soto, 2006). Also, studying the factors related to HRQL at 6 months, the same authors observed that depression, assessed by the 28-item General Health Questionnaire, a previous history of Coronary Heart Disease (CHD), or the associated comorbidity had a negative effect on quality of life, with a worse clinical course in these patients when compared with those without these conditions.

	BASELINE N=175		3 MONTHS N=80		6 MONTHS N=47		p	p^1	p^2	Partial eta-squared
	Mean	SD	Mean	SD	Mean	SD				
PF	61.9	28.9	66.9	27.9	63.4	30.0	0.67	0.41	1.00	0.004
RP	53.2	48.5	70.7	41.8	72.8	42.6	0.04	0.14	0.13	0.085
BP	56.6	29.1	60.5	27.4	67.5	25.6	0.01	0.89	0.02	0.148
GH	57.9	19.9	65.7	19.5	65.4	18.6	0.01	0.00	0.01	0.155
VT	59.7	30.7	69.7	27.4	68.3	26.7	0.04	0.09	0.13	0.084
SF	74.5	34.4	83.7	28.3	83.5	30.2	0.09	0.24	0.28	0.060
RE	76.6	39.8	80.1	39.1	84.4	36.0	0.27	1.00	0.82	0.026
MH	64.9	18.4	67.8	21.5	67.7	17.9	0.19	0.48	0.58	0.036
PCS	40.6	12.1	44.4	9.7	44.5	11.4	0.01	0.03	0.04	0.122
MCS	47.9	10.9	49.8	11.9	50.2	9.7	0.15	0.75	0.46	0.043

Table 2. Mean (SD) of SF-36 dimensions at baseline and during follow-up. PF: physical functioning; RP: role physical; BP: body pain; GH: general health. VT: vitality; SF: social functioning; RE: role emotional; MH: mental health; PCS: physical component summary; MCS: mental component summary. ANOVA test with the Bonferroni test for post hoc comparisons. p: comparison at three times; p^1: comparison between baseline and 3 months; p^2: comparison between baseline and 6 months. No significant differences were observed between 3 months and 6 months. Partial eta-squared: as an effect size estimator that describes the proportion of variability that exists in each dimension of the SF-36 during the follow-up. (0.01: Small; 0.06: Medium; 0.14: Large)

This results are in agreement with Ormel et al. (Ormel et al., 2007) and Höfer et al. (Höfer et al., 2005) who found that depression and anxiety are the most significant factors influencing HRQL in patients with heart disease, and with McBurney et al. (McBurney et al., 2002), who observed that the presence of other illnesses had a negative effect on the PCS-12 seven months after an AMI, and that having more comorbidity tends to lower HRQL in all dimensions.

Dickens et al. (Dickens et al., 2011) in a prospective cohort study conducted to investigate the impact of depression on subsequent HRQL in subjects with CHD, identified a number of cognitive targets for psychological interventions in these patients, namely a perceived tendency to avoid physical activity, increased somatic awareness, perceived symptom burden, and emotional impact of heart disease. In the Dickens´ study, when the results are controlled for demographic and medical variables, depression was associated with a subsequent worse score in the physical component summary of the SF-36, but when anxiety, awareness of somatic symptoms, and negative illness perceptions were added to the regression model, depression no longer continued to be a significant independent factor. Maladaptive cardiac related health behaviour, like a high-fat diet, no regular exercise, being stressed or smoking, among others, were not related to the SF-36 physical component summary, so could not mediate the relationship between depression and the physical component summary (Baron & Kenny, 1986).

The associations between HRQL and patients' age, gender and whether or not they have undergone revascularization have been constantly studied, but the results are still inconclusive. Older age has been found to be associated with better postoperative mental health in these patients (Rumsfeld et al., 2004). However, Miller and Grindel (Miller & Grindel, 2001) reported that both preoperative health status and physiological, psychological and social recovery of older and younger patients were similar after CABG.

It has also been observed (Duenas et al., 2011) that being female negatively affects HRQL, and most studies suggest that women do not cope as well physically and psychosocially as men. However, it remains unclear why gender-related differences in HRQL exist among coronary patients (Van Jaarsveld et al., 2002).

Several authors have shown that women with coronary disease report significantly poorer physical functioning and mental health than men (Dixon et al., 2000; Ghali et al., 2002; Norris et al., 2004; Shumaker et al., 1997; Wiklund et al., 1993) and that this effect is mediated in some cases by its interaction with other variables such as a history of the illness or the mental health status. Norris et al. (Norris et al., 2007) also showed that, after adjusting for clinical and psychosocial covariables, the physical HRQL differences between men and women did not disappear. In addition, others authors have shown that smoking, regular alcohol consumption, and overweight are the most common risk factors for worse HRQL in men, while psychological distress, role pressure, and less strenuous exercise are more characteristic of women (Verbrugge, 1989).

Prior data suggest that women with cardiac disease are more likely than men to be confronted with continuing demands in the home environment, and may be more likely to neglect health care needs (Emery et al., 2004). Thus, Emery et al. hypothesized that quality of life would be more strongly associated with social support among women than among men.

Recently, a study analysing gender differences in the outcome of HRQL in coronary patients (Duenas et al., 2011), found that baseline scores in the SF-36 were lower among women. Also, the men had a better clinical course at 6 months in most of the physical dimensions, and social functioning. Meanwhile, the women only improved in the physical component summary, role physical and social functioning. This is partly in accordance with the results obtained by Emery and co-workers, (Emery et al., 2004) which show that men and women have increased scores in physical health over time, but women have significantly lower scores in physical dimensions across all assessments. Likewise, Duenas et al reported that the variables most strongly associated with an unfavourable evolution of HRQL in men were deterioration in mental health and angina frequency. Likewise, mental health was also a determining factor in the evolution of women's quality of life, although this was also affected by other variables, such as a clinical history of the disease, angina frequency and undergoing revascularization during the follow-up (Duenas et al., 2011). In this respect, it is worth highlighting that revascularization was carried out earlier in the men, which may have conditioned the worse clinical course observed in the women, who suffered higher frequencies of angina and rehospitalisation during follow-up. Hemingway et al. (Hemingway et al., 2006) and Aguado-Romero and co-workers (Aguado-Romeo et al., 2006) detail the tendency to operate less on women with coronary disease than on men, although the latter try to justify these differences by referring to limitations in their data.

Thus, other factors, such as the perception that women have a lower pre-test probability of infarction, may influence the clinician's discharge decision (Willingham & Kilpatrick, 2005) and the different attitude to treatment among women may be another determining factor.

On the other hand, several studies have found that the evolution of HRQL differs between men and women after coronary surgery. Phillips et al. (Phillips Bute et al., 2003) concluded that women do not obtain the same benefit from CABG surgery as men, and that the difference cannot be attributed to preoperative divergence. One possible explanation for this is that women's compromised HRQL is less related to cardiac health than men's, with other environmental and/or personality variables related to quality of life affecting women more than men (Phillips Bute et al., 2003).

Finally, another important factor related to the HRQL of patients with coronary disease is familial support (Rantanen et al., 2008). Patients who receive only limited support from significant others have been reported to suffer more anxiety and depressive symptoms than patients who receive more (Okkonen & Vanhanen, 2006) and patients have reported a better HRQL than their peers when they have received much social support (Bosworth et al., 2000; Woloshin et al., 1997; Yates, 1995).

Research results explaining the relationship between HRQL for CABG patients and social support have been contradictory, however, and social support received from family members and other significant others has shown no significant association with patients' functional capacity (Barry et al., 2006; Hamalainen et al., 2000). However, ready access to concrete support, does seem to correlate with positive changes in mental health (Barry et al., 2006).

3. Conclusion

HRQL is an essential primary outcome measure in coronary patients. Several instruments, both generic and specific, have proven to be of use for its assessment, showing differences between different groups of patients affected by the disease. In addition, several variables related to patients' clinical evolution and history of the disease have been shown to be related to HRQL, with worse results among women, subjects with previous history of CHD, and those with another comorbidity.

Mental health has been shown to significantly affect the evolution of HRQL in these patients. However, the systematic assessment of this variable is not common. Therefore, more emphasis needs to be placed on the systematic assessment of mental status specially in women, and the development of patient-oriented programs which reduce mental disturbances, and on providing increased social support for this at-risk population in particular.

4. References

Aguado-Romeo, M.J., Marquez-Calderon, S., Buzon-Barrera, M.L. & por los investigadores del grupo VPM-IRYSS-Andalucia. (2006). Differences between women's and men's access to interventional cardiovascular procedures at public hospitals in Andalusia (Spain). *Revista espanola de cardiologia*, Vol.59, No.8, (August 2006), pp. 785-793, ISSN 0300-8932; 0300-8932

Alonso, J., Ferrer, M., Gandek, B., Ware Jr., J.E., Aaronson, N.K., Mosconi, P., Rasmussen, N.K., Bullinger, M., Fukuhara, S., Kaasa, S. & Leplège, A. (2004). Health-related quality of life associated with chronic conditions in eight countries: Results from the International Quality of Life Assessment (IQOLA) Project. *Quality of Life Research*, Vol.13, No.2, (March 2004), pp. 283-298

Asadi-Lari, M., Packham, C. & Gray, D. (2003). Is quality of life measurement likely to be a proxy for health needs assessment in patients with coronary artery disease? *Health and Quality of Life Outcomes*, Vol.1, No.50, (October 2003), pp. 1-8

Baron, R.M. & Kenny, D.A. (1986). The moderator-mediator variable distinction in social psychological research: conceptual, strategic, and statistical considerations. *Journal of personality and social psychology*, Vol.51, No.6, (December 1986), pp. 1173-1182, ISSN 0022-3514; 0022-3514

Barry, L.C., Kasl, S.V., Lichtman, J., Vaccarino, V. & Krumholz, H.M. (2006). Social support and change in health-related quality of life 6 months after coronary artery bypass grafting. *Journal of psychosomatic research*, Vol.60, No.2, (February 2006), pp. 185-193, ISSN 0022-3999; 0022-3999

Bosworth, H.B., Siegler, I.C., Olsen, M.K., Brummett, B.H., Barefoot, J.C., Williams, R.B., Clapp-Channing, N.E. & Mark, D.B. (2000). Social support and quality of life in patients with coronary artery disease. *Quality of life research : an international journal of quality of life aspects of treatment, care and rehabilitation*, Vol.9, No.7, (November 2000), pp. 829-839, ISSN 0962-9343; 0962-9343

Brown, N., Melville, M., Gray, D., Young, T., Munro, J., Skene, A.M. & Hampton, J.R. (1999). Quality of life four years after acute myocardial infarction: Short form 36 scores compared with a normal population. *Heart*, Vol.81, (November 1999), pp. 352-358

Bryant, B. & Mayou, R. (1989). Prediction of outcome after coronary artery surgery. *Journal of psychosomatic research*, Vol.33, No.4, (January 1989), pp. 419-427, ISSN 0022-3999; 0022-3999

Caine, N., Harrison, S.C., Sharples, L.D. & Wallwork, J. (1991). Prospective study of quality of life before and after coronary artery bypass grafting. *BMJ (Clinical research ed.)*, Vol.302, No.6775, (March 1991), pp. 511-516, ISSN 0959-8138; 0959-535X

Casas Anguita, J., Ramon Repullo Labrador, J. & Pereira Candel, J. (2001). Measurements of quality of life related with health. Basic concepts and cultural adaptation. *Medicina clinica*, Vol.116, No.20, (June 2001), pp. 789-796, ISSN 0025-7753; 0025-7753

Cepeda-Valery, B., Cheong, A.P., Lee, A. & Yan, B.P. (2011). Measuring health related quality of life in coronary heart disease: The importance of feeling well. *International journal of cardiology*, Vol.149, No.1, (May 2011), pp. 4-9

Charlier, L., Dutrannois, J. & Kaufman, L. (1997). The SF-36 questionnaire: a convenient way to assess quality of life in angina pectoris patients. *Acta Cardiologica*, Vol.52, No.3, pp. 247-260, ISSN 0001-5385; 0001-5385

Dickens, C., Cherrington, A., McGowan, L. & Taylor, C.B. (2011). Do Cognitive and Behavioral Factors Mediate the Impact of Depression on Medical Outcomes in

People with Coronary Heart Disease? *Journal of cardiopulmonary rehabilitation and prevention*, Vol.31, No.2, (March 2011), pp. 105-110, ISSN 1932-751X; 1932-7501

Dixon, T., Lim, L.L., Powell, H. & Fisher, J.D. (2000). Psychosocial experiences of cardiac patients in early recovery: a community-based study. *Journal of advanced nursing*, Vol.31, No.6, (June 2000), pp. 1368-1375, ISSN 0309-2402; 0309-2402

Dougherty, C.M., Dewhurst, T., Nichol, W.P. & Spertus, J. (1998). Comparison of three quality of life instruments in stable angina pectoris: Seattle Angina Questionnaire, Short Form Health Survey (SF-36), and Quality of Life Index-Cardiac Version III. *Journal of clinical epidemiology*, Vol.51, No.7, (July 1998), pp. 569-575, ISSN 0895-4356; 0895-4356

Duenas, M., Ramirez, C., Arana, R. & Failde, I. (2011). Gender differences and determinants of health related quality of life in coronary patients: a follow-up study. *BMC cardiovascular disorders*, Vol.11, (May 2011), pp. 24, ISSN 1471-2261; 1471-2261

Duits, A.A., Boeke, S., Taams, M.A., Passchier, J. & Erdman, R.A. (1997). Prediction of quality of life after coronary artery bypass graft surgery: a review and evaluation of multiple, recent studies. *Psychosomatic medicine*, Vol.59, No.3, (June 1997), pp. 257-268, ISSN 0033-3174; 0033-3174

Dyer, M.T.D., Goldsmith, K.A., Sharples, L.S. & Buxton, M.J. (2010). A review of health utilities using the EQ-5D in studies of cardiovascular disease. *Health and Quality of Life Outcomes*, Vol.8, No.13, (January 2010), pp. 1-12

Elliott, T.E., Renier, C.M. & Palcher, J.A. (2003). Chronic pain, depression, and quality of life: correlations and predictive value of the SF-36. *Pain medicine*, Vol.4, No.4, (December 2003), pp. 331-339, ISSN 1526-2375; 1526-2375

Ellis, J.J., Eagle, K.A., Kline-Rogers, E.M. & Erickson, S.R. (2005). Validation of the EQ-5D in patients with a history of acute coronary syndrome. *Current medical research and opinion*, Vol.21, No.8, (August 2005), pp. 1209-1216

Emery, C.F., Frid, D.J., Engebretson, T.O., Alonzo, A.A., Fish, A., Ferketich, A.K., Reynolds, N.R., Dujardin, J.P., Homan, J.E. & Stern, S.L. (2004). Gender differences in quality of life among cardiac patients. *Psychosomatic medicine*, Vol.66, No.2, (April 2004), pp. 190-197, ISSN 1534-7796; 0033-3174

Failde, I., Medina, P., Ramírez, C. & Arana, R. (2009). Assessing health-related quality of life among coronary patients: SF-36 vs SF-12. *Public health*, Vol.123, No.9, (September 2009), pp. 615-617

Failde, I. & Ramos, I. (2000). Validity and reliability of the SF-36 Health Survey Questionnaire in patients with coronary artery disease. *Journal of clinical epidemiology*, Vol.53, No.4, (April 2000), pp. 359-365

Failde, I.I. & Soto, M.M. (2006). Changes in Health Related Quality of Life 3 months after an acute coronary syndrome. *BMC public health*, Vol.6, (Jan 27), pp. 18, ISSN 1471-2458; 1471-2458

Fayers, P.M. & Machin, D. (2007). *Quality of life: The assessment, analysis and interpretationof patient-reported outcomes* (2), Wiley, ISBN 13 978-0-470-02450-8, Chichester, England

Folks, D.G., Blake, D.J., Fleece, L., Sokol, R.S. & Freeman, A.M.,3rd. (1986). Quality of life six months after coronary artery bypass surgery: a preliminary report. *Southern medical journal*, Vol.79, No.4, (April 1986), pp. 397-399, ISSN 0038-4348; 0038-4348

Gandek, B., Ware, J.E., Aaronson, N.K., Apolone, G., Bjorner, J.B., Brazier, J.E., Bullinger, M., Kaasa, S., Leplege, A., Prieto, L. & Sullivan, M. (1998). Cross-validation of item selection and scoring for the SF-12 Health Survey in nine countries: Results from the IQOLA Project. *Journal of clinical epidemiology*, Vol.51, No.11, (November 1998), pp. 1171-1178

Ghali, W.A., Faris, P.D., Galbraith, P.D., Norris, C.M., Curtis, M.J., Saunders, L.D., Dzavik, V., Mitchell, L.B., Knudtson, M.L. & Alberta Provincial Project for Outcome Assessment in Coronary Heart Disease (APPROACH) Investigators. (2002). Sex differences in access to coronary revascularization after cardiac catheterization: importance of detailed clinical data. *Annals of Internal Medicine*, Vol.136, No.10, (May 2002), pp. 723-732, ISSN 1539-3704; 0003-4819

Group, World Health Organization Quality of Life (WHOQOL). (1993). Study protocol for the World Health Organization project to develop a Quality of Life. *Quality of Life Research*, Vol.2, No.2, (April 1993), pp. 153-159, ISSN 0962-9343 (Print) 0962-9343 (Linking)

Hamalainen, H., Smith, R., Puukka, P., Lind, J., Kallio, V., Kuttila, K. & Ronnemaa, T. (2000). Social support and physical and psychological recovery one year after myocardial infarction or coronary artery bypass surgery. *Scandinavian Journal of Public Health*, Vol.28, No.1, (March 2000), pp. 62-70, ISSN 1403-4948; 1403-4948

Hawkes, A.L. & Mortensen, O.S. (2006). Up to one third of individual cardiac patients have a decline in quality of life post-intervention. *Scandinavian Cardiovascular Journal*, Vol.40, No.4, (August 2006), pp. 214-218

Hemingway, H., McCallum, A., Shipley, M., Manderbacka, K., Martikainen, P. & Keskimaki, I. (2006). Incidence and prognostic implications of stable angina pectoris among women and men. *JAMA : the journal of the American Medical Association*, Vol.295, No.12, (March 2006), pp. 1404-1411, ISSN 1538-3598; 0098-7484

Hemingway, H., Nicholson, A., Stafford, M., Roberts, R. & Marmot, M. (1997a). The impact of socioeconomic status on health functioning as assessed by the SF-36 questionnaire: the Whitehall II Study. *American Journal of Public Health*, Vol.87, No.9, (September 1997), pp. 1484-1490, ISSN 0090-0036 (Print) 0090-0036 (Linking)

Hemingway, H., Stafford, M., Stansfeld, S., Shipley, M. & Marmot, M. (1997b). Is the SF-36 a valid measure of change in population health? Results from the Whitehall II Study. *BMJ (Clinical research ed.)*, Vol.315, No.7118, (November 1997), pp. 1273-1279, ISSN 0959-8138; 0959-535X

Höfer, S., Doering, S., Rumpold, G., Oldridge, N. & Benzer, W. (2006). Determinants of health-related quality of life in patients with coronary artery disease. *European Journal of Cardiovascular Prevention & Rehabilitation*, Vol.13, No.3, (June 2006), pp. 398-406, ISSN 1741-8267

Höfer, S., Benzer, W., Alber, H., Ruttmann, E., Kopp, M., Schüssler, G. & Doering, S. (2005). Determinants of health-related quality of life in coronary artery disease patients: A prospective study generating a structural equation model. *Psychosomatics*, Vol.46, No.3, (June 2005), pp. 212-223

Höfer, S., Lim, L., Guyatt, G. & Oldridge, N. (2004). The MacNew Heart Disease Health-related Quality of Life instrument: A summary. *Health and Quality of Life Outcomes*, Vol.2, No.3, (January 2004), pp. 1-8

Jenkins, C.D., Stanton, B.A., Savageau, J.A., Denlinger, P. & Klein, M.D. (1983). Coronary artery bypass surgery. Physical, psychological, social, and economic outcomes six months later. *JAMA : the journal of the American Medical Association*, Vol.250, No.6, (August 1983), pp. 782-788, ISSN 0098-7484; 0098-7484

Kaplan, R.M. (1988). Health-related quality of life in cardiovascular disease. *Journal of consulting and clinical psychology*, Vol.56, No.3, (June 1988), pp. 382-392, ISSN 0022-006X; 0022-006X

Lewin, R.J.P., Thompson, D.R., Martin, C.R., Stuckey, N., Devlen, J., Michaelson, S. & Maguire, P. (2002). Validation of the cardiovascular limitations and symptoms profile (CLASP) in chronic stable angina. *Journal of cardiopulmonary rehabilitation,* Vol.22, No.3, (June 2002), pp. 184-191

Mancuso, C.A., Peterson, M.G. & Charlson, M.E. (2000). Effects of depressive symptoms on health-related quality of life in asthma patients. *Journal of general internal medicine,* Vol.15, No.5, (May 2000), pp. 301-310, ISSN 0884-8734; 0884-8734

Marquis, P., Fayol, C. & Joire, J.E. (1995a). Clinical validation of a quality of life questionnaire in angina pectoris patients. *European heart journal,* Vol.16, No.11, (November 1995), pp. 1554-1560, ISSN 0195-668X; 0195-668X

Marquis, P., Fayol, C., Joire, J.E. & Leplege, A. (1995b). Psychometric properties of a specific quality of life questionnaire in angina pectoris patients. *Quality of life research : an international journal of quality of life aspects of treatment, care and rehabilitation,* Vol.4, No.6, (December 1995), pp. 540-546, ISSN 0962-9343; 0962-9343

Mayou, R. & Bryant, B. (1987). Quality of life after coronary artery surgery. *The Quarterly journal of medicine,* Vol.62, No.239, (March 1987), pp. 239-248, ISSN 0033-5622; 0033-5622

McBurney, C.R., Eagle, K.A., Kline-Rogers, E.M., Cooper, J.V., Mani, O.C.M., Smith, D.E. & Erickson, S.R. (2002). Health-related quality of life in patients 7 months after a myocardial infarction: Factors affecting the short form-12. *Pharmacotherapy,* Vol.22, No.12, (December 2002), pp. 1616-1622

McDowell, I. & Newell, C. (1996). *Measuring Health: A Guide to Rating Scales and Questionnaires* (2), Oxford University Press, ISBN 0-19-510371-8, New York, USA

Miller, K.H. & Grindel, C.G. (2001). Recovery from coronary artery bypass surgery: age-related outcomes. *Outcomes management for nursing practice,* Vol.5, No.3, (September 2001), pp. 127-133, ISSN 1093-1783; 1093-1783

Norris, C.M., Hegadoren, K. & Pilote, L. (2007). Depression symptoms have a greater impact on the 1-year health-related quality of life outcomes of women post-myocardial infarction compared to men. *European Journal of Cardiovascular Nursing,* Vol.6, No.2, (June 2007), pp. 92-98, ISSN 1474-5151 (Print) 1474-5151 (Linking)

Norris, C.M., Ghali, W.A., Galbraith, P.D., Graham, M.M., Jensen, L.A., Knudtson, M.L. & APPROACH Investigators. (2004). Women with coronary artery disease report worse health-related quality of life outcomes compared to men. *Health and quality of life outcomes,* Vol.2, (May 2004), pp. 21, ISSN 1477-7525; 1477-7525

Nowels, D., McGloin, J., Westfall, J.M. & Holcomb, S. (2005). Validation of the EQ-5D quality of life instrument in patients after myocardial infarction. *Quality of Life Research,* Vol.14, No.1, (February 2005), pp. 95-105

Okkonen, E. & Vanhanen, H. (2006). Family support, living alone, and subjective health of a patient in connection with a coronary artery bypass surgery. *Heart & lung : the journal of critical care,* Vol.35, No.4, (August 2006), pp. 234-244, ISSN 0147-9563; 0147-9563

Oldridge, N., Guyatt, G., Jones, N., Crowe, J., Singer, J., Feeny, D., McKelvie, R., Runions, J., Streiner, D. & Torrance, G. (1991). Effects on quality of life with comprehensive rehabilitation after acute myocardial infarction. *The American Journal of Cardiology,* Vol.67, No.13, (May 1991), pp. 1084-1089, ISSN 0002-9149; 0002-9149

Ormel, J., Von Korff, M., Burger, H., Scott, K., Demyttenaere, K., Huang, Y.Q., Posada-Villa, J., Pierre Lepine, J., Angermeyer, M.C., Levinson, D., de Girolamo, G., Kawakami, N., Karam, E., Medina-Mora, M.E., Gureje, O., Williams, D., Haro, J.M., Bromet,

E.J., Alonso, J. & Kessler, R. (2007). Mental disorders among persons with heart disease - results from World Mental Health surveys. *General hospital psychiatry*, Vol.29, No.4, (August 2007), pp. 325-334, ISSN 0163-8343 (Print) 0163-8343 (Linking)

Permanyer-Miralda, G., Alonso, J., Anto, J.M., Alijarde-Guimera, M. & Soler-Soler, J. (1991). Comparison of perceived health status and conventional functional evaluation in stable patients with coronary artery disease. *Journal of clinical epidemiology*, Vol.44, No.8, pp. 779-786, ISSN 0895-4356; 0895-4356

Phillips Bute, B., Mathew, J., Blumenthal, J.A., Welsh-Bohmer, K., White, W.D., Mark, D., Landolfo, K. & Newman, M.F. (2003). Female gender is associated with impaired quality of life 1 year after coronary artery bypass surgery. *Psychosomatic medicine*, Vol.65, No.6, (December 2003), pp. 944-951, ISSN 1534-7796; 0033-3174

Rantanen, A., Kaunonen, M., Sintonen, H., Koivisto, A.M., Astedt-Kurki, P. & Tarkka, M.T. (2008). Factors associated with health-related quality of life in patients and significant others one month after coronary artery bypass grafting. *Journal of Clinical Nursing*, Vol.17, No.13, (July 2008), pp. 1742-1753, ISSN 1365-2702; 0962-1067

Rumsfeld, J.S., Ho, P.M., Magid, D.J., McCarthy, M.,Jr, Shroyer, A.L., MaWhinney, S., Grover, F.L. & Hammermeister, K.E. (2004). Predictors of health-related quality of life after coronary artery bypass surgery. *The Annals of Thoracic Surgery*, Vol.77, No.5, (May 2004), pp. 1508-1513, ISSN 0003-4975; 0003-4975

Shumaker, S.A. & Berzon, R.A. (1995). *The International assessement of health related quality of life: Theory, Translation, Measurement and Analysis* (1), Rapid Communications of Oxford Ltd., ISBN 1-85650-004-7, New York, USA

Shumaker, S.A., Brooks, M.M., Schron, E.B., Hale, C., Kellen, J.C., Inkster, M., Wimbush, F.B., Wiklund, I. & Morris, M. (1997). Gender differences in health-related quality of life among postmyocardial infarction patients: brief report. CAST Investigators. Cardiac Arrhythmia Suppression Trials. *Women's health (Hillsdale, N.J.)*, Vol.3, No.1, (Spring 1997), pp. 53-60, ISSN 1077-2928; 1077-2928

Soto Torres, M., Marquez Calderon, S., Ramos Diaz, I., Barba Chacon, A., Lopez Fernandez, F. & Failde Martinez, I. (2004). Health-related quality of life in coronary heart disease compared to norms in Spanish population. *Quality of life research : an international journal of quality of life aspects of treatment, care and rehabilitation*, Vol.13, No.8, (October 2004), pp. 1401-1407, ISSN 0962-9343; 0962-9343

Soto, M., Failde, I., Marquez, S., Benitez, E., Ramos, I., Barba, A. & Lopez, F. (2005). Physical and mental component summaries score of the SF-36 in coronary patients. *Quality of life research : an international journal of quality of life aspects of treatment, care and rehabilitation*, Vol.14, No.3, (April 2005), pp. 759-768, ISSN 0962-9343; 0962-9343

Spertus, J.A., Winder, J.A., Dewhurst, T.A., Deyo, R.A., Prodzinski, J., McDonell, M. & Fihn, S.D. (1995). Development and evaluation of the Seattle Angina Questionnaire: A new functional status measure for coronary artery disease. *Journal of the American College of Cardiology*, Vol.25, No.2, (February 1995), pp. 333-341

Stanton, B.A., Jenkins, C.D., Savageau, J.A. & Thurer, R.L. (1984). Functional benefits following coronary artery bypass graft surgery. *The Annals of Thoracic Surgery*, Vol.37, No.4, (April 1984), pp. 286-290, ISSN 0003-4975; 0003-4975

Tavella, R., Air, T., Tucker, G., Adams, R., Beltrame, J.F. & Schrader, G. (2010). Using the Short Form-36 mental summary score as an indicator of depressive symptoms in patients with coronary heart disease. *Quality of life research : an international journal of quality of life aspects of treatment, care and rehabilitation*, Vol.19, No.8, (October 2010), pp. 1105-1113, ISSN 1573-2649; 0962-9343

Thompson, D.R. & Yu, C.-M. (2003). Quality of life in patients with coronary heart disease-I: Assessment tools. *Health and Quality of Life Outcomes*, Vol.1, No.42, (September 2003), pp. 1-5

Thompson, D.R. & Roebuck, A. (2001). The measurement of health-related quality of life in patients with coronary heart disease. *The Journal of cardiovascular nursing*, Vol.16, No.1, (October 2001), pp. 28-33

Urzúa M, A. (2010). Health related quality of life: Conceptual elements. *Revista Médica de Chile*, Vol.138, No.3, (March 2010), pp. 358-365

Van Jaarsveld, C., Sanderman, R., Ranchor, A., Ormel, J., van Veldhuisen, D. & Kempen, G. (2002). Gender-specific changes in quality of life following cardiovascular disease: a prospective study. *Journal of clinical epidemiology*, Vol.55, No.11, (November 2002), pp. 1105-1112, ISSN 0895-4356

Verbrugge, L.M. (1989). The twain meet: empirical explanations of sex differences in health and mortality. *Journal of health and social behavior*, Vol.30, No.3, (September 1989), pp. 282-304, ISSN 0022-1465; 0022-1465

Ware, J.E. (2000). SF-36 Health Survey update. *Spine*, Vol.25, No.24, (December 2000), pp. 3130-3139

Ware, J.E., Snow, K.K., Kosinski, M. & Gandek, B. (1993). *SF-36 Health Survey: Manual and Interpretation Guide* (1), ISBN 1891810006 (user's manual) 1891810065, Boston, USA

Wells, K.B., Stewart, A., Hays, R.D., Burnam, M.A., Rogers, W., Daniels, M., Berry, S., Greenfield, S. & Ware, J. (1989). The functioning and well-being of depressed patients. Results from the Medical Outcomes Study. *JAMA : the journal of the American Medical Association*, Vol.262, No.7, (August 1989), pp. 914-919, ISSN 0098-7484; 0098-7484

Wiklund, I., Herlitz, J., Johansson, S., Bengtson, A., Karlson, B.W. & Persson, N.G. (1993). Subjective symptoms and well-being differ in women and men after myocardial infarction. *European heart journal*, Vol.14, No.10, (October 1993), pp. 1315-1319, ISSN 0195-668X; 0195-668X

Williams, A. (1990). EuroQol - A new facility for the measurement of health-related quality of life. *Health Policy*, Vol.16, No.3, (December 1990), pp. 199-208

Willingham, S.A. & Kilpatrick, E.S. (2005). Evidence of gender bias when applying the new diagnostic criteria for myocardial infarction. *Heart (British Cardiac Society)*, Vol.91, No.2, (February 2005), pp. 237-238, ISSN 1468-201X; 1355-6037

Woloshin, S., Schwartz, L.M., Tosteson, A.N., Chang, C.H., Wright, B., Plohman, J. & Fisher, E.S. (1997). Perceived adequacy of tangible social support and health outcomes in patients with coronary artery disease. *Journal of general internal medicine*, Vol.12, No.10, (October 1997), pp. 613-618, ISSN 0884-8734; 0884-8734

Yates, B.C. (1995). The relationships among social support and short- and long-term recovery outcomes in men with coronary heart disease. *Research in nursing & health*, Vol.18, No.3, (June 1995), pp. 193-203, ISSN 0160-6891; 0160-6891

Yu, C.M., Li, L.S.W., Ho, H.H. & Lau, C.P. (2003). Long-term changes in exercise capacity, quality of life, body anthropometry, and lipid profiles after a cardiac rehabilitation program in obese patients with coronary heart disease. *The American Journal of Cardiology*, Vol.91, No.3, (February 2003), pp. 321-325

8

Effects of Dietary Fiber Intake on Cardiovascular Risk Factors

Sara Arranz[1,2], Alex Medina-Remón[2,3],
Rosa M. Lamuela-Raventós[2,3] and Ramón Estruch[1,2,*]
*[1]Department of Internal Medicine, Hospital Clinic,
Institut d'Investigacions Biomédiques August Pi i Sunyer (IDIBAPS),
University of Barcelona, Barcelona,
[2]CIBEROBN Fisiopatología de la Obesidad y la Nutrición and RETIC RD06/0045
Alimentación Saludable en la Prevención Primaria de Enfermedades Crónicas:
la Red Predimed, Instituto de Salud Carlos III,
[3]Nutrition and Food Science Department, CeRTA, INSA, Pharmacy School,
University of Barcelona, Barcelona,
Spain*

1. Introduction

A healthy dietary pattern is characterized by a high consumption of non-refined grains, legumes, nuts, fruits and vegetables; relatively high intake of total fat, mainly derived from olive oil; moderate to high intake of fish and poultry; dairy products (usually as yogurt or cheese) in small amounts; low consumption of red meat and meat products; and moderate alcohol intake, usually in the form of red wine with meals (Willett et al., 1995). Therefore, a high consumption of fiber-rich foods is one of the characteristic features of a healthy diet. Dietary fiber (DF) has received much attention in nutritional epidemiology. Observational studies have consistently shown that DF intake is associated with reduced cardiovascular risk, including ischemic heart disease (Rimm et al., 1996a; Todd et al., 1999; Liu et al., 2002; Mozaffarian et al., 2003a) and stroke (Ascherio et al., 1998; Oh et al., 2005; Salmeron et al., 1997)), and a lower risk of diabetes (Meyer et al., 2000; Liu, 2003b). Clinical trials have also suggested that DF supplementation has beneficial effects on risk factors, such as blood pressure, serum lipids, insulin sensitivity and diabetic metabolic control (Streppel et al., 2005b; Brown et al., 1999; Anderson et al., 2000; Chandalia et al., 2000a; Ludwig et al., 1999).

1.1 Dietary fiber: Definition and classification

The role of DF in nutrition and health is well established (Anderson et al., 1990; Englyst, Wiggins, & Cummings, 1982). Knowledge of the beneficial effects of high DF diets toward the prevention of cardiovascular diseases and several types of cancer, as well as the inclusion of DF supplements in slimming diets, has led to the development of a large and

---

* Corresponding Author

yielding market for DF-rich products. Commonly consumed products include traditional foods (meat, dairy products, breakfast cereals, biscuits, breads, etc.) enriched with different amounts of fiber from various sources, as well as dietary supplements including tablets, capsules, etc.

Traditionally, DF referred to plant cell wall components that are not digestible by human or other mammalian gastrointestinal tract enzymes, but that may be degraded by anaerobic bacteria in the colon (Trowell, 1972). The recognition that polysaccharides added to foods, notably hydrocolloids, could have similar effects to those originating from plant cell walls led to a redefinition of dietary fiber to include "polysaccharides and lignin that are not digested in the human small intestine" (Trowell et al., 1976).

Non-starch polysaccharides (NSP) are the main constituents of DF and include a host of different polymers, highly variable in terms of molecular size and structure, as well as in monomeric composition. The main classes of non-starch polysaccharides are cellulose, hemicelluloses, pectins, and other hydrocolloids. However, some authors (Saura-Calixto F, 1988) have reported that a significant part of the starch content in foods, namely, resistant starch (RS) escapes digestion and absorption in the human small intestine, along with other dietary substances not included in the DF definition such as protein, oligosaccharides and certain polyphenolic compounds (Cummings & Macfarlane, 1991; Bravo, 1998; Saura-Calixto F, 1988; Asp et al., 1996; Prosky, 1999).

In general, the definition and delimitation of DF has been much debated and related both to physiological considerations and to methods that can be used for DF analysis in foods (Asp, van Amelsvoort, & Hautvast, 1996; Englyst, H.N. and Hudson, G.J., 1996; Englyst & Englyst, 2005; Englyst, Liu, & Englyst, 2007; IoM (Institute of Medicine), 2005; FAO/WHO (Food and Agriculture Organization/World Health Organization), 1998; EFSA (European Food Safety Authority), 2007).

Therefore, DF constitutes a heterogeneous group of compounds. The components included in DF can be classified according to their chemical properties, such as their ability to dissolve in water (soluble vs. insoluble fibers), their ability to be fermented by the colonic microflora (fermentable vs. non-fermentable fibers), or their viscosity (viscous vs. non-viscous fibers) (Slavin et al., 2009) (see Figure 1).

Thus, cellulose is insoluble in water, whereas pectins and hydrocolloids, such as guar gum and mucilages, may form highly viscous water solutions. RS is insoluble and indigestible due to its physical form or enclosure in cellular structures, whereas resistant oligosaccharides are readily soluble in water but do not form viscous solutions. The terms "soluble" and "insoluble" DF have been used in the literature to differentiate between viscous, soluble types of fiber (e.g. pectins) and insoluble components such as cellulose. The distinction was mainly based on their different physiological effects. However, this differentiation is method-dependent, and solubility does not always predict physiological effects.

According to this controversy, the U.S. Food and Nutrition Board (FNB) defines "total DF" as the sum of "DF", consisting of non-digestible carbohydrates and lignin that are intrinsic and intact in plants, and "functional fiber", consisting of isolated, non-digestible carbohydrate components with demonstrated beneficial physiological effects in humans (IoM (Institute of Medicine), 2005). The rationale behind this differentiation is that there is epidemiological evidence for the beneficial effects of foods naturally high in DF, such as whole-grain cereals, some fruits and vegetables, and that DF can be regarded as a marker of such foods. The argument that the term "dietary fiber" should be restricted to non-starch polysaccharides of cell wall origin (Englyst, K.N. & Englyst, H.N., 2005; Englyst, K.N. Liu, & Englyst, H.N., 2007) has a similar rationale. Consequently, according to the FNB, documentation of the beneficial effects of added, functional fiber is required for inclusion in "total dietary fiber".

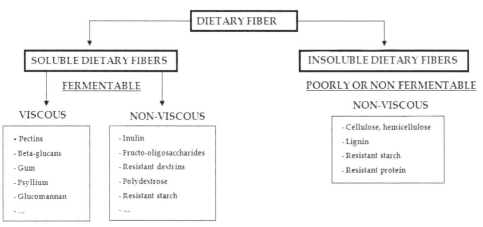

Fig. 1. Classification of dietary fiber according to chemical properties.

Based on this opinion, DF is defined as non-digestible carbohydrates plus lignin and it can be divided into different types:

-   Non-starch polysaccharides (NSP) - cellulose, hemicelluloses, pectins, hydrocolloids (i.e. gums, mucilages, -glucans).
-   Resistant oligosaccharides - fructo-oligosaccharides (FOS), galacto-oligosaccharides (GOS), other resistant oligosaccharides.
-   Resistant starch - consisting of physically enclosed starch, some types of raw starch granules, retrograded amylose, chemically and/or physically modified starches.
-   Lignin associated with the dietary fiber polysaccharides.

1.2 Methods for analysis of dietary fiber

Enzymatic-gravimetric or enzymatic-chemical methods for DF cover NSP, analytically resistant starch and lignin. However, as DF is a mixture of chemically heterogeneous carbohydrate components, several analytical methods are currently required to measure all fractions. Methods measuring only NSP (Englyst, H.N. & Hudson, G.J., 1996) give lower estimates than methods for total dietary fiber in foods containing resistant starch, and/or lignin. On the other hand, methods determining DF, including resistant starch, measure mainly retrograded amylose, resistant to the enzymes used in the assay. Finally, resistant oligosaccharides and inulin are not included in any of the current methods for total DF, and therefore need to be measured separately and subsequently added to the total fiber estimate (Cho et al., 1997; Champ et al., 2001, 2003)

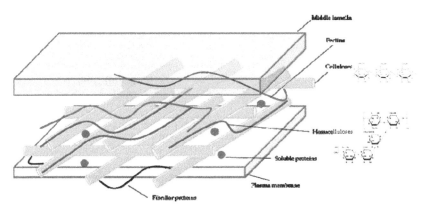

Fig. 2. The components that are part of the primary structure of the plant cell wall.

Total DF (TDF) can also be analysed by a combined enzymatic and gravimetric method, as the sum of insoluble DF (IDF) and soluble DF (SDF) which has been described in section 32.1.17 of the AOAC International Official Methods of Analysis (see Figure 3) based on previous work by Prosky et al. (Prosky et al., 1988). Another enzymatic-chemical method accepted for official action by the AOAC for the determination of TDF is one based on assays for components of TDF - neutral sugars, uronic acid residues and Klason lignin (section 45.4.11 AOAC). Starch is removed enzymatically and soluble polymers are precipitated with ethanol. Precipitated and insoluble polysaccharides are hydrolyzed using sulfuric acid and the released neutral sugars are quantitated as alditol acetates using gas-liquid chromatography. Uronic acids in the acid hydrolysate are determined by colorimetry. Klason lignin is determined gravimetrically.

However, other authors (Mañas & Saura-Calixto, 1995) have reported some methodological errors associated with precipitation and the enzymatic steps of the AOAC method. Subsequently, Saura-Calixto et al. (2000) proposed an alternative methodology to the AOAC definition of DF that measure the "indigestible fraction" (IF) of foods. The proposed method is an attempt to quantify, in a single analysis, the major non-digestible components in plant foods. This method is based on a concept of the IF that includes the main food constituents with nutritional relevance not available in the small intestine. In this method, samples are analyzed as eaten (fresh, boiled, or fried) and analytical conditions (pH, temperatures, incubation times) are close to physiological ones.

1.3 Dietary fiber content in foods

As we have mentioned before, DF occurring in foods and food products can be considered to consist mainly of cellulose, hemicelluloses, pectic substances, hydrocolloids (gums and mucilages), resistant starches, and resistant oligosaccharides.

SDF includes pectin, beta-glucans, inulin, fructans, oligosaccharides, some hemicelluloses, guar and gums. Food sources rich in SDF include legumes, vegetables, fruits, oat bran and pysllium seeds. IDF includes hemicellulose, cellulose, resistant starch and lignin. The main source of this kind of DF is whole grain. Vegetables and fruits contain both soluble and insoluble fiber, but depending on the vegetable and fruit type or maturity, the soluble to insoluble fiber ratio may vary.

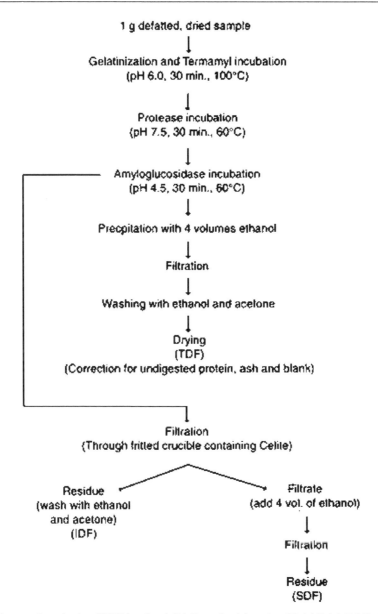

1 g defatted, dried sample

↓

Gelatinization and Termamyl incubation
(pH 6.0, 30 min., 100°C)

↓

Protease incubation
(pH 7.5, 30 min., 60°C)

↓

Amyloglucosidase incubation
(pH 4.5, 30 min., 60°C)

↓

Precipitation with 4 volumes ethanol

↓

Filtration

↓

Washing with ethanol and acetone

↓

Drying
(TDF)
(Correction for undigested protein, ash and blank)

↓

Filtration
(Through fritted crucible containing Celite)

Residue
(wash with ethanol
and acetone)
(IDF)

Filtrate
(add 4 vol. of ethanol)

↓

Filtration

↓

Residue
(SDF)

Fig. 3. Scheme of analysis of TDF by the AOAC method (section 32.1.17of AOAC, 1995).

Table 1 includes data of soluble and IDF content in some DF rich foods analyzed according to AOAC methodology. The most complete database on DF content is the USDA National Nutrient Database for Standard Reference, Release 23 (USDA). Other institutions such as FAO have also published a database on food composition, INFOODS Food Composition Database for Biodiversity (FAO).

Fiber Food Source	Insoluble DF *	Soluble DF *	Total DF
Vegetables, raw			
Broccoli, raw	0.44	3.06	3.50
Cabbage, green, raw	0.46	1.79	2.24
Carrots, raw	0.49	2.39	2.88
Cauliflower, raw	0.47	2.15	2.62
Cucumber, raw, with peel	0.20	0.94	1.14
Lettuce, iceberg, raw	0.10	0.88	0.98
Onion, mature, raw	0.71	1.22	1.93
Pepper, sweet, green, raw	0.53	0.99	1.52
Tomatoes, red, ripe, raw	0.15	1.19	1.34
Spinach, raw	0.77	2.43	3.20
Beans, green, fresh, microwaved	1.38	2.93	4.31
Carrots, fresh, microwaved	1.58	2.29	3.87
Peas, green, froz., microwaved	0.94	2.61	3.54
Potato, white, boiled, w/o skin	0.99	1.06	2.05
Fruits			
Apple (Red delicious), raw, ripe w/skin	0.67	1.54	2.21
Avocado (Calfornia, Haas), raw, ripe	2.03	3.51	5.53
Bananas, raw, ripe	0.58	1.21	1.79
Grapefruit, raw, white, ripe	0.58	0.32	0.89
Grapes, raw, ripe	0.24	0.36	0.6
Mango, raw, ripe	0.69	1.08	1.76
Nectarine, raw, ripe, w/skin	0.98	1.06	2.04
Oranges (Navel), raw, ripe	1.37	0.99	2.35
Orange juice, retail, from concentrate	0.28	0.03	0.31
Peaches, raw, ripe, w/skin	1.31	1.54	2.85
Pears, raw, ripe, w/skin	0.92	2.25	3.16
Pineapple, raw, ripe	0.04	1.42	1.46
Plum, raw, ripe, w/skin	1.12	1.76	2.87
Prunes, pitted	4.50	3.63	8.13
Watermelon, raw, ripe	0.13	0.27	0.40
Baked products			
Bread, wheat	1.26	2.13	3.38

Fiber Food Source	Insoluble DF *	Soluble DF *	Total DF
Bread, whole-wheat	1.26	4.76	6.01
Bread, rye	1.62	2.84	4.46
Bread, reduced-calorie, white	1.01	8.46	9.47
Cereal grains and pasta			
White rice, long grain, cooked	0.00	0.34	0.34
Spaghetti, cooked	0.54	1.33	2.06
Cornflakes	4.28	0.5	3.78
Brown rice, long grain, cooked	0.44	2.89	3.33
Corn, sweet, white, cooked, boiled, drained, without salt	0.62	3.32	3.94
Oat bran, cooked	0.42	1.23	1.65
Legumes			
Chick peas, canned, drained	0.41	5.79	6.19
Cowpeas, canned, drained	0.43	4.11	4.53
Lentils, dry, cooked, drained	0.44	5.42	5.86
Pinto beans, canned, drained	0.99	5.66	6.65
Red kidney beans, can, drained	1.36	5.77	7.13
Split peas, dry, cooked, drained	0.09	10.56	10.65

Table 1. List of food with their insoluble, soluble, and total fiber content (g/100 g edible food portion as eaten). * Data from Li et al., (Liu et al., 2002) and Marlett et al. (Marlett et al., 1992). Soluble and insoluble DF fractions were analyzed according to the AOAC Method 991.43.

1.4 Dietary fiber intake

Typical intakes of carbohydrates and DF are presented for children and adolescents in 19 countries and for adults in 22 countries in Europe included in the EFSA Panel on Dietetic Products, Nutrition, and Allergies (EFSA Journal 2010). The data refer to individual based food consumption surveys conducted from 1994 onwards. Most studies comprise national representative population samples. The data were derived from national reports and from a published overview (Elmadfa, 2009).

The National Academies Press also published in their web (www.nap.edu) the book titled "Dietary Reference Intakes for Energy, Carbohydrate, Fiber, Fat, Fatty Acids, Cholesterol, Protein, and Amino Acids (Macronutrients)" in which Chapter 7 entitled "Dietary, Functional, and Total Fiber" summarizes the DF intake in the American population shown in the USDA database.

Table 2 shows the DF intake in the United States and European population adapted from the two most referenced databases (USDA and EFSA).

Life stage group	Total dietary fiber intake (USDA) g/day [a]	Total dietary fiber intake (EFSA) g/day [b]
Infants		
0–6 month	ND	ND
7–12 month	ND	ND
Children		
1–3 year	19	12–15
4–8 year	25	11–20
Males		
9–13 year	31	13–27
14–18 year	38	15–33
19–34 year	38	16–26
35-64 year	30	17–27
Females		
9–13 year	26	13–25
14–18 year	26	14–27
19–34 year	25	15–24
35-64 year	21	15–26

[a] Dietary reference intake values reported by the USDA (see www.nap.edu)
[b] Dietary Reference intake values reported by the EFSA (EFSA Panel on Dietetic Products, Nutrition, and Allergies (NDA), 2010).
ND = Not determinable due to lack of data of adverse effects in this age group and concern with regard to the lack of ability to handle excess amounts.

Table 2. Dietary reference intakes of dietary fiber in United States and European population.

2. Main effects of dietary fiber

The physiological effects of DF result from its chemical and physical properties. Degradability, molecular weight, viscosity, particle size, cation exchange properties, organic acid absorption, and water-holding capacity are examples of such properties. Degradability enables the utilization of fiber in intestinal fermentation by colonic bacteria. Fermentation decreases the fecal pH and increases the bacterial biomass leading to an increase in faecal output and the production of gases and short-chain fatty acids (SCFAs). Viscous or soluble fibers form a gel by binding water and thereby decrease the gastric emptying rate and rate of absorption of glucose, triglycerides, and cholesterol. Large particle size and water holding capacity decrease transit time by increasing faecal bulk, which prevents constipation and dilutes carcinogenic compounds in the alimentary tract. Physicochemical properties are specific to different fibers and can change during cooking or digestion.

It is well known that DF plays important roles in the health of humans and in meeting the nutritional needs of animals. Much of the recent literature is focused on the ability of certain DF types to affect different physiological systems. Part of that research aims to understand how DF influences the characteristics and fermentation patterns of the intestinal microbiome in humans (Meyer & Stasse-Wolthuis, 2009; Roberfroid et al., 2010). Consequently, it is possible to understand the prebiotic function of fibers using new DNA sequencing procedures that permit complete characterization of the bacterial populations (microbiome). One of the products of fermentation, butyrate, is able to regulate gene transcription which affects cell proliferation, differentiation, and apoptosis of colon cells (Wilson et al., 2010; Crim et al., 2008). The overall goals of these studies are to determine why some individuals are more at risk to develop diseases and some animals are more efficiently using their food for production purposes, as well as to identify dietary modifications that improve animal production efficiency and human health.

3. Mechanisms of the beneficial effects of dietary fiber

Clinical recommendations for DF are routinely provided to improve gastrointestinal function, increasing laxation and reducing diverticular disease (Hall et al., 2010). In addition, an increase in the consumption of foods containing fiber is recommended to reduce obesity, type 2 diabetes mellitus (T2DM), cardiovascular disease and some cancers.

In this section we describe the mechanisms by which DF achieves its health effects focused on cardiovascular risk factors.

3.1 Body weight

DF can modulate body weight by various mechanisms, including promoting satiation, decreasing absorption of macronutrients, and altering the secretion of gut hormones.

Fiber rich foods usually have lower energy content, which contributes to a decrease into the energy density of the diet. Foods rich in fiber need to be chewed longer, leading to an increase in the time needed to eat the food and in the feeling of satiety. A number of studies (Slavin, 2005; Howarth et al., 2001a; Pereira & Ludwig, 2001) have shown that different DF affect subjective appetite, acute energy intake, long-term energy intake and body weight differently. The physicochemical properties of fibers may contribute to this variation. Fibers which make up viscous solutions and are more soluble and fermentable also delay the passage of food from the stomach to the duodenum and contribute to an increase in satiety and a decrease in energy intake. In the intestine, incorporation of fiber may complicate the interactions between digestive enzymes and their substrates, thereby slowing down the absorption of nutrients. It is also important to note that the effects of DF consumption on body weight may be related to different gut hormones which regulate satiety, energy intake and/or pancreatic functions (Aleixandre & Miguel, 2008).

3.2 Hypocholesterolemic action

The hypocholesterolemic action of fiber is partly mediated by a lower absorption of intestinal bile acid because of interruption of the enterohepatic bile acid circulation, thus increasing fecal bile acid loss, and its synthesis in liver (Morgan et al., 1993; Anderson et al., 1984). The physicochemical properties of soluble fiber result in important modifications in volume, bulk and viscosity in the intestinal lumen, which alter the metabolic pathways of hepatic cholesterol and lipoprotein metabolism, also resulting in the lowering of plasma LDL cholesterol. Other studies suggest that DF increases the enzymatic activity of cholesterol-7-αhydroxylase, the major regulatory enzyme in the hepatic conversion of cholesterol to bile acids (Roy et al., 2002) contributing to a higher depletion of hepatic cholesterol. Jones and co-workers (Jones et al., 1993) described a reduction in hepatic lipogenesis stimulated by insulin. It has also been suggested that the fermentation of DF by the intestinal microflora could modify the short chain fatty acid production thereby reducing acetate and increasing propionate synthesis. This, in turn, reduces the endogenous synthesis of cholesterol, fatty acids and very low density lipoproteins (Wolever et al., 1995; Wong et al., 2006).

Traditional dietary patterns, characterized by high fiber content, have been associated with lower rates of coronary disease. However, it should be taken into account that foods rich in fiber are also usually rich in a wide range of other bioactive substances which have a clear role in the prevention of cardiovascular disease (Craig, 1997; Hu & Willett, 2002; Buttriss & Benelam, 2010). Likewise, the beneficial effect of diets enriched in fiber on the lipid profile could also be explained by the fact that these diets are traditionally low in fat (especially saturated fat) and promote satiety and, therefore, help to protect against overweight and obesity (Mann, 2007).

3.3 Glucose tolerance and insulin sensitivity

Some studies have shown that soluble fiber plays an important role in controlling postprandial glycemic and insulin responses because of its effect on gastric emptying and macronutrient absorption from the gut (Slavin et al., 1999). Surprisingly, prospective studies have found that insoluble fiber, but not soluble fiber, is inversely related to the incidence of T2DM. In contrast, in postprandial studies, meals containing sufficient quantities of β-glucan, psyllium, or guar gum have decreased insulin and glucose responses in both healthy individuals and patients with T2DM. Diets enriched sufficiently in soluble fiber may also improve overall glycemic control in T2DM.

The association between the consumption of low dietary glycemic index (GI) foods and a lower risk of T2DM has been reported in several prospective studies (Salmeron et al., 1997), generally suggesting a preventive role of low GI diets. One of the largest was the 16-year follow-up of the Nurses' Health Study from 1980 including 3300 incident cases of type 2 diabetes, where the association between high glycemic load and the risk of developing T2DM was confirmed (Hu et al., 2001). A more recent meta-analysis of 37 prospective observational studies reported that diets with a high GI independently increased the risk of T2DM, providing protection similar to or higher than whole grains or fiber (Barclay et al., 2008). Similarly, a recent Cochrane database review concluded that low-GI diets can improve glycemic control in diabetic patients (Thomas & Elliott, 2009). However, not all investigators have reported similar findings: A well designed, controlled trial in well-controlled T2DM without oral antidiabetic therapy or insulin showed no effect on glycated hemoglobin, although a reduction in C-reactive protein and postprandial glucose was observed (Wolever et al., 2008).

To date, the physiopathologic mechanisms that explain the beneficial effects of fiber on glycemic control have still not been clearly delimited.

3.4 Blood pressure

Observational and experimental studies have reported that increased DF was associated with a lower risk of hypertension or lower self-reported blood pressure (BP), in both normotensive and hypertensive subjects (Ascherio et al., 1992; Beilin, 1994; He & Whelton, 1999). Subjects consuming a vegetarian diet are generally at lower risk of developing hypertension. However, it is unknown whether this can be ascribed to the high fiber content of the diet because vegetarians—apart from differences in lifestyle— also have higher intakes of potassium, magnesium, and polyunsaturated fatty acids and a lower intake of saturated fat.

The differences observed in BP response might be explained by fiber dose, type of fiber consumed, or better compliance with dietary supplements than with high-fiber diets (He & Whelton, 1999).

3.5 C-reactive protein

C-reactive protein (CRP) is a marker of acute inflammation recently recognized as an independent predictor of future cardiovascular disease and diabetes.

Several studies have reported that DF intake is inversely associated with serum concentrations of CRP (Butcher & Beckstrand, 2010; Oliveira et al., 2009). The mechanisms of change in CRP levels as a result of DF intake are still largely unknown; possibilities include DF slowing the absorption of glucose, fiber-rich meal modulation of cytokine responses blunting oxidative stress and inflammation, and the production of anti-inflammatory cytokines by gut flora exposed to fiber.

4. Epidemiological studies

Several limitations are common to all prospective studies examining the relationship between foods and nutrients and disease risk. The lack of consistency in the methods used for the measurement of different classes and subgroups of dietary fiber, especially the NSP, complicates comparisons between the results of studies and their extrapolation into nutritional recommendations. However, prospective epidemiological studies provide strong evidence for a protective role of wholegrain cereals, fruits and vegetables and dietary patterns characterized by relatively high intakes of such foods.

While a high consumption of DF derived from cereals is also associated with a reduced risk of cardiovascular disease, it is not clear whether this cardioprotection can entirely be attributed to the polysaccharides per se. Even the best prospective studies cannot conclusively eliminate the possibility of residual confounding, thus recommendations regarding the intake of carbohydrates in relation to cardiovascular disease also depend on the intervention studies described below.

4.1 Body weight

Large prospective studies have reported that consumption of DF is inversely associated with weight and weight gain. A high intake of DF may assist weight loss because of the incomplete digestion and absorption of energy from this type of carbohydrates and the bulky nature of high-fiber foods, with increased demands on chewing and subsequent distension and delayed emptying of the stomach, promoting satiety and thereby curtailing energy intake.

Reviews of randomized trials in adults have shown weight loss in a majority of studies with no differences between fiber types or between fiber occurring in foods or in supplements

(Pereira & Ludwig, 2001; Howarth et al., 2001a). Results from seven prospective cohort studies show an inverse relationship between weight gain and baseline intake or change in fiber intake among adults during follow-up periods of up to 12 years (Lairon, 2007; Koh-Banerjee et al., 2004).

The CARDIA (The Coronary Artery Risk Development in Young Adults) study, a multicenter population-based cohort study carried out over 10 years, examined 2909 young individuals to determine the relationship between total dietary fiber intake and plasma insulin concentrations, weight and other cardiovascular disease risk factors. After adjusting for BMI and multiple dietary and potential non-dietary confounders, the study reported an inverse association between total fiber intake, plasma insulin concentrations and body weight gain (Ludwig et al., 1999) suggesting that fiber may play an important role in the prevention of insulin resistance and obesity. Individuals consuming higher amounts of fiber had a lower weight gain compared to those consuming lower amounts, independently of the level of total fat consumed. Similarly, in the Nurses' Health Study cohort Liu (2003) showed that women in the highest quintile of DF intake had a 49% lower risk of major weight gain than women in the lowest quintile.

Kromhout et al. (2001) investigated the association between DF and indicators of body fat in a cross-cultural study of 16 cohorts of 12 763 middle-aged men in seven countries, between 1958 and 1964. The average DF intake was inversely related to population average subscapular skinfold thickness and body mass index.

Alfieri et al. (1995) assessed the total fiber intake by means of 3-day food records in 3 population groups (one normal, one moderately and one severely obese group). These authors showed that fiber intake was significantly higher in the normal weight group and was inversely associated with BMI after adjusting for several potential confounders. Recently, new research conducted as part of the PREDIMED study has also shown a significant inverse relationship between TDF consumption and body mass index or abdominal circumference (Estruch et al., 2009).

In an observational study looking at the effect of overall diet on body composition in obese and lean subjects it was demonstrated that lean men and women had significantly higher fiber intake versus obese males and females (27.0 g/d and 22.7 g/d vs. 22.0 g/d and 15.0 g/d respectively) (Miller et al., 1994). These results were supported in another study with a cohort of over 5000 subjects, which showed that higher fiber intake is associated with a lower body mass index (BMI) in both men and women (Appleby et al., 1998).

In a prospective cohort with 252 premenopausal, non-smoker women free from serious disease, Tucker & Thomas (2009) conducted a study to determine whether changes in fiber intake (total, soluble, and insoluble) influence the risk of gaining weight and body fat over time (20 months). Increasing DF significantly reduces the risk of women gaining weight and fat. For each 1 g increase in total fiber consumed, weight decreased by 0.25 kg ($P = 0.0061$) and fat decreased by 0.25 percentage point ($P = 0.0052$). Controlling for potential confounders did not affect the relationships, except for changes in energy intake, which weakened the associations by 24-32%. Soluble and insoluble fibers were borderline predictors of changes in weight and fat.

Studies on children eating mixed diets do not indicate adverse effects on growth due to high fiber intake. On the other hand, there are studies indicating that DF intake can contribute to lowering the risk of obesity in this population group (Edwards & Parrett, 2003).

In conclusion, increased intake of DF, both from naturally fiber-rich foods and added fiber or fiber supplements, has been shown to be related to improved weight maintenance in adults and sustained weight reduction in overweight subjects. Estimated intakes associated with this effect in adults are in the order of >25 g DF per day (from wholegrain cereals, fruit and vegetables).

4.2 Hypocholesterolemic action

DF has a potentially important effect on lipids and lipoproteins when consumed in plant foods or as supplements. Viscous subgroups of DF, including pectins, b-glucans, glucomannans, guar and psyllium, which are generally water soluble, all lower total and LDL cholesterol between 5 and 10 g/day, lowering LDL by about 5% (Truswell, 2002).

A cross-sectional epidemiological data, based on the EURODIAB Complications Study, which included over 2000 patients in 31 European centers, showed an inverse association between DF intake and HbA_{1c} and LDL cholesterol (in men only) and a positive association with HDL cholesterol in men and women (Toeller et al., 1999).

In an analysis of dietary factors and cardiovascular risk performed in a sample of 3,452 Swiss adults, it was observed that a healthy diet characterized by high consumption of DF was associated with lower rates of serum triglycerides and higher HDL-c (Berg et al., 2008). A 10-year study of a cohort of 2,909 healthy adults aged between 18 and 30 showed a strong negative association between fiber intake and blood pressure and levels of triglyceride, HDL cholesterol, LDL cholesterol, and fibrinogen even after adjusting for confounding factors (Ludwig et al., 1999). In a cohort of 316 Japanese-Brazilian subjects, a decrease of 12.5 mg/dl was observed in the serum total cholesterol levels ($P < 0.05$) for each increase of 10 g in the consumption of DF intake in a 7- year follow up (de Castro et al., 2006). Wu et al. (2003) studied a cohort of 573 adults aged between 40 and 60 and found and inverse relationship between the ratio of TC/HDL-c and the total intake of DF ($P = 0.01$); the ratio of TC/HDL-c has been proposed as a good indicator of cardiovascular risk.

Van Dam RM, et al. (2003) performed a cross-sectional study of 19,750 randomly selected men and women aged 20-65 y from 3 Dutch municipalities. Three dietary factors were identified: Cosmopolitan pattern (rich in fried vegetables, salad); traditional pattern (rich red meat) and refined pattern (rich sugar-beverages and white bread). A higher adherence to the Cosmopolitan pattern was significantly associated with lower blood pressure and higher HDL-c concentrations; the traditional dietary pattern was associated with higher blood pressure and higher concentrations of HDL cholesterol, total cholesterol, and glucose; and the refined dietary pattern was associated with higher total cholesterol concentrations.

Whole grain was also inversely associated with total cholesterol (P for trend = 0.02), LDL cholesterol (P for trend = 0.04), and 2-h glucose (P for trend = 0.0006) in a cross-sectional analysis of 1516 community-dwelling participants in the Baltimore Longitudinal Study of Aging. Associations between cereal fiber and anthropometrics and plasma lipids were similar (Newby et al., 2007).

In conclusion, viscous types of DF mainly from fruits, vegetables and whole grains may contribute to reducing total and LDL-cholesterol concentrations. The effects are limited to amounts usually consumed from foods.

4.3 Glycemic index and Type 2 diabetes mellitus

Glycemic control is of crucial importance in the management of T2DM. Few intervention studies have investigated the effects of fiber intake on measures of glucose tolerance or insulin sensitivity, but recent observations have shown the favourable effects of a diet with abundant fiber-rich foods, particularly whole grain, bran and germ intake, on the risk of T2DM (Murakami et al., 2005; Krishnan et al., 2007; Schulze et al., 2007; de Munter et al., 2007).

In the Nurses' Health Study, wholegrain consumption appeared to be protective for T2DM. When comparing the highest and lowest quintiles of intake, the age and energy adjusted relative risk was 0.62 (95% CI: 0.53, 0.71). Further adjustment for other risk factors did not appreciably alter this risk estimate (Liu et al., 2000; Salmeron, et al., 1997) virtually identical risk reduction was observed among men participating in the Health Professionals Study (Fung et al., 2002). A relative risk of 0.63 was reported in association with three or more servings/day of wholegrain. In the Iowa Women's Health Study, postmenopausal women in the upper quintile of wholegrain consumption (more than 33 servings per week) were 20% less likely to develop T2DM than those in the lowest quintile (fewer than 13 servings per week) (Meyer et al., 2000). Cereal fiber appears to be associated with a protective dose–response effect that is present after controlling for a range of potentially confounding factors. The role of whole grains and DF in diabetes has been reviewed in detail by Venn and Mann (Venn & Mann, 2004).

Two large cross-sectional studies, using validated food frequency questionnaires to assess nutrient intake and either the frequently sampled intravenous glucose tolerance test or homoeostasis model assessment for insulin resistance, found that intake of DF was inversely associated with the probability of having insulin resistance (Lau et al., 2005; Liese et al., 2005) and it was possible to demonstrate that fiber was associated with increased insulin sensitivity even after adjustment for body mass index.

During 8 years of follow-up (1995-2003) 1964 incident cases of T2DM were reported in a prospective cohort study including 41,186 participants of the Black Women's Health Study without a history of diabetes or CVD. Daily consumption of whole grain was associated with a lower risk of T2DM compared with consumption less than once a week. After mutual adjustment, the hazard ratio was 0.73 (0.63-0.85; P for trend = 0.0001) for whole grains (van Dam et al., 2006).

Krishnan S et al. (2007) examined the association of glycemic load, GI, and cereal fiber with risk of T2DM in 59000 black women with T2DM, CVD or cancer from the Black Women's Health Study. During 8 years of follow-up, there were 1,938 incident cases of diabetes. GI was positively associated with the risk of diabetes: the incidence rate ratios (IRR) for the highest quintile relative to the lowest was 1.23 (95% CI, 1.05-1.44). Cereal fiber intake was inversely associated with the risk of T2DM with an IRR of 0.82 (95% CI, 0.70-0.96) for the highest *vs.* the lowest quintiles of intake. Stronger associations were seen among women with a body mass index lower than 25: IRRs for the highest *vs.* the lowest quintile were 1.91

(95% CI, 1.16-3.16) for GI (P =0.12) and 0.41 (95% CI, 0.24-0.72) for cereal fiber intake (P= 0.05).

In conclusion, increasing intakes of foods rich in DF are associated with a reduced risk of developing T2DM. DF intakes associated with favorable effects are about 25 to 30 g per day, although the contribution of DF per se to this effect remains to be established.

4.4 Blood pressure

Increased DF has been associated with a lower risk of hypertension, and a meta-analysis of clinical studies of fiber supplementation also supports an inverse association between fiber and blood pressure.

In a cross-sectional study, Lairon D et al. (2007) determined the quintiles of fiber intake from dietary record, separately for 2532 men and 3429 women. The highest total DF and insoluble DF intakes were associated with a significantly ($P < 0.05$) lower risk of overweight and elevated waist-to-hip ratio, BP, plasma apolipoprotein (apo) B, apo B:apo A-I, cholesterol, triacylglycerols, and homocysteine. Fiber from cereals was associated with a lower body mass index, BP, and homocysteine concentration; fiber from vegetables with a lower BP and homocysteine concentration; and fiber from fruit with a lower waist-to-hip ratio and BP. Fiber from dried fruit or nuts and seeds was associated with a lower body mass index, waist-to-hip ratio, and fasting apo B and glucose concentrations.

Estruch et al. (2009) analyzed 772 cardiovascular high-risk subjects (age 69±5 years). On randomization they were assigned to a low-fat diet or two recommendations for increasing vegetable, fruit and legume intake. Body weight, waist circumference and mean systolic and diastolic BP significantly decreased across the quintiles of fiber intake ($P<0.005$).

In a meta-analysis of randomized placebo-controlled trials to estimate the effect of fiber supplementation on BP overall and in population subgroups, fiber supplementation (average dose, 11.5 g/d) changed systolic BP by –1.13 mm Hg (95% CI: –2.49 to 0.23) and diastolic BP by –1.26 mm Hg (–2.04 to –0.48). Reductions in BP tended to be greater in older (>40 years) and in hypertensive populations than in younger and in normotensive subjects (Streppel et al., 2005).

4.5 Cardiovascular disease

Many epidemiological studies have evaluated the effects of DF on the risk of coronary heart disease (CHD) (Rimm et al., 1996; Todd et al., 1999; Liu et al., 2002; Mozaffarian et al., 2003). Most likely, as assessed in prospective studies, DF intake with the usual diet is a marker of healthy food choices with an overall cardiovascular benefit, while changing the diet to increase DF at late stages, when clinical consequences of atherosclerosis have developed, may not be protective.

A meta-analysis, involving four of the largest studies published, suggested a 28% reduction in the risk of CHD on comparing individuals in the highest and lowest quintiles of intake of whole grains (relative risk 0.72, 95% confidence intervals: 0.48, 0.94) (Anderson, 2003).

After adjustment for cardiovascular risk factors, in the Iowa Women's Health Study the relative risks for cardiovascular disease were 1.0, 0.96, 0.71, 0.64 and 0.70 in ascending quintiles of whole grain intake, P <0.02 (Jacobs et al., 1998). The Nurses' Health Study (Liu et al., 2000) observed risk reductions of magnitude similar to those observed for CHD (relative risk 0.69, 95% CI: 0.50, 0.98 when comparing the highest relative to the lowest quintile of intake of whole grains).

The suggestion that reduced cardiovascular risk principally results from consumption of wholegrain rather than DF was supported by findings from the Iowa Women's Health Study. CHD rates were compared in women consuming similar amounts of cereal fiber from either predominantly refined grain sources or predominantly wholegrains. After adjustments, all-cause mortality was significantly lower, and CHD appreciably (though not statistically significantly) reduced among the latter group (Jacobs et al., 2000).

In the Nurses' Health Study and the Health Professionals' Study (Hu et al., 2000; Fung et al., 2001), factor analysis was used to examine the association between CHD and the two major dietary patterns identified: "western" characterized by higher intakes of red and processed meats, sweets and desserts, French fries and refined grains and 'prudent' characterized by higher intakes of fruit, vegetables, legumes, fish, poultry and wholegrains. After adjustment for cardiovascular risk factors, the prudent diet score was associated with relative risks of 1.0, 0.87, 0.79, 0.75 and 0.70 from the lowest to the highest quintiles. Conversely, the relative risks across increasing quintiles of the western pattern score were 1.0, 1.21, 1.35, 1.40 and 1.64. The patterns were also related to biochemical markers of CHD.

The effect of DF may be largely explained by fiber derived from wholewheat, rye or pumpernickel breads, in a multicenter study among 3588 men and women aged 65 years or older and free of known CVD at baseline (Mozaffarian et al., 2003). During a mean follow-up of 8.6 years, there were 811 incident CVD events. After adjustment for different confounder factors, cereal fiber consumption was inversely associated with incident CVD (P for trend=0.02), with 21% lower risk (HR: 0.79; 95% CI: 0.62-0.99) in the highest quintile of intake, compared with the lowest quintile. In similar analyses, neither fruit fiber intake (P for trend=0.98) nor vegetable fiber intake (P for trend=0.95) were associated with incident CVD.

Furthermore, in a combined analysis of 10 prospective cohort studies conducted in the USA and Europe Pereira et al. (2004) showed a 25% decrease in the risk of CHD for each 10 g increase in fiber intake, after adjusting for several dietary and cardiovascular confounding factors. A relative risk of 0.90 (95% CI: 0.77, 1.07 that is not statistically significant) was reported for total CHD events for each 10 g/day increase in cereal fiber. When considering CHD deaths, the relative risk, 0.75 (95% CI: 0.63, 0.91) was statistically significant, the association being independent of a number of dietary factors and other cardiovascular risk factors.

Recently, Streppel et al. (2008) also observed that CHD mortality and all-cause mortality were reduced by 17% and 9%, respectively for every additional 10 g of DF per day, with no clear associations for different types of DF.

4.6 Inflammatory markers

CRP is an inflammatory marker useful in the prediction of coronary events. Results from recent epidemiologic studies have consistently shown an inverse association between DF intake and plasma CRP levels. In a recent study, both increasing fiber intake by about 30 g/day from a diet rich in fiber or from a supplement reduced the levels of CRP.

Jenkins et al. (2003) reported reduced CRP levels in hyperlipidaemic patients consuming a high carbohydrate diet rich in viscous fiber-containing foods. However, the diets were also high in nuts (almonds), plant sterols and soy proteins, and it is therefore impossible to disentangle separate effects. A recent study (Kasim-Karakas et al., 2006) found that when carbohydrate replaced a substantial proportion of dietary fat under eucaloric conditions, the levels of several inflammatory markers increased along with an increase in triglycerides.

Data from the Massachusetts Hispanic Elders Study (Gao et al., 2004) obtained from 445 Hispanic and 154 non-Hispanic white elders showed that greater frequency of fruit and vegetable intake, which are reach in fiber, was associated with lower CRP and homocysteine concentrations. With each additional serving of fruit and vegetable intake, the risk of having high CRP (>10 mg/l) and homocysteine concentrations decreased by 21% and 17%, respectively.

The relation between DF and CRP was examined from 1999 to 2000 in 3,920 participants in the National Health and Nutrition Examination Survey (Ajani, Ford, & Mokdad, 2004). DF intake was inversely associated with serum CRP concentrations: The adjusted odds ratio for increased CRP levels (>3 mg/l) was 0.59 (P = 0.006) for the highest quintile of fiber intake compared with the lowest. The results were not affected after exclusion of persons with diabetes, cancer, CVD, or CRP levels >10 mg/l. The results of Ajani et al. confirmed the previous findings (King et al., 2003).

5. Clinical trials

Most of the data available on disease prevalence and events are from epidemiological studies. However, it is necessary to also resort to clinical trials to test effects of different types and sources of DF on cardiovascular risk factors taking into account a specific population.

5.1 Body weight

Although epidemiological data and mechanistic studies support the contention that fiber has beneficial effects on body weight regulation; there has been inconsistent data from randomized controlled clinical trials that have evaluated how body weight is affected by supplementing fiber in the diet (Rodriguez-Moran et al., 1998; Birketvedt et al., 2000; Pittler & Ernst, 2001).

In a systematic review, Howarth et al. (2001) analyzed several clinical trials conducted in small and heterogeneous population samples over relatively short periods of time (from 1 to 12 months). The findings were that the intake of 12 g fiber/day resulted in a decrease of 10% in energy intake and a body weight loss of 1.9 kg over 3.8 months, with this effect on body weight loss being greater in obese subjects.

Esposito et al. (2004) explored the possible mechanisms underlying a dietary intervention and randomized 180 patients (99 men, 81 women) with the metabolic syndrome to a Mediterranean-style diet (instructions about increasing daily consumption of whole grains, vegetables, fruits, nuts, and olive oil) versus a cardiac prudent diet with fat intake less than 30%. After 2 years, body weight decreased more in the intervention group than in the control group, even after controlling for weight loss, inflammatory markers, such as IL-6, IL-7, IL-18, and CRP.

In randomized placebo-controlled studies, 176 overweight or obese men and women were included to receive either active fiber substance or placebo during a five-week observation period. The fiber supplements consisted of the viscous fibers glucomannan (Chrombalance), glucomannan and guar gum (Appe-Trim) and glucomannan, guar gum and alginat (Glucosahl). All fiber supplements plus a balanced 1200 kcal diet induced a significant weight reduction more than placebo and diet alone, during the observation period (Birketvedt et al., 2005).

Salas-Salvador et al. (2008) evaluated the effect of a mixed fiber supplement on body-weight loss, in 200 overweight or obese patients in a parallel, double-blind, placebo-controlled clinical trial. Weight loss tended to be higher after both doses of fiber (-4.52 ± 0.56 and -4.60 ± 0.55 kg) than placebo (-0.79 ± 0.58 kg); the differences in changes between groups were not statistically significant. Postprandial satiety increased in both fiber groups compared to the placebo. Estruch et al. (2009) analyzed 772 cardiovascular high-risk subjects that were assigned to a low-fat diet or two recommendations for increasing the intake of vegetables, fruit and legumes. Body weight, waist circumference and BP significantly decreased across the quintiles of fiber intake ($P=0.04$).

In a dietary intervention involving 107 overweight and obese children it was shown that low GI diets are more effective in reducing weight than low-fat diets (Spieth et al., 2000). The BMI of subjects assigned to the low GI diet reduced significantly in comparison to those on the low-fat diet across all three tertiles (<28.3 kg/m^2, 28.3–34.9 kg/m^2 and >34.9 kg/m^2). The mean overall reduction was 1.53 kg/m^2 vs. 0.06 kg/m^2 ($P < 0.001$). Another study showed that low GI diets result in the greatest reduction in fat mass, especially in women (McMillan-Price et al., 2006).

5.2 Serum lipids

Several studies have shown that a high consumption of DF, particularly soluble fiber (pectin, guar gumm, β-glucans, glucomannan, and psyllium), significantly decreases serum levels of total and LDL cholesterol (Anderson, 2000; Brighenti, 2007). Other clinical trials support the hypocholesterolemic effects of soluble fiber derived both from supplements or fiber derived from foods in patients at high risk of cardiovascular disease.

In a double-blind placebo-controlled study, Rodríguez-Morán M et al., (1998) determined the plasma-lowering effects of *Plantago psyllium*, as an adjunct to dietary therapy, on lipid and glucose levels, in patients with T2DM. The study included 125 subjects undergoing a 6-week period of diet counseling followed by a 6-week treatment period in which *Plantago psyllium* or placebo was given in combination with a low fat diet. No significant changes were observed in the patient's in either group. Fasting plasma glucose, total cholesterol, LDL-c, and triglyceride levels, showed a significant reduction ($P < 0.05$), whereas HDL-c increased significantly ($P < 0.01$) following *Psyllium* treatment.

A meta-analysis carried out by Brown et al. (1999) indicates that the effects of different types of viscous fibers on TC concentrations are modest. These results were obtained from 67 experimental metabolic studies carried out on 2,990 subjects showing that for each gram of soluble fiber added to the diet, the TC and the LDL-c concentration decreased by 1.7 mg/dL and 2.2 mg/dL, respectively.

In a meta-analysis of 8 controlled trials, it was observed that the hypolipidemic effects of physillium in hypocholesterolemic individuals already consuming a low-fat diet achieved reductions with diet only. Results confirm that *Psyllium* significantly lowers an additional 4% of serum total and cholesterol and an additional 7% relative of LDL-c concentrations in comparison to a placebo group consuming a low fat diet (Anderson, 2000).

In a randomized, crossover study Maki KC et al. (2007) compared the effects of consuming high-fiber oat and wheat cereals on postprandial metabolic profiles in healthy men. Twenty-seven subjects received oat (providing 5.7 g/day beta-glucan) or wheat (control) cereal products, in random order, incorporated into their usual diets for two weeks. Peak triglyceride concentration was lower after oat vs. wheat cereal consumption. Mean area under the triglyceride curve also tended to be lower.

In a recent parallel, double-blind, placebo-controlled clinical trial, 200 overweight or obese patients were randomized to receive a mixed dose of soluble fiber (3 g *Plantago ovata husk* and 1 g glucomannan) or a placebo twice or three times daily in the context of an energy-restricted diet for a period of 16 weeks. Differences in plasma LDL-c changes between the groups were significant, with greater reductions in the two fiber supplemented groups in comparison to the placebo (Salas-Salvado et al., 2008).

Insoluble fiber, such as that from wheat or cellulose, has not been reported to have any significant effect on blood cholesterol (Jenkins et al., 2000; Sola et al., 2007), possibly because of the presence, along with DF, of several bioactive and antioxidant phytochemical substances in foodstuffs (Salas-Salvado et al., 2006) or because of the effect that fiber has on blood pressure, body weight and postprandial glycemia or insulin levels.

5.3 Glycemic index and type 2 diabetes mellitus

On glycemic control, several randomized controlled trials have been performed to determine the effect of DF on insulin sensitivity, blood glucose control and hypoglycemic episodes. However, all were short-term studies. A whole grain diet led to a postprandial improvement in insulin sensitivity when compared to a refined grain diet. Plasma glucose concentrations were significantly lower for the high fiber diet than for the low-fiber diet. In clinical studies using fiber supplements, it appears that only soluble fiber plays a significant role in reducing postprandial glycemia. However, prospective epidemiological studies have shown that insoluble fiber, but not soluble fiber, from natural food sources was inversely related to the risk of diabetes.

Giacco and co-workers (Giacco et al., 2000) carried out a 6-month randomized parallel study comparing a diet containing 50 g/d of soluble fiber with a diet containing only 15 g/d of fiber. Thirty-two patients (intervention group) and 31 patients (control group) were randomized to follow a high-fiber or low-fiber diet for a 24-week period. This study confirmed the potential for around 40 g/d DF (half of the soluble type from legumes, fruits and vegetables) to improve glycemic control. They found an improvement in the daily blood glucose profile and the HbA_{1c} levels, as well as a marked reduction in the number of hypoglycemic events.

Chandalia et al. (2000) also demonstrated that high-fiber diets contributed to better metabolic control in 13 T2DM diabetic patients. In a cross-over study, patients were randomized to a diet containing a moderate amount of fiber (8 g of soluble fiber and 16 g insoluble fiber) or to a diet containing a high amount of fiber (25 g of soluble fiber and 25 g insoluble fiber). Plasma glucose concentrations were significantly lower for the high fiber than for the low-fiber diet.

In a controlled 6-week study, overweight hyperinsulinaemic adults consumed diets providing 55% energy from carbohydrate and 30% from fat, Pereira et al. (Pereira et al., 2002) observed that insulin sensitivity measured by a euglycemic hyperinsulinaemic clamp was appreciably improved in the wholegrain compared with the refined grain diet. Fasting insulins and area under the 2-h insulin curve were lower, despite body weight not being significantly different in the two diets. In this intervention, carbohydrates were derived from predominantly wholegrain or refined grain cereals, with DF content of the wholegrain diet 28 g compared with 17 g on the refined grain diet. DF was predominantly from cereal sources. Total carbohydrate and fat and fat sources were virtually identical in the two diets. Rye bread has also been shown to improve insulin sensitivity in overweight and obese women too (Juntunen et al., 2003).

Likewise, Weicker and co-workers (Weickert et al., 2006) used the same method to measure insulin sensitivity in overweight and obese women and found that this increased after 3 days of a diet containing bread enriched with insoluble fiber compared to another diet containing white bread

In a recent 6-month parallel, randomized clinical trial composed of 210 patients with T2DM the patients were randomized to either a high cereal fiber diet (GI = 80.8) or a low GI diet (GI = 69.6). The low GI diet resulted in statistically significant reductions in fasting plasma glucose and HbA$_{1c}$ (Jenkins et al., 2008). The results of this study confirm the notion that high fiber diets in a low GI setting are more effective in managing and preventing T2DM in comparison with high fiber diets that have medium or high GI.

A recent meta-analysis of randomized controlled trials looking at the effect of legumes on glycemic markers concluded that legumes as part of a high fiber diet significantly reduce fasting blood glucose and glycated proteins (Sievenpiper et al., 2009).

5.4 Inflammatory markers

In hyperlipidemic patients a reduction was founded in CRP levels (28% vs. baseline) following a whole diet approach, which was low in saturated fat and included viscous fibers, almonds, soy protein, and plant sterols being comparable to statin therapy (33% reduction of CRP levels) and independent of changes in body weight. The diet also induced a reduction in lipids that was comparable to lovastatin therapy (Jenkins et al., 2003). They reported reduced CRP levels in hyperlipidemic patients consuming a high carbohydrate diet rich in viscous fiber-containing foods. However, the diets were also high in nuts (almonds), plant sterols and soy proteins, and it was therefore impossible to disentangle separate effects.

Kasim-Karakas et al. (2006) found that when carbohydrates replaced a substantial proportion of dietary fat under eucaloric conditions in post-menopausal women, the levels of several inflammatory markers increased along with an increase in triglycerides. However, when the participants consumed the 15% fat diet *ad libitum* under free living conditions, they lost weight and triglyceride and the levels of inflammatory markers decreased. In another study, Estruch et al. (2009) analyzed 772 cardiovascular high-risk subjects concluding that plasma concentrations of CRP decreased in parallel with increasing DF (P=0.04).

A review of seven clinical trials of at least 2 weeks in duration, with an increased and measurable consumption of DF, reported significantly lower CRP concentrations of 25-54% with increased DF consumption with dosages ranging between 3.3-7.8 g/MJ. The seventh trial with *Psyllium* fiber supplementation failed to lower CRP levels significantly in overweight/obese individuals. Weight loss and altered fatty acid intakes were present in most of the studies (North et al., 2009). The mechanisms are inconclusive but may involve the effect of DF on weight loss, and/or changes in the secretion, turnover or metabolism of insulin, glucose, adiponectin, interleukin-6, free fatty acids and triglycerides.

6. Conclusions

Based on epidemiological and clinical studies that have attributed important health effects to fiber, several organizations such as the American Dietetic Association and the Institute of Medicine recommend an intake of 14 g of DF per 1,000 kcal, or 25 g/day for adult women and 38 g/day for adult men, to protect against the risk of CHD and T2DM and improved weight maintenance. However, in most Western countries, the current intakes of DF are below those recommended with, for instance, an average consumption of 19 and 16 g per day for men and women, respectively. In order to improve the DF intake of the population, national dietary guidelines usually recommend the consumption of high-fiber foods.

Since no biomarker of DF intake is available, food frequency questionnaire (FFQ) data is the only source of information on food consumption, including DF. FFQs are known to contain measurement errors, a reason why energy intake should be included as a covariate in the models to achieve the equivalent of an isoenergetic diet and thereby overcome this problem.

The evidence available shows that the intake of foods that are high in fiber has clear benefits regarding lipid profile and other cardiovascular risk factors. Although some studies of fiber supplements have shown positive effects on the lipid profile, the number of adults who adhere to the use of fiber supplements tends to be low. Likewise, these effects are modest when compared with a whole foods approach that encourages the consumption of fiber-rich foods.

Epidemiologic studies show that intact fruit, vegetables, whole grains, nuts and legumes, all of which are rich in potentially cardioprotective components, protect the body from cardiovascular diseases and mortality. There is debate in relation to cereals that are especially rich in insoluble fiber, but some studies have shown an inverse association between their intake and blood pressure. However, in clinical studies, only soluble viscous fiber has been demonstrated to have metabolic advantages. This paradox can be explained by the fact that food rich in fiber contains other phytochemical compounds that have been demonstrated to modulate inflammation, oxidation, insulin resistance and cholesterol metabolism.

Consequently, a Mediterranean-style diet rich in fiber-rich foods should be recommended to reduce the risk of cardiovascular disease.

7. Acknowledgments

The authors are grateful for the support granted by the Spanish Minister of Health (RETIC G03/140 and RD06/0045), the Spanish Minister of Science and Innovation (AGL2010-22319-C03-02), the FIS 070473, Centro Nacional de Investigaciones Cardiovasculares (CNIC06) and CIBEROBN that is an initiative of Instituto de Salud Carlos III, Spain. Sara Arranz received support from the Sara Borrell postdoctoral program with reference CD10/00151 supported by the Instituto de Salud Carlos III, Spain.

8. References

Ajani, U. A., Ford, E. S., & Mokdad, A. H. (2004). Dietary fiber and C-reactive protein: findings from national health and nutrition examination survey data. *The Journal of nutrition, 134*(5), 1181-1185.

Aleixandre, A., & Miguel, M. (2008). Dietary fiber in the prevention and treatment of metabolic syndrome: a review. *Critical reviews in food science and nutrition, 48*(10), 905-912.

Alfieri, M. A., Pomerleau, J., Grace, D. M., & Anderson, L. (1995). Fiber intake of normal weight, moderately obese and severely obese subjects. *Obesity research, 3*(6), 541-547.

Anderson, J. W. (2003). Whole grains protect against atherosclerotic cardiovascular disease. *The Proceedings of the Nutrition Society, 62*(1), 135-142.

Anderson, J. W. (2000). Dietary fiber prevents carbohydrate-induced hypertriglyceridemia. *Current atherosclerosis reports, 2*(6), 536-541.

Anderson, J. W. et al. (2000). Cholesterol-lowering effects of psyllium intake adjunctive to diet therapy in men and women with hypercholesterolemia: meta-analysis of 8 controlled trials. *The American Journal of Clinical Nutrition, 71*(2), 472-479.

Anderson, J. W., Deakins, D. A., Floore, T. L., Smith, B. M., & Whitis, S. E. (1990). Dietary fiber and coronary heart disease. *Critical reviews in food science and nutrition, 29*(2), 95-147.

Anderson, J. W., Story, L., Sieling, B., Chen, W. J., Petro, M. S., & Story, J. (1984). Hypocholesterolemic effects of oat-bran or bean intake for hypercholesterolemic men. *The American Journal of Clinical Nutrition, 40*(6), 1146-1155.

Appleby, P. N., Thorogood, M., Mann, J. I., & Key, T. J. (1998). Low body mass index in non-meat eaters: the possible roles of animal fat, dietary fibre and alcohol. *International journal of obesity and related metabolic disorders : journal of the International Association for the Study of Obesity, 22*(5), 454-460.

Ascherio, A. et al. (1992). A prospective study of nutritional factors and hypertension among US men. *Circulation, 86*(5), 1475-1484.

Ascherio, A. et al. (1998). Intake of potassium, magnesium, calcium, and fiber and risk of stroke among US men. *Circulation, 98*(12), 1198-1204.

Asp, N. G., van Amelsvoort, J. M., & Hautvast, J. G. (1996). Nutritional implications of resistant starch. *Nutrition research reviews, 9*(1), 1-31.

Barclay, A. W. et al. (2008). Glycemic index, glycemic load, and chronic disease risk--a meta-analysis of observational studies. *The American Journal of Clinical Nutrition, 87*(3), 627-637.

Beilin, L. J. (1994). Vegetarian and other complex diets, fats, fiber, and hypertension. *The American Journal of Clinical Nutrition, 59*(5 Suppl), 1130S-1135S.

Berg, C. M. et al. (2008). Food patterns and cardiovascular disease risk factors: the Swedish INTERGENE research program. *The American Journal of Clinical Nutrition, 88*(2), 289-297.

Birketvedt, G. S., Aaseth, J., Florholmen, J. R., & Ryttig, K. (2000). Long-term effect of fibre supplement and reduced energy intake on body weight and blood lipids in overweight subjects. *Acta Medica (Hradec Kralove) / Universitas Carolina, Facultas Medica Hradec Kralove, 43*(4), 129-132.

Birketvedt, G. S., Shimshi, M., Erling, T., & Florholmen, J. (2005). Experiences with three different fiber supplements in weight reduction. *Medical science monitor : international medical journal of experimental and clinical research, 11*(1), PI5-8.

Bravo, L. (1998). Polyphenols: chemistry, dietary sources, metabolism, and nutritional significance. *Nutrition reviews, 56*(11), 317-333.

Brighenti, F. (2007). Dietary fructans and serum triacylglycerols: a meta-analysis of randomized controlled trials. *The Journal of nutrition, 137*(11 Suppl), 2552S-2556S.

Brown, L., Rosner, B., Willett, W. W., & Sacks, F. M. (1999). Cholesterol-lowering effects of dietary fiber: a meta-analysis. *The American Journal of Clinical Nutrition, 69*(1), 30-42.

Butcher, J. L., & Beckstrand, R. L. (2010). Fiber's impact on high-sensitivity C-reactive protein levels in cardiovascular disease. *Journal of the American Academy of Nurse Practitioners, 22*(11), 566-572.

Buttriss, J. L., & Benelam, B. (2010). Nutrition and health claims: the role of food composition data. *European journal of clinical nutrition, 64 Suppl 3*, S8-13.

Champ,M., Kozlowski,F. and Lecannu,G. (2001). In-vivo and in-vitro methods for resistant starch measurement. In McCleary,B., Prosky,L., *Advanced dietary fibre technology.*(pp. 106-119)Blackwell Science, Oxford.

Champ,M., Langkilde,A.M., Brouns,F., Kettlitz,B. and Le Bail Collet,Y. (2003). Advances in dietary fiber characterization. 1. Definition of dietary fiber, physiological relevance, health benefits and analytical aspects. *Nutrition Research Reviews*, 16, 71-82.

Chandalia, M., Garg, A., Lutjohann, D., von Bergmann, K., Grundy, S. M., & Brinkley, L. J. (2000). Beneficial effects of high dietary fiber intake in patients with type 2 diabetes mellitus. *The New England journal of medicine, 342*(19), 1392-1398.

Cho, S., DeVries, J. and Prosky, L. (1997). Dietary fiber analysis and applications. *AOAC International*, Gaithersburg, Maryland.

Craig, W. J. (1997). Phytochemicals: guardians of our health. *Journal of the American Dietetic Association, 97*(10 Suppl 2), S199-204.

Crim, K. C. et al. (2008). Upregulation of p21Waf1/Cip1 expression in vivo by butyrate administration can be chemoprotective or chemopromotive depending on the lipid component of the diet. *Carcinogenesis, 29*(7), 1415-1420.

Cummings, J. H., & Macfarlane, G. T. (1991). The control and consequences of bacterial fermentation in the human colon. *The Journal of applied bacteriology, 70*(6), 443-459.

de Castro, T. G., Gimeno, S. G., Ferreira, S. R., Cardoso, M. A., & Japanese Brazilian Diabetes Study Group. (2006). Association of dietary fiber with temporal changes in serum cholesterol in Japanese-Brazilians. *Journal of nutritional science and vitaminology, 52*(3), 205-210.

de Munter, J. S., Hu, F. B., Spiegelman, D., Franz, M., & van Dam, R. M. (2007). Whole grain, bran, and germ intake and risk of type 2 diabetes: a prospective cohort study and systematic review. *PLoS medicine, 4*(8), e261.

Edwards, C. A., & Parrett, A. M. (2003). Dietary fibre in infancy and childhood. *The Proceedings of the Nutrition Society, 62*(1), 17-23.

EFSA (European Food Safety Authority). (2007). Statement of the Scientific Panel on Dietetic Products, Nutrition and Allergies related to dietary fibre.

EFSA Panel on Dietetic Products, Nutrition, and Allergies (NDA). (2010). Scientific Opinion on Dietary Reference Values for carbohydrates and dietary fibre. *8(3)*, 1462.

Elmadfa, I. (2009). European Nutrition and Health Report 2009. Preface. *Forum of nutrition, 62*, vii-viii.

Englyst, H. N., Wiggins, H. S., & Cummings, J. H. (1982). Determination of the nonstarch polysaccharides in plant foods by gas- liquid chromatography of constituents sugars as alditol acetates. *107*, 307-318.

Englyst, H.N. and Hudson, G.J. (1996). The classification and measurement of dietary carbohydrates. *57*, 15-21.

Englyst, K. N., & Englyst, H. N. (2005). Carbohydrate bioavailability. *The British journal of nutrition, 94*(1), 1-11.

Englyst, K. N., Liu, S., & Englyst, H. N. (2007). Nutritional characterization and measurement of dietary carbohydrates. *European journal of clinical nutrition, 61 Suppl 1*, S19-39.

Esposito, K. et al. (2004). Effect of a mediterranean-style diet on endothelial dysfunction and markers of vascular inflammation in the metabolic syndrome: a randomized trial. *JAMA : the journal of the American Medical Association, 292*(12), 1440-1446.

Estruch, R. et al. (2009). Effects of dietary fibre intake on risk factors for cardiovascular disease in subjects at high risk. *Journal of epidemiology and community health, 63*(7), 582-588.

FAO. INFOODS Food Composition Database for Biodiversity, Available from: <http://www.fao.org>

FAO/WHO (Food and Agriculture Organization/World Health Organization). (1998). Carbohydrates in human nutrition. Report of a Joint FAO/WHO expert consultation.

Fung, T. T. et al. (2002). Whole-grain intake and the risk of type 2 diabetes: a prospective study in men. *The American Journal of Clinical Nutrition, 76*(3), 535-540.

Fung, T. T., Willett, W. C., Stampfer, M. J., Manson, J. E., & Hu, F. B. (2001). Dietary patterns and the risk of coronary heart disease in women. *Archives of Internal Medicine, 161*(15), 1857-1862.

Gao, X., Bermudez, O. I., & Tucker, K. L. (2004). Plasma C-reactive protein and homocysteine concentrations are related to frequent fruit and vegetable intake in Hispanic and non-Hispanic white elders. *The Journal of nutrition, 134*(4), 913-918.

Giacco, R. et al. (2000). Long-term dietary treatment with increased amounts of fiber-rich low-glycemic index natural foods improves blood glucose control and reduces the number of hypoglycemic events in type 1 diabetic patients. *Diabetes care, 23*(10), 1461-1466.

Hall, J., Hammerich, K., & Roberts, P. (2010). New paradigms in the management of diverticular disease. *Current problems in surgery, 47*(9), 680-735.

He, J., & Whelton, P. K. (1999). Effect of dietary fiber and protein intake on blood pressure: a review of epidemiologic evidence. *Clinical and experimental hypertension (New York, N.Y.: 1993), 21*(5-6), 785-796.

Howarth, N. C., Saltzman, E., & Roberts, S. B. (2001). Dietary fiber and weight regulation. *Nutrition reviews, 59*(5), 129-139.

Hu, F. B. et al. (2001). Diet, lifestyle, and the risk of type 2 diabetes mellitus in women. *The New England journal of medicine, 345*(11), 790-797.

Hu, F. B., Rimm, E. B., Stampfer, M. J., Ascherio, A., Spiegelman, D., & Willett, W. C. (2000). Prospective study of major dietary patterns and risk of coronary heart disease in men. *The American Journal of Clinical Nutrition, 72*(4), 912-921.

Hu, F. B., & Willett, W. C. (2002). Optimal diets for prevention of coronary heart disease. *JAMA : the journal of the American Medical Association, 288*(20), 2569-2578.

IoM (Institute of Medicine). (2005). Dietary reference intakes for energy, carbohydrate, fiber, fat, fatty acids, cholesterol, protein, and amino acids.

Jacobs, D. R.,Jr, Meyer, K. A., Kushi, L. H., & Folsom, A. R. (1998). Whole-grain intake may reduce the risk of ischemic heart disease death in postmenopausal women: the Iowa Women's Health Study. *The American Journal of Clinical Nutrition, 68*(2), 248-257.

Jacobs, D. R., Pereira, M. A., Meyer, K. A., & Kushi, L. H. (2000). Fiber from whole grains, but not refined grains, is inversely associated with all-cause mortality in older women: the Iowa women's health study. *Journal of the American College of Nutrition, 19*(3 Suppl), 326S-330S.

Jenkins, D. J., Kendall, C. W., Axelsen, M., Augustin, L. S., & Vuksan, V. (2000). Viscous and nonviscous fibres, nonabsorbable and low glycaemic index carbohydrates, blood lipids and coronary heart disease. *Current opinion in lipidology, 11*(1), 49-56.

Jenkins, D. J. et al. (2003). Effects of a dietary portfolio of cholesterol-lowering foods vs lovastatin on serum lipids and C-reactive protein. *JAMA : the journal of the American Medical Association, 290*(4), 502-510.

Jenkins, D. J. et al. (2008). Effect of a low-glycemic index or a high-cereal fiber diet on type 2 diabetes: a randomized trial. *JAMA : the journal of the American Medical Association, 300*(23), 2742-2753.

Jones, P. J., Leitch, C. A., & Pederson, R. A. (1993). Meal-frequency effects on plasma hormone concentrations and cholesterol synthesis in humans. *The American Journal of Clinical Nutrition, 57*(6), 868-874.

Juntunen, K. S., Laaksonen, D. E., Poutanen, K. S., Niskanen, L. K., & Mykkanen, H. M. (2003). High-fiber rye bread and insulin secretion and sensitivity in healthy postmenopausal women. *The American Journal of Clinical Nutrition, 77*(2), 385-391.

Kasim-Karakas, S. E., Tsodikov, A., Singh, U., & Jialal, I. (2006). Responses of inflammatory markers to a low-fat, high-carbohydrate diet: effects of energy intake. *The American Journal of Clinical Nutrition, 83*(4), 774-779.

King, D. E., Egan, B. M., & Geesey, M. E. (2003). Relation of dietary fat and fiber to elevation of C-reactive protein. *The American Journal of Cardiology, 92*(11), 1335-1339.

Koh-Banerjee, P. et al. (2004). Changes in whole-grain, bran, and cereal fiber consumption in relation to 8-y weight gain among men. *The American Journal of Clinical Nutrition, 80*(5), 1237-1245.

Krishnan, S. et al. (2007). Glycemic index, glycemic load, and cereal fiber intake and risk of type 2 diabetes in US black women. *Archives of Internal Medicine, 167*(21), 2304-2309.

Kromhout, D., Bloemberg, B., Seidell, J. C., Nissinen, A., & Menotti, A. (2001). Physical activity and dietary fiber determine population body fat levels: the Seven Countries Study. *International journal of obesity and related metabolic disorders : journal of the International Association for the Study of Obesity, 25*(3), 301-306.

Lairon, D. (2007). Dietary fiber and control of body weight. *Nutrition, metabolism, and cardiovascular diseases : NMCD, 17*(1), 1-5.

Lau, C. et al. (2005). Dietary glycemic index, glycemic load, fiber, simple sugars, and insulin resistance: the Inter99 study. *Diabetes care, 28*(6), 1397-1403.

Liese, A. D. et al. (2005). Dietary glycemic index and glycemic load, carbohydrate and fiber intake, and measures of insulin sensitivity, secretion, and adiposity in the Insulin Resistance Atherosclerosis Study. *Diabetes care, 28*(12), 2832-2838.

Liu, S. (2003). Whole-grain foods, dietary fiber, and type 2 diabetes: searching for a kernel of truth. *The American Journal of Clinical Nutrition, 77*(3), 527-529.

Liu, S., Buring, J. E., Sesso, H. D., Rimm, E. B., Willett, W. C., & Manson, J. E. (2002). A prospective study of dietary fiber intake and risk of cardiovascular disease among women. *Journal of the American College of Cardiology, 39*(1), 49-56.

Liu, S., Manson, J.E., Stampfer, M.J., Rexrode, K.M., Hu, F.B., Rimm, E.B. & Willett, W.C. (2000). Whole grain consumption and risk of ischemic stroke in women: A prospective study. *JAMA : the journal of the American Medical Association, 284*(12), 1534-1540.

Ludwig, D. S. et al. (1999). Dietary fiber, weight gain, and cardiovascular disease risk factors in young adults. *JAMA : the journal of the American Medical Association, 282*(16), 1539-1546.

Maki, K. C., Davidson, M. H., Witchger, M. S., Dicklin, M. R., & Subbaiah, P. V. (2007). Effects of high-fiber oat and wheat cereals on postprandial glucose and lipid responses in healthy men. *International journal for vitamin and nutrition research.Internationale Zeitschrift fur Vitamin- und Ernahrungsforschung.Journal international de vitaminologie et de nutrition, 77*(5), 347-356.

Manas, E., & Saura-Calixto, F. (1995). Dietary fibre analysis: methodological error sources. *European journal of clinical nutrition, 49 Suppl 3*, S158-62.

Mann, J. (2007). Dietary carbohydrate: relationship to cardiovascular disease and disorders of carbohydrate metabolism. *European journal of clinical nutrition, 61 Suppl 1*, S100-11.

Marlett, J. A. (1992). Content and composition of dietary fiber in 117 frequently consumed foods. *Journal of the American Dietetic Association, 92*(2), 175-186.

McMillan-Price, J. et al. (2006). Comparison of 4 diets of varying glycemic load on weight loss and cardiovascular risk reduction in overweight and obese young adults: a randomized controlled trial. *Archives of Internal Medicine, 166*(14), 1466-1475.

Meyer, D., & Stasse-Wolthuis, M. (2009). The bifidogenic effect of inulin and oligofructose and its consequences for gut health. *European journal of clinical nutrition, 63*(11), 1277-1289.

Meyer, K. A., Kushi, L. H., Jacobs, D. R.,Jr, Slavin, J., Sellers, T. A., & Folsom, A. R. (2000). Carbohydrates, dietary fiber, and incident type 2 diabetes in older women. *The American Journal of Clinical Nutrition, 71*(4), 921-930.

Miller, W. C., Niederpruem, M. G., Wallace, J. P., & Lindeman, A. K. (1994). Dietary fat, sugar, and fiber predict body fat content. *Journal of the American Dietetic Association, 94*(6), 612-615.

Morgan, L. M., Tredger, J. A., Shavila, Y., Travis, J. S., & Wright, J. (1993). The effect of non-starch polysaccharide supplementation on circulating bile acids, hormone and metabolite levels following a fat meal in human subjects. *The British journal of nutrition, 70*(2), 491-501.

Mozaffarian, D., Kumanyika, S. K., Lemaitre, R. N., Olson, J. L., Burke, G. L., & Siscovick, D. S. (2003). Cereal, fruit, and vegetable fiber intake and the risk of cardiovascular disease in elderly individuals. *JAMA : the journal of the American Medical Association, 289*(13), 1659-1666.

Murakami, K., Okubo, H., & Sasaki, S. (2005). Effect of dietary factors on incidence of type 2 diabetes: a systematic review of cohort studies. *Journal of nutritional science and vitaminology, 51*(4), 292-310.

National Academies Press, Available from: <www.nap.edu>

Newby, P. K., Maras, J., Bakun, P., Muller, D., Ferrucci, L., & Tucker, K. L. (2007). Intake of whole grains, refined grains, and cereal fiber measured with 7-d diet records and associations with risk factors for chronic disease. *The American Journal of Clinical Nutrition, 86*(6), 1745-1753.

North, C. J., Venter, C. S., & Jerling, J. C. (2009). The effects of dietary fibre on C-reactive protein, an inflammation marker predicting cardiovascular disease. *European journal of clinical nutrition, 63*(8), 921-933.

Oh, K. et al. (2005). Carbohydrate intake, glycemic index, glycemic load, and dietary fiber in relation to risk of stroke in women. *American Journal of Epidemiology, 161*(2), 161-169.

Oliveira, A., Rodriguez-Artalejo, F., & Lopes, C. (2009). The association of fruits, vegetables, antioxidant vitamins and fibre intake with high-sensitivity C-reactive protein: sex and body mass index interactions. *European journal of clinical nutrition, 63*(11), 1345-1352.

Pereira, M. A. et al. (2002). Effect of whole grains on insulin sensitivity in overweight hyperinsulinemic adults. *The American Journal of Clinical Nutrition, 75*(5), 848-855.

Pereira, M. A., & Ludwig, D. S. (2001). Dietary fiber and body-weight regulation. Observations and mechanisms. *Pediatric clinics of North America, 48*(4), 969-980.

Pereira, M. A. et al. (2004). Dietary fiber and risk of coronary heart disease: a pooled analysis of cohort studies. *Archives of Internal Medicine, 164*(4), 370-376.

Pittler, M. H., & Ernst, E. (2001). Guar gum for body weight reduction: meta-analysis of randomized trials. *The American Journal of Medicine, 110*(9), 724-730.

Prosky, L. (1999). Inulin and oligofructose are part of the dietary fiber complex. *Journal of AOAC International, 82*(2), 223-226.

Prosky, L., Asp, N. G., Schweizer, T. F., DeVries, J. W., & Furda, I. (1988). Determination of insoluble, soluble, and total dietary fiber in foods and food products: interlaboratory study. *Journal - Association of Official Analytical Chemists, 71*(5), 1017-1023.

Rimm, E. B., Ascherio, A., Giovannucci, E., Spiegelman, D., Stampfer, M. J., & Willett, W. C. (1996). Vegetable, fruit, and cereal fiber intake and risk of coronary heart disease among men. *JAMA : the journal of the American Medical Association, 275*(6), 447-451.

Roberfroid, M. et al. (2010). Prebiotic effects: metabolic and health benefits. *The British journal of nutrition, 104 Suppl 2*, S1-63.

Rodriguez-Moran, M., Guerrero-Romero, F., & Lazcano-Burciaga, G. (1998). Lipid- and glucose-lowering efficacy of Plantago Psyllium in type II diabetes. *Journal of diabetes and its complications, 12*(5), 273-278.

Roy, S., Freake, H. C., & Fernandez, M. L. (2002). Gender and hormonal status affect the regulation of hepatic cholesterol 7alpha-hydroxylase activity and mRNA abundance by dietary soluble fiber in the guinea pig. *Atherosclerosis, 163*(1), 29-37.

Salas-Salvado, J., Bullo, M., Perez-Heras, A., & Ros, E. (2006). Dietary fibre, nuts and cardiovascular diseases. *The British journal of nutrition, 96 Suppl 2*, S46-51.

Salas-Salvado, J. et al. (2008). Effect of two doses of a mixture of soluble fibres on body weight and metabolic variables in overweight or obese patients: a randomised trial. *The British journal of nutrition, 99*(6), 1380-1387.

Salmeron, J., Manson, J. E., Stampfer, M. J., Colditz, G. A., Wing, A. L., & Willett, W. C. (1997). Dietary fiber, glycemic load, and risk of non-insulin-dependent diabetes mellitus in women. *JAMA : the journal of the American Medical Association, 277*(6), 472-477.

Saura-Calixto F. (1988). Effect of condensed tannins in the analysis of dietary fiber in carob pods. *53*, 1769-1771.

Saura-Calixto, F., Garcia-Alonso, A., Goni, I., & Bravo, L. (2000). In vitro determination of the indigestible fraction in foods: an alternative to dietary fiber analysis. *Journal of Agricultural and Food Chemistry, 48*(8), 3342-3347.

Schulze, M. B., Schulz, M., Heidemann, C., Schienkiewitz, A., Hoffmann, K., & Boeing, H. (2007). Fiber and magnesium intake and incidence of type 2 diabetes: a prospective study and meta-analysis. *Archives of Internal Medicine, 167*(9), 956-965.

Sievenpiper, J. L. et al. (2009). Effect of non-oil-seed pulses on glycaemic control: a systematic review and meta-analysis of randomised controlled experimental trials in people with and without diabetes. *Diabetologia, 52*(8), 1479-1495.

Slavin, J. L. (2005). Dietary fiber and body weight. *Nutrition (Burbank, Los Angeles County, Calif.), 21*(3), 411-418.

Slavin, J. L., Martini, M. C., Jacobs, D. R.,Jr, & Marquart, L. (1999). Plausible mechanisms for the protectiveness of whole grains. *The American Journal of Clinical Nutrition, 70*(3 Suppl), 459S-463S.

Slavin, J. L., Savarino, V., Paredes-Diaz, A., & Fotopoulos, G. (2009). A review of the role of soluble fiber in health with specific reference to wheat dextrin. *The Journal of international medical research, 37*(1), 1-17.

Sola, R. et al. (2007). Effects of soluble fiber (Plantago ovata husk) on plasma lipids, lipoproteins, and apolipoproteins in men with ischemic heart disease. *The American Journal of Clinical Nutrition, 85*(4), 1157-1163.

Spieth, L. E. et al. (2000). A low-glycemic index diet in the treatment of pediatric obesity. *Archives of Pediatrics & Adolescent Medicine, 154*(9), 947-951.

Streppel, M. T., Arends, L. R., van 't Veer, P., Grobbee, D. E., & Geleijnse, J. M. (2005). Dietary fiber and blood pressure: a meta-analysis of randomized placebo-controlled trials. *Archives of Internal Medicine, 165*(2), 150-156.

Streppel, M. T., Ocke, M. C., Boshuizen, H. C., Kok, F. J., & Kromhout, D. (2008). Dietary fiber intake in relation to coronary heart disease and all-cause mortality over 40 y: the Zutphen Study. *The American Journal of Clinical Nutrition, 88*(4), 1119-1125.

Thomas, D., & Elliott, E. J. (2009). Low glycaemic index, or low glycaemic load, diets for diabetes mellitus. *Cochrane database of systematic reviews (Online), (1)*(1), CD006296.

Todd, S., Woodward, M., Tunstall-Pedoe, H., & Bolton-Smith, C. (1999). Dietary antioxidant vitamins and fiber in the etiology of cardiovascular disease and all-causes mortality: results from the Scottish Heart Health Study. *American Journal of Epidemiology, 150*(10), 1073-1080.

Toeller, M., Buyken, A. E., Heitkamp, G., de Pergola, G., Giorgino, F., & Fuller, J. H. (1999). Fiber intake, serum cholesterol levels, and cardiovascular disease in European individuals with type 1 diabetes. EURODIAB IDDM Complications Study Group. *Diabetes care, 22 Suppl 2*, B21-8.

Trowell, H. (1972). Ischemic heart disease and dietary fiber. *The American Journal of Clinical Nutrition, 25*(9), 926-932.

Trowell, H., Southgate, D. A., Wolever, T. M., Leeds, A. R., Gassull, M. A., & Jenkins, D. J. (1976). Letter: Dietary fibre redefined. *Lancet, 1*(7966), 967.

Truswell, A. S. (2002). Cereal grains and coronary heart disease. *European journal of clinical nutrition, 56*(1), 1-14.

Tucker, L. A., & Thomas, K. S. (2009). Increasing total fiber intake reduces risk of weight and fat gains in women. *The Journal of nutrition, 139*(3), 576-581.

USDA. National Nutrient Database for Standard Reference, Release 23, Available from: <http://www.ars.usda.gov>

van Dam, R. M., Grievink, L., Ocke, M. C., & Feskens, E. J. (2003). Patterns of food consumption and risk factors for cardiovascular disease in the general Dutch population. *The American Journal of Clinical Nutrition, 77*(5), 1156-1163.

van Dam, R. M., Hu, F. B., Rosenberg, L., Krishnan, S., & Palmer, J. R. (2006). Dietary calcium and magnesium, major food sources, and risk of type 2 diabetes in U.S. black women. *Diabetes care, 29*(10), 2238-2243.

Venn, B. J., & Mann, J. I. (2004). Cereal grains, legumes and diabetes. *European journal of clinical nutrition, 58*(11), 1443-1461.

Weickert, M. O. et al. (2006). Cereal fiber improves whole-body insulin sensitivity in overweight and obese women. *Diabetes care, 29*(4), 775-780.

Willett, W. C. et al. (1995). Mediterranean diet pyramid: a cultural model for healthy eating. *The American Journal of Clinical Nutrition, 61*(6 Suppl), 1402S-1406S.

Wilson, A. J. et al. (2010). Apoptotic sensitivity of colon cancer cells to histone deacetylase inhibitors is mediated by an Sp1/Sp3-activated transcriptional program involving immediate-early gene induction. *Cancer research, 70*(2), 609-620.

Wolever, T. M. et al. (2008). Low glycaemic index diet and disposition index in type 2 diabetes (the Canadian trial of carbohydrates in diabetes): a randomised controlled trial. *Diabetologia, 51*(9), 1607-1615.

Wolever, T. M., Spadafora, P. J., Cunnane, S. C., & Pencharz, P. B. (1995). Propionate inhibits incorporation of colonic [1,2-13C]acetate into plasma lipids in humans. *The American Journal of Clinical Nutrition, 61*(6), 1241-1247.

Wong, J. M., de Souza, R., Kendall, C. W., Emam, A., & Jenkins, D. J. (2006). Colonic health: fermentation and short chain fatty acids. *Journal of clinical gastroenterology, 40*(3), 235-243.

Wu, H., Dwyer, K. M., Fan, Z., Shircore, A., Fan, J., & Dwyer, J. H. (2003). Dietary fiber and progression of atherosclerosis: the Los Angeles Atherosclerosis Study. *The American Journal of Clinical Nutrition, 78*(6), 1085-1091.

9

"Recognizing Hunger" – A Training to Abate Insulin Resistance, Associated Subclinical Inflammation and Cardiovascular Risks

Mario Ciampolini
Università di Firenze,
Italy

1. Introduction

1.1 Background

People cannot share subjective sensations with others as they do with sounds and figures. Subjective sensations guide the intake. In this chapter, subjective sensations of hunger that induce intake, become objective (verifiable by others, reproducible and comparable) by the association with measurements of blood glucose concentration (BG). This is possible after about two weeks of training with BG measurements. Subjective sensations become thus a meal by meal information tool on energy balance. Respecting the arousal of the validated sensation before any intake was useful to treat infants with chronic non-specific diarrhea (Ciampolini et al. 1990). In a health policy for cardiovascular risk prevention, for a suppression of subclinical inflammation and for a decrease or maintenance of a stable body weight, treating functional intestinal disorders means treating a reversible condition like insulin resistance to prevent irreversible events. Functional intestinal disorders are also capable to give valid motivation to patients for training (see further "Training to...").

Subjective signals that promote intake are reported by many researchers (Harshaw, 2008). In past investigations, we suggested subjects to find a subjective target (initial hunger, IH) before intake on the first day, and measuring blood glucose concentration as a marker of this target on the first and subsequent days (Ciampolini & Bianchi, 2006a).

In our experience, less than 10% of healthy people report never perceiving any kind of hunger. No perception may depend on insulin resistance or non-insulin dependent diabetes (NIDD). With the word hunger, all over the world, healthy subjects report gastric pangs or sensations of gastric emptiness. In other circumstances, the subject's definition is inadequate. Subjects trained to "hunger recognition" were able to assess current value of blood glucose with a fairly low estimation error from measurement (Figure 1) both when they either recognized or denied hunger (Figure 2, Ciampolini & Bianchi, 2006a). Subjects who denied hunger, reported mental and/or physical sensations of weakness. They reported these sensations from 10% to 45% of instances of eating induction. In these instances, animals actually show a decrease of resting metabolic rate (RMR). In this report, with the term "initial hunger" (IH) we indicate gastric, physical and mental sensations that are associated with a low error of estimation of BG measurement after training (Ciampolini & Bianchi, 2006a).

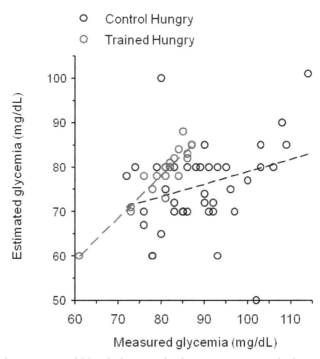

Fig. 1. Estimated *vs.* measured blood glucose of subjects reporting to be hungry at the final laboratory investigative session.

Hollow red circles, trained hungry subjects (n = 18); hollow black circles, control (untrained) hungry subjects (n = 42). Linear correlation was significant for the trained data (dashed red line; r = 0.92; p = 0.0001) but not for the control data (dashed black line; r = 0.29, p = 0.06). (By kind permission of the Authors: Ciampolini & Bianchi, 2006a).

We named intake adaptation to IH arousal before meals three times a day as initial hunger meal pattern (IHMP) (Ciampolini et al. 2010°; 2010b; Ciampolini & Sifone, 2011). This is a meal pattern based on "recognizing hunger". We use these two simple words in this report to be more evocative than by using the term IHMP. We chose the assessment of the validated sensation and of BG measurement before meals for six reasons: first, because before meals people sometimes recognise definite hunger sensations, and are able to validate them through BG measurement (Ciampolini & Bianchi, 2006a). Second, a BG measurement (as well as validated hunger sensations, initial hunger, IH) is an evaluation of either sufficiency or excess of energy intake at previous meal, and is useful in planning meal sizes (Ciampolini et al. 2010; 2010b; Ciampolini & Sifone, 2011). Third, 7 day-food-diary reporting consecutive 21 BG measurements and meal compositions may prove to be a highly effective educational instrument to evaluate intake meal by meal as suggested in point two. Fourth, a mean of pre-meal BG sequence informs on lowest mean energy availability for the body. "Mean BG" is a metabolic characterization of an individual, energy meal pattern (fifth), which is standard in metabolic time and allows comparisons and classifications better than daily energy intake (Ciampolini & Sifone, 2011). Sixth, mean BG measures the blood function of providing energy to body tissues (Ciampolini & Sifone, 2011).

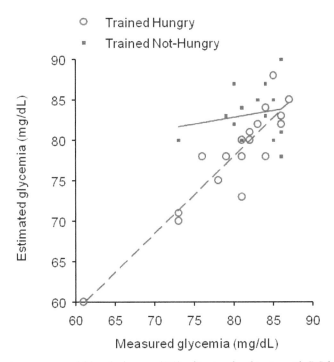

Fig. 2. Estimated *vs* measured blood glucose (BG) of trained subjects with BG below 87
mg/dL at the final session.
The highest BG measured in trained hungry subjects was 87 mg/dL. Below this value of measured BG,
18 subjects reported to be hungry (hollow red circles) and 14 subjects were not hungry (filled red
squares). The errors in estimation (estimated BG value less measured one) showed no significant
difference between the two groups. (By kind permission of the Authors: Ciampolini & Bianchi, 2006a).

Meal adaptation to "recognizing hunger" decreased mean BG, metabolic risks, insulin
resistance and overweight in the trained group compared to control subjects (Ciampolini et
al. 2010b). The global response in mean BG and the global improvement overlooks differences
in single meal patterns, insulin sensitivity and health at recruitment and in response to
training. If mean BG is maintained as a personal habit, the differences may explain huge risk
differences that can be personally felt and corrected by "recognizing hunger".

1.2 Investigation aims

After suspension of food intake and initial identification of the first sensation of hunger, can
a subject show a stable recognition of the same hunger sensation by coincidence between BG
estimation and measurement? Can a subject maintain a meal rhythm based on recognition
of the same subjective sensation (IH)? Can few subjects maintain the rhythm before any
training? Can the trained rhythm decrease metabolic risk factors? Can prevent malnutrition
and slightly depressed BG? Can decrease body weight in overweight people and in subjects
with insulin resistance? The demonstration of these effects show that the achieved rhythm
(mean BG) is homeostatic rather than being an artifact, i.e. maintains a BG that is constant and

both sufficient for activity and body weight maintenance, and effective in risk prevention. Informed people may approximate this *reference* model in eating as much as they can.

1.3 Subjects

A total of 181 subjects were recruited by the Paediatric Gastroenterology Unit of Florence University, a third level referring center, between 1995 and 2000 (Ciampolini et al. 2010). Subjects were gastroenterology patients between 18 and 60 years of age with functional bowel disorders, a self recovering disease. Subjects showed no morphological, physical or biochemical signs of organic disease. Subjects with impaired glucose tolerance (fasting plasma-glucose > 115 mg/dL (6.4 mmol/l)), as well as subjects suffering from non-insulin dependent diabetes mellitus (NIDDM), celiac, inflammatory bowel, liver, heart, brain and kidney diseases were excluded from recruitment. At end of investigation, 149 completed the protocol. 120 served for the metabolic study. All 149 were used for the body weight study. Informed consent was obtained from all participants. The local Hospital Ethics Committee approved the study in compliance with the Helsinki Declaration.

2. Metabolic study on 120 subjects

2.1 Design

All 120 subjects who completed the protocol were fully assessed at recruitment (before training), clinically only after the first 7 weeks of training, and completely at the end of the investigation (total investigation 5 months). In 31 control subjects, we investigated whether food intake is habitual, ie, maintaining the same meal pattern by "mean BG". Moreover, habits in BG maintenance may be personal, ie, sharply defined from most others. In all 120 subjects, we calculated mean confidence interval at recruitment (0.95%) for this purpose, and we stratified all 120 subjects in groups that contained subjects without significant differences in mean BG. Some subjects who had low mean BG at recruitment might fail any response to "recognizing hunger", because their meal pattern lowers mean BG to the point of imminent subjective insufficiency (see description of training) (Ciampolini et al. 2010a; 2010b; Ciampolini & Sifone, 2011). We decided to find the most significant cutoff point on the basis of individual response in mean BG (decrease), either significant or not. After finding the cutoff, we separately investigated (at recruitment and during "recognizing hunger" 5 months from recruitment, compared with controls) the association of subjects with low mean BG (LBG) and high mean BG (HBG) with insulin area under curve (AUC), and indices of insulin sensitivity and beta cell function (primary endpoints). Analyses were also performed on BG AUC, measurements of BG and insulin concentrations during oral glucose tolerance test (GTT), mean BG, and glycated hemoglobin (HbA1c) values (secondary endpoints). Data are presented post hoc division. Data without division have also been published and are not reported here (Ciampolini et al. 2010b).

2.2 Assessment of metabolic and health conditions

Additional analyses were performed on energy balance, cardiovascular status, well-being, and nutrition. i) Energy balance during the 5-month investigation interval was assessed through measurement of arm and leg skin-fold thickness changes, by measurements of body weight and body mass index (BMI) and by assessment of reported energy and vegetable intake (Ciampolini et al. 1987; Ciampolini et al. 1990; Ciampolini & Bianchi, 2006a; Ciampolini et al. 2010; 2010b; Ciampolini & Sifone, 2011) ii) Cardiovascular status was assessed by systolic and diastolic blood pressures, plasma LDL cholesterol/HDL cholesterol ratio, triglycerides, and HDL cholesterol. iii) Structured interviews ascertained the number of days in which each of five functional symptoms (diarrhea, vomiting, headache, epigastric or abdominal pain) occurred during the previous three months (Ciampolini et al. 1987; Ciampolini et al. 1990). The hours of daily physical activity and time spent in bed reported in the seven-day diary were also assessed. iv) Nutrition was assessed by monitoring blood hemoglobin (Hb), mean cellular volume (MCV), transferrin saturation, plasma ferritin, zinc, folates, and vitamin B12 (Ciampolini et al. 1990).

2.3 Training to "recognizing hunger"

The trained group exercised regularly under tutorial assistance for seven weeks, and maintained the new strategies of food consumption and energy expenditure for further three months without any assistance. On the first day, subjects suspended food intake until arousal of a sensation of hunger, generally epigastric hunger (Ciampolini & Bianchi, 2006a). Meal consumption delayed two hours in average, 0 - 48 hours in range. At first arousal subjects memorized the sensation, measured BG by a portable instrument (See, please later) and consumed a meal. The energy content was calibrated to a further hunger arousal before the planned, subsequent mealtime. After 3 – 14 days of this training, subjects became aware of current BG state before meals by sensations (Ciampolini et al. 2010; 2010b; Ciampolini & Sifone, 2011). After showing association with constant BG, we named the three sensations of epigastric hunger, physical or mental weakness as "Initial Hunger" (IH). IH was maintained pre-meal, adjusting meal sizes, composition or timing of food intake. After a few days of trials and errors, and sometimes irregular mealtimes, subjects were able to arrange their intake so that IH appeared before the usual three mealtimes per day with an average error of half-an-hour in 80% of instances in adults and 90% in children ("recognizing hunger" or initial hunger meal pattern, IHMP) (Ciampolini et al. 1987; Ciampolini et al. 1990; Ciampolini & Bianchi, 2006a; Ciampolini et al. 2010; 2010b; Ciampolini & Sifone, 2011; Ciampolini et al. 2001; Ciampolini, 2006b). Thus, subjects chose BG the first day on hunger sensations, in subsequent days learned the food amount per meal, and confirmed the chosen sensation as reference for intake by showing the same BG attainment before each meal. Both control (N = 31) and trained (N = 89) subjects had the same information on food energy contents, on recommended vegetable intake and physical activity amount per day.

2.4 BG measurements

Subjects measured by themselves capillary blood by glucometer (a portable device for whole blood glucose measurement: Glucocard Memory; Menarini Diagnostics; Florence, Italy) within the 15 minutes before each meal. Accuracy of measurements by the glucometer was validated against periodic measurements by hospital autoanalyzer. Subjects avoided BG measurements taken less than 1 hour after consuming even few grams of food, after changes in ambient temperature, after physical activity such as walking or cycling, or being feverish, or under psychic stress because BG in these circumstances is higher than 1 hour after cessation of the transient metabolic condition (Ciampolini & Bianchi, 2006a). Seven-day home diaries reported BG measurements before the three main meal times, energy and vegetable intake, hours in bed and hours spent during physical and outdoor activities (weekly mean and SD) and presence or absence of pre-prandial sensation of epigastric hunger (Ciampolini et al. 1987; Ciampolini et al. 1990; Ciampolini et al. 2001; Ciampolini & Bianchi, 2006a; Ciampolini, 2006b; Ciampolini & Sifone, 2011). Subjects compiled the diaries before training, after seven weeks and at the end of investigation. Our previous studies include more details on validation of BG estimation compared to BG measurements; comparison of energy intake and total energy expenditure as assessed by doubly labelled water in infants (Ciampolini, 2006b); glycated hemoglobin (HbA1c); methods for anthropometric measurements, structured interviews, and relevant clinical blood tests.

2.5 Preliminary findings and subgrouping

2.5.1 Stratification of 120 subjects by significant differences in mean pre-prandial BG

At recruitment, mean BG was distributed from 64.5 to 109.9 mg/dL in all 120 subjects, but the mean confidence interval (95%) of diary measurements around mean BG was ± 3.84 mg/dL. In Figure 3, all 120 subjects were stratified in ten groups by increasing mean BG at recruitment. Each of ten stratifications included subjects who showed no difference in mean for BG (P > 0.05), but excluded subjects who had significant differences (Armitage & Berry, 1994).

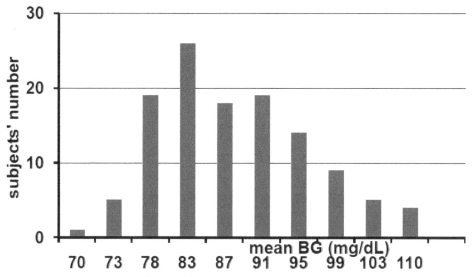

Fig. 3. Increasing sequence of mean blood glucose (mean BG) of all 120 trained and control subjects divided in 10 strata (columns) by significance of differences in mean BG at recruitment.
Strata consist of subjects with no significant difference in mean BG inside the stratum. Moreover each stratum excludes subsequent subjects whose mean BG is significantly higher than that of the first subject in the stratum. Column height shows the first component. Mean blood glucose reported in sequentially increasing order at recruitment, not in linear correlation with segment length on the x-axis scale. (By kind permission of the Authors: Ciampolini & Sifone, 2011).

2.5.2 Stability of mean BG in 31 control subjects

31 control subjects maintained a stable mean BG after 5 months (from 85.2 ± 8.1 mg/dL to 85.3 ± 7.6 mg/dL). The absolute pre/post change (increase or decrease) was 6.0 ± 4.6 mg/dL with a confidence interval (95%) from 3.1 mg/dL to 8.9 mg/dL.

2.5.3 LBG and HBG subgroups by response to "recognizing hunger"

Figure 4 shows the increasing mean BG sequence in 89 trained subjects and their response to "recognizing hunger" training. Significant decrease of mean BG by the end of the investigation occurred mainly in subjects with high mean BG at recruitment, whereas mean BG remained relatively constant in subjects with low BG at recruitment. A cutoff value (demarcation point) of mean BG that most significantly divided these two subgroups was identified, being 81.8 mg/dL (Figure 4: mean BG changes: post-minus pre-values as a function of the BG means at recruitment). 34 subjects below this "cutoff" (demarcation point) formed the low BG (LBG) subgroup. 55 subjects over this cutoff formed the high mean BG subgroup (HBG). Similarly, the BG value of 81.8 mg/dL was used to divide control subjects into LBG and HBG control subgroups (Tables 1 and 2).

2.6 Results from subgroups and discussion

2.6.1 Clinical events

About one third of subjects already maintained a mean LBG by free personal choice at recruitment. Others, motivated by bowel disorders, considered compliance as difficult before training and easy after training. Yet, the easy maintenance and the rapid recovery allowed sustained compliance. The functional disorder was significantly associated with high mean BG (and insulin resistance etc.) in HBG subjects, and possibly with high standard deviation of BG in LBG subjects (Table 2). In infants we suggested that positive balance of energy stimulates a diarrheic feedback (Ciampolini et al. 1990; Ciampolini et al. 1996). In the trained HBG group (Table 3), the decreases in days with abdominal pain or stomach-ache, were significant and significantly larger than in the control HBG group. In a national assistance design of risk prevention, recurrences of bowel disorder are sufficiently diffuse and sufficiently disturbing to motivate balance correction (training "recognizing hunger") and to improve insulin sensitivity in large part of population.

2.6.2 Stressful states

A large number of evidence shows an association between the emotional state of central nervous system and high levels of serotonin, cortisol, cortisol releasing factor and glucose in blood and/or mucosa (De Giorgio & Camilleri, 2004; Gershon, 1999; Spiller, 2008; Bischoff et al. 2009; van den Wijngaard et al. 2010; Wang et al. 2003; Lal et al. 2001; Ohman & Simrén, 2010; Spiller, 2008). These factors activate mast cells (Sand et al. 2009) and disrupt motility, secretion and absorption in mucosa (Dinan et al. 2006; Rana, 2009).

Persistence of these biological, infective stimuli and/or psychophysical stresses modify activity of monocytes, macrophages and mast cells, and together alter the neuro-endocrine system, and increase intestinal permeability. Bacterial biofilms may develop inside the alimentary canal and produce endotoxins that invade blood and all tissues (Ciampolini et al.

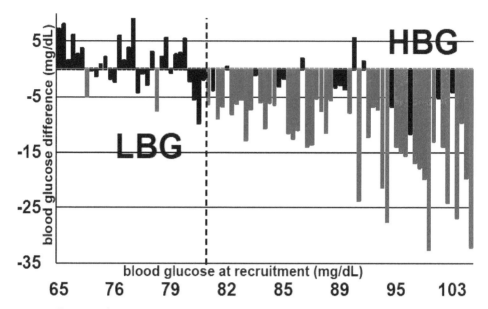

Fig. 4. Difference after training versus value in mean blood glucose for each trained subject at recruitment.

Column height shows 5-month post less pre mean blood glucose difference from 7d-diary in each trained subject. Significant decreases in red and not significant changes in black. Mean blood glucose reported in sequentially increasing order at recruitment, not in linear correlation with segment length on the x-axis scale. The dashed division indicates the most significant division between subjects who showed no mean blood glucose decrease after training (LBG group, n = 34 subjects) and those who showed significant decrease of mean blood glucose (HBG group, n = 55 subjects; χ2 analysis: P = 0.00001). This threshold blood glucose (demarcation point) is 81.8 mg/dl (4.5 mmol.l) at recruitment. (By kind permission of the Authors Ciampolini & Sifone, 2011).

1996). Locally, an inflammatory process develops in mucosa and may persist for months and years. (Tornblom et al. 2002; Ohman, L. & Simrén, 2010; Spiller, 2008). Locally, the process is minimal, because of intestinal tolerance (Brandtzaeg et al. 1989). Inside the intestine, a minority (10% - 20%) of bacterial species are immunogenic although being incapable of promoting a general illness such as Salmonella species do (van der Waaij et al. 1996). Immunogenic bacteria induce a huge biological activity of human immune system and a deep functional alteration (Reaven, 2006; Festa et al. 2000). Body tissues develop a pro-inflammatory state (subclinical inflammation, a synonym) that is sterile, ineffective and dangerous for body tissues in the intestine, vascular bed and elsewhere (Reaven, 2006; Festa et al. 2000). The invasion of body tissues by bacterial products and endotoxins sustains subclinical inflammation and causes the slow progression of many chronic diseases.

The start of the subclinical inflammatory process is controversial. Stress is associated with a condition of high BG and insulin resistance. This condition is causally associated with a "pro-inflammatory state" or "subclinical inflammation". General acceptance of this causal association took unfortunately 80 years (Kylin, 1923; Randle et al. 1963; Festa et al. 2000; Reaven, 2006). Stressed people may eat as usually, and even more, disregarding any hunger

"Recognizing Hunger" – A Training to Abate Insulin Resistance, Associated Subclinical
Inflammation and Cardiovascular Risks

167

or signs of low BG (Robbins & Fray, 1980; Flaa et al. 2008). This meal pattern can maintain intestinal disorders for years (Zwaigenbaum et al.1999), and may contribute to current epidemic of insulin resistance, obesity (Flaa et al. 2008), subclinical inflammation and vascular diseases (Reaven, 2006; Festa et al. 2000; Kahna et al. 2005; Cefalu, 2005; Moller & Flier, 1991; Mather & Verma, 2005; Weiss et al. 2004). On the contrary, "recognizing hunger" prescribes transient suspension of intake during stress and in the subsequent hours until BG lowering (Table 7). Implementation of "recognizing hunger" definitely stopped intestinal disorders in adults (Table 3) and relapses in children (Ciampolini et al. 1987; Ciampolini et al. 1990; Ciampolini et al. 1991; Ciampolini et al. 1994; Ciampolini et al. 1996; Ciampolini et al. 2000; Ciampolini & Sifone, 2011).

2.6.3 Subjective and objective assessments

The training was subjective. Subjects learned to recognize IH in the first day and adapted intake to the arousal of this target sensation three times a day. The BG association checked the consistency of the recognition ("recognizing hunger").

	Low BG group				High BG group			
	Control		Trained		Control		Trained	
	Recruit-ment	After 5 mo.	Recruit-ment	After 5 mo.	Recruit-ment	After 5 mo.	Recruit-ment	After 5 mo.
Number of subjects and Gender	8 F + 4 M		21 F +13 M		6 F + 13 M		25 F + 30 M	
Schooling (years)[1]	12.0±3.2		12.9±2.7		9.8±4.4		11.4±3.7	
Age (years)[1]	28.3±8.2		32.2±8.5		30.5±9.2		32.8±11.4	
BMI	21.8±3.4	21.9±3.1	22.6±3.3	22.0±2.7**,b	22.4±5.1	23.0±4.1	23.2±4.0	22.1±3.4**,a***,b
Weight (Kg)	57.5±8.4	57.7±8.9	62.4±11.1	60.8±9.9*,b	60.9±12.2	62.9±8.4	65.2±13.4	62.7±12.1**,a***,b
Arm skin-fold thickness (mm)	15.6±9.8	15.7±9.5	15.4±8.4	13.3±6.4*,b	14.9±10.2	13.9±7.2	16.4±7.9	12.8±6.0*,a*,b
Leg skin-fold thickness (mm)	21.7±13.5	21.7±13.4	20.1±10.8	17.3±8.0**,b	20.0±11.8	18.6±9.4	22.5±11.4	17.5±8.8*,a,**,b

Values are expressed as means ± SD. [1], values at the beginning of the study. Asterisks indicate a significant difference (Student's t-test: *, $P < 0.05$; **, $P < 0.01$; ***, $P < 0.001$) on pre/post difference $vs.$ respective control group (a), or $vs.$ value of the same group at recruitment (b).

Table 1. Group composition and effects of training on anthropometry in low and high BG subjects.

.	Low BG group				High BG group			
	Control		Trained		Control		Trained	
	Recruit-ment	After 5 mo.	Recruit-ment	After 5 mo.	Recruit-ment	After 5 mo.	Recruit-ment	After 5 mo.
Mean pre-meal BG (mg/dL)	76.9 ± 3.4	79.1±3.5	76.6±3.7	77.2±4.2	90.4±5.3	89.2±6.9	91.6±7.7***,c	81.0±7.7 ***,a ***,b
BG diary SD (mg/dL) [1]	7.6±2.3	8.7±1.7**b	6.8±3.0	5.4±2.3 *,a **,b	9.0±3.3	9.3±3.9	9.4±4.8**,c	6.6±2.6**,a ***,b
Glycated Hb (%)	4.38±0.29	4.53±0.35	4.50±0.30	4.43±0.31	4.65±0.38	4.83±0.39	4.81±0.44***, c	4.56±0.47 ***,a ***,b
Insulin AUC^2 (mU L^{-1}3h^{-1})	192±106	243±133	180±98	183±83*,a	222±81	215±98	244±138*,c	164±92**,a ***,b
Insulin peak (mU L^{-1})	66±30	83±41	62±44	58±30	75±33	68±36	79±46**,c	54±29*,a ***,b
Insulin sens. (index)^3	14.6±7.2	11.8±5.8	15.9±8.3	15.7±9.0	6,0±2.2	6,8 ± 3,9	5.9±3.3***,c	9.8±5.6**,a ***,b
Insulingenic index [4]	0.9 ±0.6	0.8±0.6	0.9±0.9	1.0±0.7	1.1±1.2	0.7±0.7	1.0±0.7	1.4±1.1*a *,b
BG AUC (mg/dL)	547±117	542±126	548±73	537±81	627±101	598±107	639±98***,c	567±91***, b
BG peak (mg/dL)	124±25	124±30	119±22	122±24	136±22	128±27	145±27***,c	128±27***, b
Energy intake (kcal/d)	1803±567	1565±677	1568±612	1303±590***, b	1887±599	1703±557	1872±655*,c	1251±470 ***,a ***,b
Meals per day^5	3.7±0.7	3.8±0.6	3.8±0.6	3.5±0.5**,b	4.0±0.7	3.9±0.7	3.9±0.7	3.7±0.7***, b
Vegetable intake (g/d)	272±265	292±223	388±257	492±217*,b	127±128	166±218	287±223*,c	392±251**, b
Fruit intake (g/d)	183±177	188±205	233±152	334±315	183±133	147±113	214±150	290±219*,a *,b

[1] diary SD refers to the mean of the mean BG standard deviations of 21 measurements reported by each of 7d diary.

[2] AUC = area under GTT curve.

[3] Whole body insulin sensitivity index (Matsuda & DeFronzo, 1999).

[4] Insulinogenic index of beta cell function (Wiesli et al. 2004).

[5] Meal was an event of higher intake than 20 kcal.

Values are expressed as mean ± SD. Peak values include different observations from those at 30' during GTT. *Asterisks* indicate a significant difference (Student's *t*-test: *, P < 0.05; **, P < 0.01; ***, P < 0.001) on pre/post difference *vs.* respective control group (*a*), or *vs.* the value of the same group at recruitment (*b*), or *vs.* the value of LBG trained group at recruitment (*c*).

Table 2. Effects of training on metabolic and intake parameters in low and high BG subjects

We assume that a week sequence of BG measurements before meals shows the least energy availability to body cells in that week, and the mean value at this metabolic moment represents the standardized parameter that we needed in the evaluation of habitual energy balance (meal pattern) in relation to its main function, provision of energy to body. Mean BG was maintained as a habit in control subjects, i.e. for a longer period than a week, and was personal, at different level from one person to another. Before initial abstinence from food (before training), HBG subjects habitually forestalled the arousal of the physiological regulation mechanism and maintained positive energy balance. On the basis of the high standard deviation of BG (Table 2 and 7), the meal pattern of untrained LBG subjects was irregular from a meal to another in comparison with during "recognizing hunger", despite of null balance, of low mean BG and weight stability in a long period (see, please, later). We cannot conclude that LBG coincided with "recognizing hunger" (See, please, later).

2.6.4 Unremitting adjustment to energy expenditure

The food diary with pre-prandial BG measurements served moreover as an educational instrument. We trained (and checked) "recognizing hunger" in adjusting intake to sensations meal by meal by the reported diary. Changes in skinfold thickness, i.e. five-month energy balance, showed reliability of the reported "recognizing hunger" (Tables 1 and 7). Within this view, dieting represents a rough attempt to achieve an ideal (?) weight without understanding and implementing the necessary meal by meal adjustments to expenditure.

2.6.5 Sufficient intake by "recognizing hunger"

As regards normal-weight subjects, trained HBG but not LBG subjects showed a cumulative balance that was negative in the 5 months, and the longitudinal difference was significant in comparison with control subjects (Table 7). The significant decrease of glycated hemoglobin (Table 2) and of body weight, BMI and arm and leg skin-fold thickness in HBG group and the stability of LBG group (Table 7), confirmed the persistence of reliability throughout 5 months of this investigation, and also the meal adjustments by "recognizing hunger" to expenditure. The maintenance of previous physical activities in all trained subjects and the improvement in nutrition parameters in HBG subgroup (Table 3) demonstrate that meals taken by trained subjects were sufficient to meet energy needs. This confirms earlier controlled, randomised studies in children with chronic non-specific diarrhea, in which daily activity was preserved and body weight increased normally after seven months, 4 years and 12 years of complying with a pediatric adaptation of the present training (Ciampolini et al. 1990).

We adapted "recognizing hunger" to infants, and the initial request of children substituted initial hunger (Initial Request Meal Pattern, IRMP) (Ciampolini et al. 1990). In 73 infants (Ciampolini, 2006b), the cutoff at 81.2 mg/dL divided subjects with low mean BG from those with high mean BG at recruitment by the highest significance. By this division, 18 infants showed low mean BG and 55 infants showed high mean BG at recruitment. This cutoff in infants is quite similar to the cutoff (81.8 mg/dL) that we found in adults in the present chapter and to the cutoff found in prevention of non-insulin dependent diabetes in Israeli recruits (Tirosh et al. 2005).

In the same preliminary work (Ciampolini, 2006b), we reported a significant 15% – 16% decrease in RMR by respiratory calorimetry and in total daily expenditure (TDE) by doubly labeled water in 24 infants from before training to during IRMP (Ciampolini, 2006b). IRMP decreases mean BG, RMR and TDE in infants. We interpreted the three decreases during IRMP (Vs. meal pattern at recruitment) as an elimination of forestalling IH, i.e. leaving behind meal by meal positive balance and acquiring null balance in blood. Taking together the investigations on children and adults, "recognizing hunger" decreased mean BG, RMR and TDE, meal by meal positive balance in blood, insulin resistance, intestinal disorders, and vascular risks (subclinical inflammation). Table 4 has not been published, except for 6 groups. There are findings on mean BG from 9 different groups.

		Control		Trained	
		Recruitment	After 5 mo.	Recruitment	After 5 mo.
Well being trial	Vomiting (days with vom./90 days)	0.1±0.3	0.1±0.2	0.2±0.9	0.1±0.5
	Headache (days with pain/90 days)	12.3±27.8	8.8±20.9	6.2±13.4	1.9±4.9**,b
	Diarrhoea (days with diarrhoea/90 days)	2.0±0.6	0.6±1.4	5.6±15.7	0.6±2.8 **,b
	Abdominal pain (days with pain/90 days)	5.8±20.5	5.9±20.6	7.6±13.6	1.0±2.0 ***,a ***,b
	Stomach ache (days with pain/90 days)	7.3±11.0	2.2±4.6	7.5±11.4	0.5±1.9 ***,a ***,b
	Outdoor and gym hours (hours/d)	4.3±3.4	3.8±3.4	3.5±2.9	4.2±2.9 *,a
	Bedtime (hours/d)	8.4±0.7	8.3±0.9	7.91.0	7.7±1.1
Cardio vascular trial	Systolic blood pressure (mm Hg)	114.7±15.0	112.3±12.2	114.1±16.4	106.3±15.2 **,b
	Diastolic blood pressure (mm Hg)	64.7±12.1	69.2±11.0	70.4±12.6	65.5±11.5 **,a *,b
	Triglycerides (mg/dL)	87.7±65	68.0±36	73.8±30.7	71.3±33.2
	HDL cholesterol (mg/dL)	52.9±14.3	44.9±14.9	45.4±14.6	52.0±13.9 **,a **,b
	LDL cholest./HDL cholest. ratio	2.1±0.9	2.7±1.5	2.9±1.5	2.3±1.2 **,a **,b
Nutrition trial	Hemoglobin (g/dL)	13.3±0.6	13.5±0.9	13.3±1.5	13.4±1.4
	MCV (micr3)	86.9±5.5	85.6±3.7	87.4±6.5	87.2±6.4
	Transferrin Sat. (%)	45.9±17.8	43.8±15.0	37.1±16.9	40.3±17.0
	Ferritin (ng/ml)	42.7±41.8	42.4±17.3	63.1±58.5	68.4±56.6
	Zn (micrgr/dL)	86.0±29.2	80.1±14.5	77.8±24.4	81.9±20.7
	Folates ng/ml	7.9±4.4	8.3±4.3	9.6±4.6	11.3±4.9
	B12 (pg/ml)	567±465	438±149	544±262	590±264

*, suppressed for Bonferroni correction. **, ***, a and b symbols as in Table 2.

Table 3. Effects of training on well-being, cardiovascular, and nutrition parameters in HBG groups.

2.6.6 Diabetes prevention

It is interesting that insulin production decreases with increasing non-insulin dependent diabetes (NIDD) duration and HbA1c height (Wiesli et al. 2004). In this investigation, the HBG control subgroup decreased insulinogenic index of beta cell function whereas the HBG trained subgroup increased it (Table 2). The difference between control and trained subgroups was significant, this implies higher insulin production, preservation of beta cell function and the possibility of an innovative therapy designed to preserve or even improve functional beta-cell mass by "recognizing hunger" (Wiesli et al. 2004). In a longitudinal investigation of 13,163 subjects a fasting plasma glucose of $\geq$ 87 mg/dL (4.8 mmol/l) was found to be associated with an increased risk of non insulin-dependent diabetes (NIDD) in men compared to those whose fasting plasma glucose was < 81 mg/dL (4.5 mmol/l) (Tirosh et al. (2005). Assessment and classification of meal habits allows correction toward metabolic risk decrease as in Framingham studies (Singer et al. 1992).

Training [1]	Before	After
34 adults (BMI from 17 to 40)[2]	76.6 ± 3.7 2	77.2 ± 4.2
12 adults, ctrl[2]	76.9 ± 3.4	No training
18 diarrheic infants	77.1 ± 3.8	75.2 ± 6.9
9 normalweight adults, ctrl	77.3 ± 3.9	No training
26 normalweight adults, [2]	76.5 ± 3.9	76.7 ± 4.1
8 overweight adults, ctrl	77.4 ± 3.6	No training
12 overweight adults	77,1 ± 3,1	77,2 ±4,8
41 HBG adults [23]	91.7 ± 7.8	78.5 ± 6.8
41 HBG infants [4]	92,3 ± 7,7	74,7 ± 5,1

[1] Trained subjects show mean BG both before and after training. No training refers to subjects kept as control (ctrl).
[2] Mean ± SD of mean diary of 21 pre-prandial BG in a week in mg/dL, (present report, subchapter 2).
[3] 41 of 55 adults of mixed body mass index (BMI) and mean BG > 81.8 mg/dL at recruitment who significantly decreased mean BG after training "recognizing hunger" (present report, subchapter 2).
[4] 41 of 55 HBG infants of 73 recruited for diarrhea, who showed arm skin-fold thickness on 15th percentile of normal reference. They significantly decreased mean BG from > 81.1 mg/dL, the level at recruitment. Further 18 of 73 diarrheic infants appear in the third line.

Table 4. Occurrence of low mean blood glucose (LBG) either by free, spontaneous choice (Before) or after training (After) "recognizing hunger" in 9 different groups

2.6.7 Diabetes treatment

In this report, "recognizing hunger" either prevented or cured insulin resistance and NIDD in young, clinically healthy, adults with "normal" BG. A condition of insulin sensitivity suppresses subclinical inflammation (pro-inflammatory state) and the associated functional disorders and evolving vascular diseases (Reaven, 2006; Festa et al. 2000; Kahna et al. 2005; Cefalu, 2005; Moller & Flier, 1991; Mather & Verma, 2005; Weiss et al. 2004). "Recognizing hunger" might be helpful also to some people with NIDD. Unfortunately, "recognizing hunger" contrasts the currently prevailing idea of constancy in time of daily energy intake. NIDD patients may have no hunger sensation at all. Absent arousal of hunger yet facilitates low energy intake. As an extreme example, two meals per day of 50 grams of fish and salad, 100 kcal per meal produced rapid and large weight loss and recovery of hunger sensations after adequate weight loss. Some of these lowered weight people may show low estimation error of BG after training "recognizing hunger" (Ciampolini & Bianchi, 2006a). The low error validates "recognizing hunger", and prevents regaining body weight (Table 7),(Ciampolini et al. 2010; 2010b; Ciampolini & Sifone, 2011). Thus, adaptation of "recognizing hunger" to treating aged people with fully developed NIDD requires further investigation, and suggests that current treatment practices shall survive for part of patients.

2.6.8 Prevention of vascular diseases

In tables 2 and 3, the untrained meal pattern of HBG subjects was positively associated with energy intake, mean BG, insulin resistance, glycated hemoglobin, diastolic blood pressure, high LDL to HDL cholesterol ratio, and low HDL cholesterol. Briefly, these associations form the 'metabolic syndrome, which is strongly associated with development of bacteria in small intestine (Ciampolini et al. 1996), high absorption of microbial antigens (Brandtzaeg et al. 1989; Kinugasa et al. 2000; Perez et al. 2007), subclinical inflammation and vascular diseases (Reaven, 2006; Festa et al. 2000; Kahna et al. 2005; Cefalu, 2005; Moller & Flier, 1991; Mather & Verma, 2005; Weiss et al. 2004). Subclinical inflammation develops in blood and on endothelia, and may become clinically relevant in every tissue for local presence of additional inflammatory factors. Bronchitis becomes respiratory distress, and ankle trauma becomes local arthritis. "Recognizing hunger" was associated with lowering the habitual BG and disappearing of metabolic syndrome and risks of vascular disease. "Recognizing hunger" decreased body weight in normal weight adults who were insulin resistant, and in overweight adults (BMI > 25)."Recognizing hunger" decreased insulin resistance index, HbA1c, and increased the insulinogenic index of beta cell function in 55 HBG of 89 trained subjects as compared to control subjects. In future investigations on the risks due to high blood pressure, "recognizing hunger" and achievement of insulin sensitivity may prove far better than drug control of blood pressure and thrombotic tendency.

2.6.9 "Recognizing hunger" fading and overlapping over HBG

Mean BG had little absolute change (13.2% ± 10.1% of the range at recruitment in mean BG in the 120 investigated subjects: 64.5 mg/dL to 109.9 mg/dL) in control subjects over 5 months. The division of all 120 subjects in ten strata at recruitment was a classification of associated meal pattern. Subjects chose "recognizing hunger" at the lowest level of BG availability during the day. No surprise if "recognizing hunger" largely coincides with LBG meal patterns. The point of mean inversion was at 81.8 mg/dL. However, 27 out of 89 subjects further persisted at HBG level at final investigation although 15 out of 27 were within LBG limits after seven weeks training. Six of the 27 subjects were engaged in heavy handwork during cool winters. The six subjects had a mean BG of 86.4 ± 4.0 mg/dL that showed no difference from 87.1 ± 5.3 mg/dL in 21 out of all 27 other subjects. They reported pre-prandial IH and were insulin sensitive (Table 5). IH developed in these heavy outdoor workers at higher levels than 81.8 mg/dL for high expenditure (Table 5). The division between compliance and no compliance with "recognizing hunger" is statistically strong at

"Recognizing Hunger" – A Training to Abate Insulin Resistance, Associated Subclinical
Inflammation and Cardiovascular Risks

173

81.8 mg/dL, but single subjects who actually comply with "recognizing hunger" may show higher mean BG than 81.8 mg/dL, an overlapping over HBG.

	6 HBG [1]	21 HBG [2]
Mean Blood glucose (mg/dL)	86.4 ± 4.0	87.1 ± 5.3
Final insulin AUC (mU L^{-1}3h^{-1})	124 ± 26	207± 99 **
Final blood glucose AUC (mg dL^{-1}3h^{-1})	536 ± 56	601 ± 82 *
Insulin Sensitivity Index	11.4 ± 2.9	6.68 ± 4.0 ***
Beta cell Function Index	1.29 ± 0.66	1.43 ± 1.22

*, **, *** symbols as in Table 2.
[1] Six HBG subjects reported to make heavy handwork all day in outdoor environment during cold winter and to practice "recognizing hunger". No significant differences in the five parameters from recruitment. At recruitment mean BG = 86.9±5.3 mg/dL.
[2] 21 HBG subjects included 15 that were LBG after seven weeks training (clinical assessment) and six who had higher mean BG than 100 mg/dL at recruitment.

Table 5. Effects of heavy outdoor work[1] in 27 trained subjects who remained with high BG at investigation end.

3. Body weight study on 149 subjects

3.1 Effects of "recognizing hunger"

The study on 120 adults included 30 overweight (OW) subjects. This number was not sufficient to draw separate conclusions on responses of LBG and HBG OW subjects to "recognizing hunger". We had however treated and investigated also OW subjects who had not performed blood examinations. We thus could add 29 OW subjects to the 120 subjects that we reported up to now (Table 6). We trained these OW subjects and collected 7-d-food intake diaries like in previous investigation. We randomized 90 NW subjects separately from 59 who were OW to the control and the trained groups. We assigned both control and trained, NW and OW subjects to LBG and HBG subgroups on the basis of diary mean BG. The cutoff was 81.8 mg/dL (Figure 4) (Ciampolini et al. 2010a; Ciampolini & Sifone, 2011).

"Recognizing hunger" (IHMP) led to loss of weight in subjects who are either OW or who are of NW with HBG (Table 7). In NW LBG subjects, weight was maintained (Ciampolini et al. 2010a). The division between normal-weight and overweight people is based on a significant increase of vascular diseases over the limit of 25 for BMI. About 20% of people below 25 BMI is at increased risk for vascular diseases (Colditz, 2004; Weiss et al. 2004). The present report is in agreement with this statement: forty of 55 HBG subjects were NW and insulin-resistant (Table 2 and 7). Maintenance of high BG and of the associated insulin resistance provokes the increased risk, although subjects may have a small fat increase, insufficient to overcome the limit of 25 BMI, and insufficient to be classified as overweight (Table 7). Insulin resistance is a sort of fattening that remains below 25 BMI in lean subjects, and is thus un-apparent even by an esthetical evaluation. People with thin bones and thin muscles are at high risk of intentional fat accumulation (and associated insulin resistance). They may increase subcutaneous fat to improve their figure, and become insulin-resistant by remaining NW or even thin!

174 Cardiovascular Risk Factors: Recent Developments

NORMAL-WEIGHT

	Low BG group				High BG group			
	Control		Trained		Control		Trained	
	Baseline	After 5 mo.	Baseline	After 5 mo.	Baseline	After 5 mo.	Baseline	After 5 mo.
Number of subjects and gender	5 F + 4 M		16 F +10 M		3 F + 12 M		19 F + 21 M	
Schooling[1]	11.8±3.5		13.3±2.9		10.3±4.7		11.2±3.8	
Age[1]	27.9±8.2		31.0±8.9		29.3±2.5		29.7±8.9	
Subjects showing BG decrease[2]	0/9 (0.0%)		3/26 (11.5%)		6/15 (40.0%)		33/40 (82.5%)**,a	
BG group mean pre-meal[3]	77.3±3.9	79.8±3.7	76.5±3.9	76.7±4.1	90.7±5.2	89.7±6.6	91.4±7.7	80.1±6.6 ***,a***,b
Subjects < 81.8 mg/dL[4]	9	7	26	22	0	1	0	25***,a
Vegetable intake[5]	228±217	238±226	403±273	504±235	133±151	142±158	247±240	368±246 *,a**,b
Fruit intake[5]	150±122	146±75	246±162	376±346	161±91	143±123	201±157	291±218 *,a*,b

OVER-WEIGHT

	Low BG group				High BG group			
	Control		Trained		Control		Trained	
	Baseline	After 5 mo.	Baseline	After 5 mo.	Baseline	After 5 mo.	Baseline	After 5 mo.
Number of subjects and gender	6 F + 2 M		9 F +3 M		7 F + 6 M		14 F + 12 M	
Schooling[1]	11.8±3.0		12.3±2.6		10.6±4.0		11.9±3.3	
Age[1]	32.8 ±12.7		35.0±6.7		34.3±15,4		37.5±15.3	
Subjects showing BG decrease[2]	1/8 (12.5%)		2/12 (16.7%)		2/13 (15.4%)		22/26 (84.6%)***,a	
BG group mean pre-meal[3]	77.4±3.6	81,8±6.9	77,1±3,1	77,2±4,8	90,9±7,1	93,9±4,8	91,3±6,5	79,6±7.5 ***,a***,b
Subjects < 81.8 mg/dL[4]	8	5	12	10*,a	0	0	0	19***,a
Vegetable intake[5]	194±95	373±232	333±169	514±197	278±225	460±284 *,b	247±160	420±224 ***,b
Fruit intake[5]	138±121	182±219	214±138	223±124	226±168	167±121	225±116	286±191

Values are expressed as means ± SD. [1], years at the beginning of the study. [2],Number of subjects who significantly decreased mean pre-meal diary BG . [3],Mean pre-meal of diary blood glucose, mg/dL, LBG = lower than 81.8 mg/dL. HBG = higher than 81.8 mg/dL [4], Number of subjects who fell into the LBG at end of the study. [5], grams/d. *Asterisks* indicate significant differences (Student's *t*-test or Yates test: *, P < 0.05; **, P < 0.01; ***, P < 0.001) *vs.* respective control group values based on "post – pre" measurements (*a*), or *vs.* baseline values of the same group (*b*).

Table 6. Normal- and over-weight groups divided by low and high mean pre-meal diary blood glucose (BG). Composition and compliance at baseline and at investigation end.

3.2 Possible mechanisms and explanations

We suggested above (background) that IH may begin an important afferent arm of a physiological regulation mechanism that provides meal-by-meal feedback on energy need thus optimizing energy intake (Ciampolini et al. 1996). Subjects who are overweight and those who are normal-weight but have pre-meal HBG forestalled this homeostatic mechanism. Restoring the homeostatic mechanism would explain our finding that "recognizing hunger" (IHMP) leads to loss of weight in OW and NW HBG subjects but not in NW LBG subjects (Ciampolini et al. 2010a).

3.3 Training period and 7-day diaries

Implementation of "recognizing hunger" was associated with significant decrease of mean weekly BG as compared to control subjects. Glycated haemoglobin reflects the average BG over a 4 month period (Singer et al. 1992) and the lowered glycated haemoglobin (table 2) and significant weight loss observed in this study are unlikely to have occurred in the final week. These data suggest that awareness of IH indeed preceded final diary BG measurements, and was not significantly affected by it.

NORMAL-WEIGHT								
	Low BG group				High BG group			
	Control		Trained		Control		Trained	
	Baseline	After 5 mo.	Baseline	After 5 mo.	Baseline	After 5 mo.	Baseline	After 5 mo.
Energy intake[1]	1794±587	1660±732	1518±586	1357±628	2034±528	1886±417	1852±697	1270±457 **,a***,b
Diary BG SD[2]	8,0±2,4	9,1±1,7	6,3±3,0	5,2±1,8 **,a*,b	8,6±2,2	8,5±2,4	9,1±3,9	6,6±2,5 **,a***,b
BMI[3]	20.3±1,7	21.0±2.8	21.1±1.8	20.7±1.6	20.2±2.3	21.4±2.1	21.8±2.4	20.7±1.9 ***,a***,b
Weight[4]	55.2±7.7	57.0±9.6	57.9±7.8	57.0±7.6	57.5±6.9	60.9±6.4	61.4±10.4	58.9±9.6 ***,a***,b
Arm skinfold thickness[5]	12.9±5.3	14.7±7.7	12.6±6.6	11.3±5.0	11.3±4.3	11.7±4.2	14.1±7.0	11.6±5.7 **,a***,b
Leg skinfold thickness[5]	17.9±8.7	18.6±11.0	17.6±9.3	15.9±7.7	16.0±6.6	15.6±6.5	20.4±10.3	16.2±8.4 **,a***,b
OVER-WEIGHT								
Energy intake[1]	1611±471	1257±629	1618±616	950±448**,b	1799±701	1343±489 *,b	1820±570	1123±503 ***,b
Diary BG SD[2]	9.1±4.5	8.2±2.6	7.9±2.9	4,8±2.0 **,b	8.7±4.2	9.4±4.5	10.4±5.4	7.1±4.0 **,a**,b
BMI[3]	29.1±7.9	28.9±7.6	27,9±2.0	26.5±1.9 *,a***,b	29.2±3.9	27.8±4.2 *,b	29.0±4.1	26.5±4.0 ,a*,***b
Weight[4]	74.5±18.3	74.1±17.9	77.0±9.5	73.0±9.1 *,a***,b	77.1±16.2	73.7±15.9 *,b	78.5±10.6	71.8±10.7 *,a***,b
Arm skinfold thickness[5]	25.3±10.8	23.3±8.7 **,b	25.9±7.0	21.8±6.4 *,b	25.5±9.9	19.6±6.8	25.7±10.2	19.09±8.2 ***,b
Leg skinfold thickness[5]	33.7±13.7	30.3±12.6 **,b	32.5±12.1	26.6±10.3 ***,b	34.9±13.1	29.4±9.8** ,b	31.9±13.1	24.4±10.3 ***,b

[1] Kcal/d. [2], mg/dL; diary SD refers to BG SD of 21 measurements reported by each of 7d diary. [3] body weight kg/square height meters. [4] Kg [5] mm. *Asterisks* indicate significant differences as in Table 1.

Table 7. Effects of training (IHMP) on diary reports and anthropometry in normal- and over-weight groups divided by low and high mean pre-meal BG.

3.4 Clinical and research implications: Advantages over conventional dieting

3.4.1 Restraint approach

Control subjects were encouraged to lose weight and can be considered to represent a conventional restraint approach to dieting. Although control OW HBG subjects significantly lost weight in the first two months, they significantly increased their energy intake and BG during the last three months of the study and lost no further weight. This is consistent with a "restrained" eating pattern. Control OW LBG subjects showed a mean pre-meal BG just at 81.8 mg/dL at the end of the study indicating that without training, their meals remained partly conditioned, thus explaining firstly, their overweight status, and secondly, their failure to lose weight. Thus the findings in the two control OW subgroups (LBG and HBG) are consistent with the fact that restraint-type dieting tends to give short term results that are not sustained.

Weight cycling is a well-described phenomenon (Colditz, 2004). In the first phase of the cycle intake is conditioned or non-homeostatic. This leads to positive energy balance and weight increase. In the second phase OW subjects restrain their eating to lose weight. Most likely, the OW LBG subgroup was in this second phase at baseline. In the post-absorptive state, OW subjects have been shown to mobilise three times greater amounts of energy from reserve tissues to blood compared to NW subjects (Corcoran et al. 2007). By attending to preprandial arousal of IH, trained OW LBG subjects had to adjust meal energy intake downwards sufficiently to take into account the increased availability of energy owing to postabsorptive energy release, hence their lower energy intake (about 300 kcal per day) compared to trained LBG NW subjects (Table 7). During established application of "recognizing hunger", OW subjects reported that, provided meals were not delayed, their hunger was of no greater intensity nor more prolonged than NW subjects. Moreover, despite significantly higher body weight and lower energy intake than NW LBG subjects, trained OW LBG subjects showed the same mean preprandial BG as trained NW subjects (Table 6 and 7). These findings have at least three important clinical and research implications:

Trained OW subjects do not need to endure more prolonged or more intense hunger than trained NW subjects in order to lose weight.

The IHMP ("recognizing hunger") allows loss of weight without compromising energy availability for day-to-day energy need. The input of fatty acids from fat tissues to blood is limited in the overweight. Diets with lower mean content than 900 kcal a day may yield insufficient energy for body functions. That preprandial BG in the OW LBG group was the same as the NW LBG group indicates that in the OW LBG group a sufficiently high BG concentration was maintained for immediate energy needs. SD of diary BG in trained OW groups significantly decreased and regressed to that of NW groups further suggesting that under the IHMP ("recognizing hunger") OW groups adapted energy intake to metabolic need. In the absence of energy deprivation, less cycling of intake among trained OW groups would be expected.

An important subgroup exists (NW HBG) who appear NW by BMI criteria but who may nevertheless be at risk of weight related complications since they lose weight and decrease BG to a concentration comparable to the LBG group when trained to "recognizing hunger" (Tables 5 and 6).

3.4.2 Food composition approach (increased vegetables)

After 5 months, no significant difference was found in vegetable intake between control and trained subjects. At the end of the study controls did not attain significantly lower BG or body weight than the trained group although they had been encouraged to lose weight. This implies that high vegetable intake alone is insufficient in preventing conditioned meals and lowering high BG (Tables 6 and 7).

3.4.3 Advantages of immediate feedback

Subjects following the IHMP ("recognizing hunger") receive meal-by-meal subjective feedback from physiological signals (Ciampolini et al. 1996). These signals map closely to BG and allow subjects to eat in an unconditioned manner without self-imposed restraint or the necessity to seek any particular goal weight. The resulting improved energy balance leads to loss of weight. "Normal weight" is an artificial construct based on population statistics and may not apply to a given individual. Recommendations of goal weight may be unhelpful for some subjects to whom the goal may seem arbitrary and daunting especially if it is to be achieved by dietary restraint. The IHMP ("recognizing hunger") obviates the need for pursuit of a statistical norm and allows each individual to find his or her physiological norm.

This approach could thus prove useful in the clinical setting since it removes major obstacles to weight loss – the need for restraint, the need for dietary change, and the need to attain an arbitrary weight goal.

3.5 General interpretation

Even before any training, a consistent minority maintains a meal pattern that is similar to "recognizing hunger", and is similarly associated with improved insulin sensitivity (Table 2) and normal weight (Table 7) (Ciampolini et al. 2010; 2010b; Ciampolini & Sifone, 2011). Others may easily and reliably learn "recognizing hunger" (IHMP) to improve insulin sensitivity and lose weight, and can easily maintain this meal pattern below the age of 60 years. The IHMP ("recognizing hunger") could therefore be an important tool in the clinical management of overweight and obese patients and could have implications for health policy in the prevention of a wide range of metabolic and vascular disorders.

4. Conclusions

People share sounds and figures with other people but not subjective sensations. Subjective sensations guide the intake, but nobody knows sensations reported from others. Present investigation validated initial hunger (IH) by BG, and created a rhythm of meals at the arousal of IH, which decreased vascular risks. A three-times- daily meal pattern ("recognizing hunger" or IHMP) was associated with low mean blood glucose (LBG) and sustained regression of overweight and of the fat excess that is associated with insulin resistance, metabolic syndrome, subclinical inflammation and vascular diseases. Post hoc division of NW and OW subjects into subgroups with mean pre-meal BG either lower or higher than 81.8 mg/dL suggests body weight maintenance in NW subgroup with low mean BG and decrease in those who were either OW or HBG NW. The method was more effective than restraint-type dieting in a 5 month trial. IH, validated by BG, may represent the recovery of a vital afferent arm of the body's homeostatic energy regulation system allowing sustained self-regulation of energy intake.

Present findings suggest that the current epidemic of insulin resistance and overweight may have its origin in the non-cognizance of hunger – the physiological signals of energy insufficiency to body cells. Lack of a subjective limit in intake (a similar limit to arousal of initial hunger) explains current epidemic of insulin resistance and overweight, This may owe to forestalling such signals in early life and subsequent reinforcement of this behavior pattern. Training "recognizing hunger" rationalized the arousal of the subjective, validated limit in order to acquire and maintain energy homeostasis in blood, and decrease vascular risks. The achieved rhythm (mean BG) is homeostatic rather than being an artifact, i.e. maintains a BG that is constant and both sufficient for activity and body weight maintenance, and effective in the prevention and treatment of diabetes and obesity and a range of associated disorders and thus lessen the high economic burden of health services in industrialized societies.

5. Acknowledgments

The author wish to thank Laura Chiesi and Stefania Bini MD for dietary analyses, Riccardo Bianchi, David Lovell-Smith, Andrea Giommi (Statistics professor) and Stella Zagaria for technical support and insights, Stephen Buetow, Tim Kenealy, Chris Harshaw, Simon Thornton, Kent Berridge, James Gibbs, Charlotte Erlanson-Albertsson and Michael Hermanussen for helpful insights on earlier drafts of this paper. This research was supported by the Italian Ministry of University, Research, Science and Technology grants for the years 1998–2002 and ONLUS Nutrizione e Prevenzione, Firenze for years 2003–2008. The authors declare that they have no competing interests.

6. List of abbreviations

IHMP: Initial hunger meal pattern = "Recognizing Hunger"
AUC: area under curve at GTT
BMI: body mass index (body weight in kg/square height in m)
BG: blood glucose concentration (glycemia)
GTT: oral glucose tolerance test
HBG: high mean BG (> 81.8 mg/dL)
LBG: low mean BG (< 81.8 mg/dL)
NIDD: non-insulin dependent diabetes
Mean BG: mean of 21 pre-prandial blood glucose measurements reported by 7 day diary
Diary-BG standard deviation: Mean pre-meal blood glucose standard deviation reported by 7 day diary
BG estimation: During training: writing the expected BG value in the minute before measuring the blood sample by glucometer. After training and validation: evaluating one's own current BG value without measurement.

7. References

Armitage, P. & Berry, G. (1994). Statistical Methods in Medical Research, Blackwell, Oxford, UK, 3rd edition.
Brandtzaeg, P. et al. (1989). Immunobiology and immunopathology of human gut mucosa: humoral immunity and intreaepithelial lymphocytes. Gastroenterology, 97, 1562-1584.

"Recognizing Hunger" – A Training to Abate Insulin Resistance, Associated Subclinical
Inflammation and Cardiovascular Risks

179

Bischoff, S.C. et al. (2009). Role of serotonin in intestinal inflammation: knockout of serotonin reuptake transporter exacerbates 2,4,6-trinitrobenzene sulfonic acid colitis in mice. Am. J. Physiol. Gastrointest. Liver Physiol., 296, G685-G695.

Cefalu, W.T., (2005). Glycemic Control and Cardiovascular Disease – Should We Reassess Clinical Goals?. N. Engl. J. Med., 353, 2707-2709.

Ciampolini, M. et al. (1987). Internal stimuli controlled lower calorie intake: effects after eight months in toddler's diarrhoea. Ital. J. Gastroenterology, 19, 201–204.

Ciampolini, M. et al. (1990). Normal Energy intake range in children with chronic nonspecific diarrhea: association of relapses with the higher level. J. Pediatric Gastroenterology and Nutrition, 11, 342–350.

Ciampolini, M. et al. (1991). Decrease in serum IgE associated with limited restriction in energy intake to treat toddler's diarrhea. Physiology and Behavior, 49, 155–160.

Ciampolini, M. et al. (1994). Same growth and different energy intake over four years in children suffering from chronic non-specific diarrhea. International J. Obesity, 18, 17–23.

Ciampolini, M. et al. (1996). Microflora persistence on duodeno-jejunal flat or normal mucosa in time after a meal in children. Physiology and Behavior, 60, 1551-1556.

Ciampolini, M. et al. (2000). Attention to metabolic hunger and its effects on Helicobacter pylori infection. Physiology and Behavior, 70, 287–296.

Ciampolini, M. et al. (2001). Attention to metabolic hunger for a steadier (SD decrease to 60%), slightly lower glycemia (10%), and overweight decrease (Abstract). Appetite, 37, 123-172.

Ciampolini, M. & Bianchi, R. (2006a). Training to estimate blood glucose and to form associations with initial hunger. Nutrition and Metabolism, 3, 42

Ciampolini, M., (2006b). Infants do request food at the hunger blood glucose level, but adults don't any more (Abstract). Appetite, 46, 345.

Ciampolini, M. et al. (2010a). Sustained self-regulation of energy intake. Loss of weight in overweight subjects. Maintenance of weight in normal-weight subjects. Nutrition and Metabolism, 7, 4

Ciampolini, M. et al. (2010b). Sustained Self-Regulation of Energy Intake: Initial Hunger Improves Insulin Sensitivity. J. Nutrition and Metabolism, Article ID 286952.

Ciampolini, M. & Sifone, M. (2011). Differences in maintenance of mean blood glucose (BG) and their association with response to "Recognizing Hunger". International J. Gen. Med., 4, 403-412

Colditz, G.A. (2004) Weight Cycling and the Risk of Developing Type 2 Diabetes among Adult Women in the United States. Obesity Res., 12, 267-274.

Corcoran, M.P. et al., (2007). Skeletal muscle lipid deposition and insulin resistance: effect of dietary fatty acids and exercise. Am. J. Clin. Nutr., 85, 662-677.

De Giorgio, R. & Camilleri, M. (2004). Human enteric neuropathies: morphology and molecular pathology. Neurogastroenterol. Motil., 16, 515-531.

Dinan,T.G. et al. (2006). Hypothalamic-pituitary-gut axis dysregulation in irritable bowel syndrome: plasma cytokines as a potential biomarker? Gastroenterology, 130, 304-311.

Festa, A. et al. (2000). Chronic subclinical inflammation as part of the insulin resistance syndrome: the Insulin Resistance Atherosclerosis Study (IRAS). Circulation, 102, 42–47.

Flaa, A. et al. (2008). Does sympathoadrenal activity predict changes in body fat? An 18-y follow-up study. Am. J. Clin. Nutr., 87, 1596-1601.

Gershon, M.D., (1999). Review article: roles played by 5-hydroxytryptamine in the physiology of the bowel. Aliment. Pharmacol. Ther., 13(Suppl 2), 15-30.

Harshaw, C. (2008). Alimentary epigenetics: A developmental psychobiological systems view of the perception of hunger, thirst and satiety. Developmental Review, 28, 541-569.

Kahna, R. et al. (2005). The metabolic syndrome (Correspondence). Lancet, 366, 1921-1922.

Kinugasa, T. et al. (2000). Claudins regulate the intestinal barrier in response to immune mediators. Gastroenterology, 118, 1001-1011.

Kylin, E. (1923). Studien ueber Hypertonie-Hyperglykamie-Hyperurikamie syndrome., Zentralblatt fur innere Medizin, 44.

Lal, S. et al. (2001). Vagal afferent responses to fatty acids of different chain length in the rat., Am. J. Physiol. Gastrointest. Liver Physiol. 281, G907-G915.

Mather, K. & Verma, S. (2005). Function determines structure in the vasculature: lessons from insulin resistance. Am. J. Physiol. Regul. Integr. Comp. Physiol., 289, R305-R306.

Matsuda, M. & DeFronzo, R.A. (1999). Insulin sensitivity indices obtained from oral glucose tolerance testing: comparison with the euglycemic insulin clamp. Diabetes Care, 22, 1462–1470,

Moller, D.E. & Flier, G.S. (1991). Insulin resistance—mechanisms, syndromes, and implications. N. Engl. J. Med., 325, 938–948.

Ohman, L. & Simrén, M. (2010). Pathogenesis of IBS: role of inflammation, immunity and neuroimmune interactions. Nat. Rev. Gastroenterol. Hepatol., 7,163-173.

Perez PF et al. (2007). Bacterial Imprinting of the Neonatal Immune System: Lessons From Maternal Cells? Pediatrics, 119, e724-e732.

Rana, S.V., (2009). Role of serotonin in gastrointestinal motility and irritable bowel syndrome. Clin. Chim. Acta., 403, 47-55.

Randle, P.J. et al. (1963). The glucose-fatty acid cycle: its role in insulin sensitivity and the metabolic disturbances of diabetes mellitus. Lancet, 93, 785-789.

Robbins, T.W. & Fray, P.J. (1980). Stress induced eating: fact, fiction or misunderstanding? Appetite, 1, 103-133.

Reaven, G.M. (2006). The metabolic syndrome: is this diagnosis necessary? Am. J. Clin. Nutr., 83, 1237–1247.

Sand, E. et al. (2009). Mast cells reduce survival of myenteric neurons in culture. Neuropharmacology, 56, 522-30.

Singer, D.E. et al. (1992). Association of HbA(1c) with prevalent cardiovascular disease in the original cohort of the Framingham Heart Study. Diabetes, 41, 202–208.

Spiller, R. (2008). Serotonin and GI clinical disorders. Neuropharmacology, 55, 1072-1080.

Tirosh, A. et al. (2005). Normal Fasting Plasma Glucose Levels and Type 2 Diabetes in Young Men. N. Engl. J. Med., 353, 1454-1462.

Tornblom, H. et al. (2002). Full-thickness biopsy of jejunum reveals inflammation and enteric neuropathy in irritable bowel syndrome. Gastroenterology, 123, 1972-1979.

van den Wijngaard, R.M. et al. (2010). Peripheral relays in stress-induced activation of visceral afferents in the gut. Auton. Neurosci.,153, 99-105.

van der Waaij, L. A. et al. (1996). In vivo IgA coating of anaerobic bacteria in human faeces. Gut, 38, 348-354

Wang, H. et al. (2003). Nicotinic acetylcholine receptor alpha7 subunit is an essential regulator of inflammation. Nature, 421, 384-388.

Weiss, M.D. et al. (2004). Obesity and the Metabolic Syndrome in Children and Adolescents. N Engl J Med, 350, 2362-2374.

Wiesli, P. et al. (2004). Islet secretory capacity determines glucose homoeostasis in the face of insulin resistance. Swiss Medical Weekly, 134, 37-38, 559–564.

Zwaigenbaum, L. et al. (1999). Highly somatizing young adolescents and the risk of depression. Pediatrics, 103, 1203-1209.

10

Mediterranean Diet and Gene-Mediterranean Diet Interactions in Determining Intermediate Cardiovascular Disease Phenotypes

Mercedes Sotos Prieto
*University of Valencia, Department of Preventive Medicine and Public Health and CIBER Fisiopatología de la Obesidad y Nutrición,
Spain*

1. Introduction

Currently, cardiovascular diseases (CVD) are one of the most important problems in the world. In fact, CVD are the first cause of death all over the world and, according to the World Health Organization (WHO), it is expected to remain so over coming years due to aging population and the increase of prevalence of CVD in countries with fewer resources.

According to European statistics, 2008 for CVD, the leading causes of death in Europe are coronary heart disease and stroke. In Europe, deaths from these diseases are 4.3 million each year. Nearly half (48%) of all deaths are due to CVD (54% of deaths in women and 43% of deaths in men). Regional variations in cardiovascular mortality have been observed both between and within countries in Europe (Sans et al., 1997; Müller et al., 2004). Coronary heart disease mortality patterns showed a clear north–east to south–west gradient in CVD mortality (1990–1992; 45–74 years age-adjusted) with the lowest rates for both men and women in France, Spain, Switzerland, and Italy (Sans et al., 1997). Many factors could be related to the different distribution (eating behaviours, life style, and genetics).

To begin with the development of this chapter it is necessary to consider firstly the health determinants to better understand and focus the aim of this chapter.

The model of health fields proposed by Latramboise in 1973 and developed in Lalonde Report in 1974 (Lalonde 1974) has revolutionized contemporary public health due to the approaching and explaining of the health levels in the populations and therefore, the way of formulating health policies. Marc Lalonde proposed a new "health field" concept that can be broken up into four broad elements: Human biology, Environment, Lifestyle, and Health Care Organization".

Of the four determinants of health, the one which is most susceptible to be modified is lifestyle. Apart from not smoking, the most important lifestyle determinants of good health are what we eat and how active we are. A healthy diet helps to maintain or improve our health. However, as we said before, the CVD are increasing all over the word, and authorities view it as one of the most serious Public Health problems in the 21st century.

CVD are complex and the risk factors that contribute to the development of CVD can be classified into different categories depending on whether they are modified or not (Posner et al., 1991, Haskell et al., 2003) and how they contribute to the development of CVD (Linton et al., 2003). Thus, on the one hand, we have not modifiable factors such as age, sex, family history and genetics. With regard to genetics, we inherit the genetic risk to develop CVD, but this risk can be modulated by other modifiable factors. In this chapter we will deeply discuss the relation between genes and environmental factors (especially diet) in the prevention of CVD (Figure 1).

On the other hand, we also have factors that are susceptible to be modified such as cholesterol concentrations, hypertension, smoking, diabetes, type of diet, obesity, sedentary lifestyle, stress and consumption of oral contraceptives. The more risk factors a person has, the higher risk of developing CVD. Some risk factors can be changed, treated or modified, and some others not. But controlling the largest possible number of risk factors through changes in lifestyle and/or drugs can reduce cardiovascular risk. Among the environmental factors associated with CVD, and as a part of one of the health determinants proposed by Lalonde, diet has a great impact on lipid metabolism, oxidative stress and the development of the atherosclerotic process (Ordovas et al., 2004) (Figure 1). Changes in eating behaviours have contributed to the growing epidemic of chronic diseases. These changes are characterized by an unbalanced diet consisting of food with a high density of energy rich in saturated fatty acids (SAF) as well as a decrease in physical activity. This process is called nutritional transition. Given these facts, researchers are trying to elucidate the best diet to prevent CVD. However, there is a widespread of controversy. Different proposals have been considered such as low-fat diet, diet low in carbohydrates and high in proteins, among others, all promoted by the acquisition of knowledge, fashion or business interests (Ordovas et al., 2004).

Traditionally, the American Heart Association (AHA) has based dietary recommendations for primary care of cardiovascular risk in a low-fat diet (Krauss MR et al, 2000). This diet is also based on reducing all types of fat so that the contribution of total fat calories should be less than 30% (of which SAF are less than 10%) and cholesterol intake less than 300 mg daily. This type of diet causes a decrease in total cholesterol (TC) and LDL-C, and a decrease or not variation in HDL-C and increases or unchanged triglycerides (TG) concentrations (Obarzanek et al., 2001; Lichtenstein et al., 2002, Howard et al., 2006). Later on, in 2005, a new version of USDA pyramid in which food groups are presented in vertical and which incorporates the concept that the diet should be tailored to individual needs came up (USDA, 2005).

After the AHA recommendations, other types of diets have been proposed such as diets rich in protein, low carb, Mediterranean diet, etc. Mediterranean diet has attracted the most interest by its great relevance regarding the protective role in primary and secondary care of CVD.

The aim of this chapter is to analyse the role of the Mediterranean diet in determining intermediate CVD phenotypes. We also review one of the most emerging topics currently: the role of gene-Mediterranean diet interactions on CVD.

2. Mediterranean diet

Due to the great incidence of CVD, Mediterranean diet has gained a considerable popularity during the last decades. The Mediterranean area is a sociocultural construction built on the

Mediterranean Diet and Gene-Mediterranean Diet Interactions in Determining
Intermediate Cardiovascular Disease Phenotypes

183

countries bordering the Mediterranean Sea. Food habits have been consolidated over the centuries and are the result of geographical and climatic factors, as well as cultural, political and religious factors of Mediterranean people. Mediterranean area is identified by characteristics based on agriculture (natural grain, olives, wine and vegetables), fishing and consumption of poultry instead of other meats.

Furthermore, Mediterranean diet includes food and cooking techniques typical of Mediterranean countries which have been gradually abandoned by western patterns.

The Mediterranean diet has been described as a model from a nutritional point of view due to the good balance that provides its food items (micronutrients, vitamins, antioxidants). Nevertheless, as well as the cooking techniques have been abandoned, in the last few years changes in lifestyle have triggered a move away from the recommended intakes in relation to several nutrients. All these changes make it even more difficult to ensure adequate intakes of vitamins and minerals. This problem could affect more to certain risk groups such us women, the elderly, children, gestating and lactating women and ill people. Knowing the extent of this reality it seems worthy to inform people and society in general about the necessary changes in the diet and about the characteristics of the Mediterranean diet which are being lost and should be restored.

2.1 Definition of the Mediterranean diet

The concept of the Mediterranean diet originated from several observational studies in the 1950s, being the most known the Seven Countries Study initiated by Ancel Keys (Ancel Keys 1970). Subsequently, several studies have associated increased longevity, lower mortality and morbidity to Mediterranean diet (Keys et al., 1986; de Lorgeril et al., 1999; Singh et al., 2002; Trichopoulou et al., 2003; Knoops et al., 2004). Taken as a whole, these studies showed that, despite a high fat intake, these populations had low rates of coronary heart disease and other vascular diseases, cancer, inflammatory and degenerative diseases, resulting in a long life expectancy. The Mediterranean dietary pattern was considered to be largely responsible for the good health observed in these regions (Keys et al., 1986). Currently, there is a great number of clinical and epidemiological studies that have shown the benefits of the Mediterranean diet. However, these effects are attributed to the traditional Mediterranean diet and not to the Westernized patterns that nowadays characterize the South European countries (Serra-Majem et al., 2004).

Although there are several variations of the Mediterranean diet, the main characteristics include high consumption (daily consumption) of vegetables, fruit, whole grain cereals and low fat dairy products; weekly consumption of fish, poultry, tree nuts and legumes; relatively low consumption of red meat (approximately twice a month) as well as moderate daily consumption of alcohol (preferably in the form of wine) normally with meals (keys et al., 1986) (Figure 1).

Most of the articles published so far on Mediterranean diet are observational studies. However, there is a lack of intervention studies that demonstrate causal relationship. Although there are few randomized controlled trials of dietary intervention with Mediterranean Diet, we have recently strong data from one large randomize control trial supporting the beneficial effects of Mediterranean diet on CVD prevention (Estruch et al., 2006).

2.2 Principal studies that focus on Mediterranean diet and cardiovascular diseases

In general, there is a predominance of observational studies related to Mediterranean Diet compared to clinical trials in the study of CVD. Thus, most of the studies are cross-sectional studies with a level III of evidence (based on the quality of evidence according to the 2nd edition of the U.S. Task Force (Harris et al., 2001)). The *ATTICA* study is the most remarkable (Pitsavos et al., 2003) and it was conducted on a representative sample of Greek men and women recruited from May 2001 to December 2002 in order to analyze cardiovascular risk factors, establish associations with lifestyle, socioeconomic factors, psychological characteristics, and assess their impact on CVD over a year, five and ten years. Several studies found a positive association between Mediterranean Diet and CVD (Tzima et al., 2007; Panagiotakos et al., 2006; Pitsavos et al., 2007).

Two other large European cohort studies (evidence level II-2) include the Greek cohort within *EPIC* (European Prospective Investigation into Cancer) (Trichopoulou et al., 2003, Slimani et al., 2002). They study the relationship between nutrition and cancer in 519,978 participants from 23 centers located in 20 European countries.

Another cohort study is the *HALE* (Knoops et al., 2004) (Healthy Ageing: Longitudinal Study in Europe). This project analyzed age-related changes and the determinants of healthy aging in terms of mortality and morbidity, and physical, mental, cognitive and social functionality in 13 European countries. Results from this study suggest that a high adherence to Mediterranean diet is associated with a reduction in both overall mortality and cardiovascular mortality.

Regarding intervention studies (level I of scientific evidence), two of the most known studies analyzing Mediterranean Diet are *PREDIMED* study (Prevention with Mediterranean diet) (Estruch et al., 2006) and *Medi-RIVAGE* study (Mediterranean Diet, Cardiovascular Risks and Gene Polymorphism) (Vincent-Baudry et al., 2005).

PREDIMED study is a multicenter, prospective, randomized, controlled trial whose goals are to assess the efficacy and safety of a Mediterranean diet in primary care of CVD. It was designed in 2002 and it is the first long-term clinical trial that recruits high-risk patients (around 7,000 participants from different regions in Spain) to follow a Mediterranean diet supplemented with virgin olive oil (VOO) (1 liter a week) or nuts (30 g per day of which 15 g almonds and 15 g walnuts).

Medi-RIVAGE study is a randomized clinical trial conducted in France on 212 women and men with at least one cardiovascular risk factor. The aims of the study are to evaluate the effect of two types of diet in the prevention of CVD and to investigate biological mechanisms and genetic polymorphisms related to metabolism. On the one hand, they study the traditional Mediterranean diet (35-38% of total energy from fat: 50% monounsaturated fatty acids (MUFA), 25% polyunsaturated fatty acids (PUFA), 25% SFA) and on the other hand, a low fat diet based on the AHA (30% of total energy from fat: 33% MUFA, 33% PUFA, 33% SFA).

With regard to studies that analyze final cardiovascular risk phenotypes, two of the most outstanding studies (level I of scientific evidence) are the Lyon Diet Heart Study and the Indio-Mediterranean Diet Heart study.

The *Lyon Diet Heart Study* (de Lorgeril et al., 1999), a randomized, controlled trial with free-living subjects (half of 600 men and women in France), tested the effectiveness of a Mediterranean-type diet (consistent with the new AHA Dietary Guidelines) on composite measures of the coronary recurrence rate after a first myocardial infarction during 46 months. Subjects in the experimental group were instructed by cardiologists and dietitians to adopt a Mediterranean-type diet. They demonstrated the effectiveness of Mediterranean diet in the secondary care of CVD. However, the intervention group with Mediterranean diet received margarine rich in alpha-linolenic fatty acid, fact that distorted the interpretation of results, as margarine is not a component of traditional Mediterranean diet. Something similar happens with the Indo-Mediterranean Diet Heart Study (Singh et al., 2002).

The *Indo Mediterranean Diet Heart* study is a randomized, single-blind trial in 1000 patients with angina pectoris, myocardial infarction, or surrogate risk factors for CVD. 499 patients were allocated to a diet rich in whole grains, fruits, vegetables, walnuts, and almonds. 501 controls consumed a local diet similar to the step I National Cholesterol Education Program (NCEP) prudent diet. They showed that an Indo-Mediterranean diet, that is rich in a-linolenic acid, might be more effective in primary and secondary prevention of CVD than the conventional step I NCEP prudent diet. However, as in the Lyon Diet Heart Study, the intervention group with Mediterranean diet increased the consumption of alpha-linolenic fatty acid from soybean and mustard oil, which are not typical from Mediterranean countries.

3. Mediterranean diet in determining intermediate cardiovascular disease phenotypes

There is a great number of studies analysing the effect of the consumption or adherence to Mediterranean diet and intermediate CVD phenotypes. In the following sections we review the studies analysing Mediterranean diet and obesity, lipid metabolism, glucose concentrations, blood pressure and inflammation. Table 1 shows the effect of Mediterranean diet on the aforementioned phenotypes.

3.1 Mediterranean diet and obesity

Currently, it is not known which is the best diet is to lose weight (low-carb, high protein, low fat diet, etc.). Consumption of nuts, and high fat diets (rich in MUFA), characteristics of the Mediterranean diet, have been traditionally associated with an increased body weight by its high contain in fats. However, recent scientific evidence does not support these data. Adherence to Mediterranean diet was inversely associated with BMI and obesity in a cross-sectional survey carried out in the northeast of Spain (Schröder et al., 2004). Obesity risk decreased in both men and women with increasing adherence to the traditional Mediterranean diet.

Results from epidemiological studies on large populations indicate that subjects who usually consume nuts have lower BMI than those who do not consume (Bes-Rastrollo et al, 2009, Garcia-Lorda et al, 2003; Schroder et al, 2004). In addition, the SUN cohort (Seguimiento Universidad de Navarra) (follow-up University of Navarra) evaluated 11,895 participants and found an inverse association between consumption of nuts and weight gain per year (Martinez-Gonzalez & Bes-Ballostro, 2011). Similarly, a recent study carried out in EPIC-PANACEA project showed that individuals with high adherence to Mediterranean diet, according to the score based on a questionnaire of adherence to Mediterranean diet (11-18 points), showed in a weight change of 20.16 kg (95% CI :20,2-20, 7 kg) 5 years and they were also 10% less likely to become overweight and obese compared with individuals with lower adherence (0-6 points) (Romaguera et al., 2010). Furthermore, a study that evaluated 497,308 individuals aged between 25-70 years in 10 European countries found that high adherence to the Mediterranean diet is associated with lower abdominal adiposity, using waist circumference as a measure (Romaguera et al., 2009).

With respect to intervention studies, it has been shown that subjects that consume daily tree nuts in their diet are less likely to gain weight (Li et al., 2010). A study evaluating the intake of almonds (42-72 g daily) in 81 patients over 6 months found that there was no significant weight gain (Fraser et al., 2002). Similarly, García-Londa et al, (2003) found that in the short term, the addition of tree nuts to diet, in amounts up to 50 g daily, does not increase weight. After one year of intervention in the PREDIMED study, beneficial effects on waist circumference were shown (Martinez-Gonzalez & Bes-Ballostro, 2011).

Finally, a meta-analysis regarding Mediterranean diet and weight loss analyzing randomize controlled trials has been recently published (Esposito et al., 2011), and it concludes that Mediterranean diet does not cause weight gain, which removes the objection to its relatively high fat content. Mediterranean diet could be a strategy to help people lose weight.

Some of the proposed mechanisms that might explain these facts are that the absorption of nuts may be incomplete, thus some of its fat content may not be absorbed by the body and would be excreted in the feces. Moreover, the consumption of nuts may have a satiating effect, producing a decrease in consumption of other foods and helping to control total energy intake. Although it still has not been proved, there may be an adaptation of the metabolism, so that energy consumption could be more efficient and get the body burn more energy, thus avoiding an accumulation of body fat (Brennan et al., 2010; Garcia-Lorda et al., 2003; Rajaram & Sabaté, 2006).

3.2 Mediterranean diet and lipid metabolism

Mediterranean diet has been largely studied in relation to lipid metabolism because of its beneficial effect on CVD. However, different results have been shown regarding a variety of studies, designs, and sample sizes. Cross-sectional studies with similar characteristics, with a sample size between 1762 and 2032 participants in Greece (ATTICA study), evaluated the adherence to Mediterranean diet and lipid profile. Thus, Tzima et al (2007) reported that subjects who are overweight (BMI 25-29.9) or obese (BMI $\geq$ 30) in the highest tertile of the Mediterranean diet score had lower total cholesterol (TC) (-13 %, P = 0.001) after adjusting for age, sex and BMI compared to the first tertile. However, there were no significant differences in triglycerides (TG) and HDL-C. This increase in the adherence to Mediterranean diet was also associated with lower total cholesterol (p <0.001) in a study carried out by Panagiotakos et al (2006). In addition to that, individuals with abdominal obesity and less physically active had lower adherence to Mediterranean diet (p = 0.008) with lower HDL-C (p <0.05) (Pitsavos et al., 2007).

Moreover, seven studies of 29 clinical trials with 3,822 subjects (2,202 assigned to Mediterranean diet and 1,903 assigned to a control diet) reported beneficial effects of adherence to Mediterranean diet on HDL-C (Papadaki & Scott, 2008; Esposito et al., 2004; Estruch et al., 2006; Esposito et al., 2003; Esposito et al., 2009; Athryros et al., 2011). A recent meta-analysis (Kastorini et al., 2011) showed that, overall, adherence to Mediterranean diet was associated with higher HDL-C levels as compared with a control diet.

Benefits in TC have also been shown in some randomized controlled trials (Estruch et al., 2006; Vincent-Baudry et al., 2005; Ambring et al., 2004). In this sense, Estruch et al., (2006) carried out a study of 3 months with individuals who had diabetes mellitus or one or more cardiovascular risk factors, which were assigned to three intervention groups (n = 257-8 / group) (2 Mediterranean diet (one supplemented with VOO and another one with 15g of almonds+15g walnuts/day) and one control diet low in fats). Regarding the lipid profile, both Mediterranean diets showed significant increase in HDL-C levels (p = <0.001 and p = 0.006, respectively) and a significant reduction (p <0.001 and p = 0.002, respectively) in the atherogenic index (TC/HDL-C) in contrast to the control group. However, only Mediterranean diet supplemented with nuts showed a significantly reduction in TC (p = 0.040) and TG (p = 0.022), compared to control. Neither of the Mediterranean diets significantly reduced LDL-C compared to the control diet (low fat diet).

Concerning TG, three observational studies reported a beneficial effect of Mediterranean diet (Chrysohoou et al., 2004; Tzima et al., 2007; Barzi et al., 2003) as compared with low adherence to Mediterrenean diet. Five interventional studies showed beneficial effects of Mediterranean diet on TG concentrations (Shai et al., 2008; Esposito et al., 2004; Estruch et al., 2006; Esposito et al., 2009; Elhayany et al., 2011), whereas other studies did not find significant differences (de Lorgeril et al., 1994; Castro et al., 2000; Michalsen et al., 2006).

Moreover, results from a crossover study during 4 weeks for each intervention (22 healthy people (12H/10M)) found an improvement in lipid profile to compare a Mediterranean diet (rich in omega 3) with a Swedish standard diet (Ambring et al., 2004). The results showed a significant decrease in TC, LDL-C, TG (17%, 22%, and 17%) in the group with Mediterranean diet. On the other hand, one non-randomize control trial carried out in Italy (47 obese women) during 4-month with an hypoenergetic Mediterranean diet together with a program of physical exercise showed a significant decrease in total cholesterol and TG concentrations. Levels of LDL-C decreased (p <0.001) after 4 months of intervention, whereas HDL-C increased (Andreoli et al., 2008). However, another study carried out in 71 healthy Canadian found a significant decrease in TC at 6 weeks of intervention (p <0.05), whereas no significant changes were observed after 12 weeks. Levels of HDL-C, LDL-C and TG were not affected after 6 or 12 weeks of intervention (Goulet et al., 2003). Different characteristics of the recruitment of individuals can influence the final results of the studies.

The relationship between nut consumption and reduced risk of CVD has been established in numerous epidemiological studies. Thus, Ros et al (2004), in a crossover study carried out in hypercholesterolemia subjects in Spain, determined whether a diet containing nuts (18% of energy) could improve markers related to endothelial function against another typical Mediterranean diet with similar energy intake, fat, protein, carbohydrates, but not MUFA intake, after 4 weeks. Estruch et al (2006) also found a significant decrease in TC (p = 0.017) and LDL-C (p = 0.010). However, no differences were found in TG concentrations and HDL-

C. Pooled analysis in 25 clinical trials to evaluate nut consumption in blood lipids showed that the most important finding is that the cholesterol-lowering effects of nut consumption are dose related and are more pronounced in subjects with higher baseline LDL-C or lower BMI. Nut consumption also lowered TG levels in subjects with hypertriglyceridemia (Sabate et al., 2010).

3.3 Mediterranean diet and glucose concentrations

The increasing incidence of type 2 diabetes throughout the world is also linked to westernized dietary patterns. Lifestyle changes are effective measures to prevent diabetes. The Mediterranean diet has also shown beneficial effects on diabetes risk and glucose concentrations.

Two observational studies reported a beneficial effect of close adherence to Mediterranean diet as compared with a control diet in lowering fasting glucose (FG) levels (Tzima et al., 2007; Panagiotakos et al., 2007).

Furthermore, Estruch et al., 2006 found that participants in the intervention group with Mediterranean diet supplemented with VOO or nuts, showed a significant reduction in FG compared with the control group (-0.39 mmol / L and -0.30 mmol / L, respectively).

In this sense, in another randomized controlled trial (Vincent-Baudry et al., 2005) with Mediterranean diet or low-fat diet, after 3 months of intervention, both diets significantly reduced blood glucose, insulinemia, insulin resistance and HOMA-IR index. Insulin levels remained significant after adjusting for BMI. However, there was no interaction between time and type of diet for any of the variables. Negative results were shown in a study that compared the intervention with Mediterranean diet rich in omega 3 versus the standard Swedish diet (Ambring et al., 2004). Recently, results from PREDIMED study also reported that, after a median follow-up of 4 years, diabetes incidence was lower in the groups with Mediterranean diet as compared with control group (10,1% in Mediterranean diet with VOO, 11% in Mediterranean diet with nuts, 17,9% in control group) (Salas-Salvado et al., 2011).

In conclusion, overall adherence to Mediterranean diet is associated with lower FG levels as compared with the control diet (Kastorini et al., 2011). Among the mechanisms associated with that decrease in glucose levels are the properties of the components of Mediterranean diet. Fiber delays gastric emptying, antioxidants increase oxidative capacity and moderate alcohol could have a role in adiponectin. As a consequence, it ends in the prevention of insulin resistance and, finally, in prevention of type 2 diabetes (Schröder, 2007).

3.4 Mediterranean diet and blood pressure

Nutritional factors and dietary patterns have been associated with hypertension. Hypertensive individuals can remarkably reduce their blood pressure through nutritional changes. Mediterranean diet has also shown beneficial effects in the prevention and control of blood pressure.

Cross-sectional studies associate the consumption of Mediterranean diet with lower systolic blood pressure (SBP). Higher adherence to Mediterranean diet was associated with lower SBP (p<0.001) (Tzima et al., 2007; Panagiotakos et al., 2006) as well as with 70% of decrease of prevalence of hypertension (Alvarez-León et al., 2006). In contrast, lower adherence was associated with increased blood pressure (BP) (Pitsavos et al., 2007). However, one study showed higher SBP in the group more closely following the Mediterranean diet in the SUN cohort in young individuals after a median follow-up of 4.2 years (Nunez-Cordoba et al., 2009). Most of the effects of the Mediterranean diet on blood pressure have been attributed to the consumption of olive oil, fruits, nuts and vegetables. Psaltopoulou et al (2004) in the Greek-EPIC cohort studied whether Mediterranean diet together or olive oil in particular reduced blood pressure in 20,343 people without a diagnosis of hypertension. In this study, the Mediterranean diet score was inversely and significantly associated with both, SBP and diastolic blood pressure (DBP), as well as the intake of olive oil, fruits and vegetables. However, Giuseppe et al (2008) found a significant and positive association of BP with the rate of adaptation to the Mediterranean diet. However, we have to consider that the study was carried out in older women (> 60 years). In the Italian EPIC Florence cohort, which include more than 10,000 non-hypertensive women aged 35-64 years, consumption of olive oil was inversely associated with DBP (Masala et al., 2008). However, with regard to DBP and Mediterranean diet as a whole, observational studies did not found significant associations (Kastorini et al., 2011).

Regarding randomized clinical trials (level I scientific evidence) in a meta-analysis, it was found that the overall adherence to Mediterranean diet was associated with lower SBP and DBP as compared with control diet (Kastorini et al., 2011). In the PREDIMED study, results showed a significant decrease in both SBP and DBP in the two groups with Mediterranean diet (one supplemented with VOO and another with nuts) as compared with control group (Estruch et al., 2006). Finally, in a non-randomized clinical trial whose aim was to evaluate the effect of a moderately hypoenergetic Mediterranean diet with an exercise program in women with overweight-obesity, DBP decreased significantly ($p < 0.001$) after two months of intervention, while the SBP was not changed significantly after four months of intervention (Andreoli et al., 2008).

In conclusion, as we mention before, the beneficial effects of the Mediterranean diet on blood pressure have been attributed to a synergy of its components, especially to fruits, vegetables, nuts and olive oil. These components are low in sodium and rich in minerals (magnesium, potassium and calcium), antioxidant, fiber, PUFA and MUFA, all of them with potentially protective properties against hypertension.

3.5 Mediterranean diet and inflammation

Obesity and other related diseases associated with CVD are caused or related to inflammation. Three of five cross-sectional studies, showed a significant decrease in inflammation markers with higher adherence to Mediterranean diet (Sotos-Prieto et al., 2010). Thus, Panagiotakos et al (2006) found significant negative association between adherence to Mediterranean diet and protein C reactive (CRP) ($p < 0.001$). Also, the highest score in the AHEI index (Alternate Healthy Eating Index) and AMED (alternate mediterranean diet index) was associated with lower inflammation biomarkers concentrations (IL-6 and CRP) (24% and 16% respectively). This study was carried out in 690 nurses, in the Nurses' Health Study (Fung et al., 2005). Moreover, subjects in the highest tertile of adherence to Mediterranean diet had 20 % lower CRP levels ($p = 0.015$) and 17% IL-6 ($p = 0.025$) (Chrysohoou et al., 2004), while the lower adherence to Mediterranean diet was associated with higher levels of CRP (> 3.0 mg / ml) (Pitsavos et al., 2007).

Salas-Salvado et al (2008), in a study that included subjects with high cardiovascular risk (339H/433M, 55-80 years), found an association between consumption of certain foods that characterized the Mediterranean pattern (fruits, cereals, VOO and nuts) with lower concentrations of inflammatory markers, especially those related to endothelial function (ICAM-1 and VCAM-1). However, participants with higher adherence to a Mediterranean diet showed no significant decrease in the inflammatory biomarkers' concentrations (CRP, IL-6, ICAM-1 and VCAM-1), although there was a statistical trend in the case of ICAM-1 and VCAM-1 ($p < 0.1$).

In two randomized controlled trials, CRP levels decreased only in the group with Mediterranean diet supplemented with VOO (-0.54 mg / L) compared with the control group (low-fat). The IL-6 decreased in both groups with Mediterranean diet (VOO and nuts), whereas it increased in the group with low-fat diet. Similarly, Esposito et al (Esposito et al., 2004), in a study conducted in Italy with 180 people with metabolic syndrome (99H, 81M), observed a significant decrease in CRP ($p = 0.01$) and IL-6 ($p = 0.04$) in the intervention group (instructed to follow a Mediterranean diet) compared with the control group (prudent diet with fat percentage <30%) after two years. By contrast, Michalsen et al (2006) found no changes in CRP levels, although there were some limitations in the study.

In a non-randomized clinical trial, plasma levels of CRP decreased significantly (6%, P <0.02) after two hours of Mediterranean diet rich in MUFA intake (Blum et al., 2006).

In conclusion, Mediterranean diet is characterized by a high consumption of fruit and vegetables. This adds other mechanistic benefits provided by their polyphenolic content to its high antioxidant content that could be linked with the prevention of inflammation. Other components of the Mediterranean diet such as VOO and red wine gather antioxidants and anti-inflammatory actions that may contribute to the healthy effects of this diet on inflammation.

	Decrease	Increase	No significant
BMI (kg/m²)	Scröder et al., 2004 Romaguera et al., 201 Bes-Ballostro et al., 2009; Garcia-Londa et al., 2003 Martinez-Gonzalez & Bes-Ballostro, 2011		
Weight gain	Fraser et al., 2002 Martinez-Gonzalez & Bes-Ballostro, 2011		
Waist circumference	Romaguera et al., 2002 Martinez-Gonzalez & Bes-Ballostro, 2011		
TC	Estruch et al.,2006 Vicent-Baudry et al., 2005 Ambring et al., 2004		
LDL-C	Vicent-Baudry et al., 2005 Ambring et al., 2004 Ros et al., 2004 Andreoli et al., 2008		Michalsen et al., 2006 Goulet et al., 2003 Estruch et al., 2006

	Decrease	Increase	No significant
HDL-C	Pitsavos et al., 2007	Estruch et al, 2006 Andreoli et al.,2008 Papadaki & Scott, 2008 Esposito et al., 2004; Esposito et al., 2003; Esposito et al., 2009; Athryros et al., 2011 Ambring et al., 2004	Michalsen et al., 2006 Goulet et al., 2003
TG	Estruch et al.,2006 Vicent-Baudry et al., 2005 Ambring et al., 2004 Ros et al., 2004 Chrysohoou et al., 2004; Tzima et al., 2007; Barzi et al., 2003 Shai et al., 2008 Esposito et al., 2004 Esposito et al., 2009 Elhayany et al., 2011 Sabate et al., 2010		Michalsen et al., 2006 de Lorgeril et al., 1994 Castro et al., 2000 Goulet et al., 2003
Glucose	Estruch et al., 2006 Vicent-Baudry et al., 2005 Andreoli et al.,2008 Panagiotakos et al., 2007 Tzima et al., 2007 Salas-Salvado et al., 2011		Ambring et al., 2004
SBP	Estruch et al., 2006 Tzima et al., 2007 Psaltopoulou et al., 2004 Panagiotakos et al., 2006	Giussepe et al., 2008 Nunez-Cordoba et al., 2009	Andreoli et al., 2008
BP	Estruch et al., 2006 Andreoli et al., 2008 Alvarez-Leon et al., 2006 Psaltopoulou et al., 2004 Pitsavos et al., 2007 Masala et al., 2008		
CRP	Estruch et al., 2006 Esposito et al., 2004 Blum et al., 2006 Fung et al., 2005 Chrysohoou et al., 2004 Panagiotakos et al., 2006	Pitsavos et al., 2007	Michalsen et al., 2006 Salas-Salvado et al., 2008
IL-6	Estruch et al., 2006 Esposito et al., 2004		Salas-Salvado et al., 2008

BMI: Body mass index; TC: Total Cholesterol; LDL-C: Low density lipoprotein cholesterol
HDL: High density lipoprotein cholesterol; TG: Triglycerides; SBP: Systolic blood pressure; BP: Blood pressure; CRP: Protein C reactive; IL-6: Interleukin 6

Table 1. Studies that analyze Mediterranean diet and variation (decrease, increase, no significant) in intermediate cardiovascular disease phenotypes.

4. Nutritional genomics

Current changes in lifestyle, in part promoted by the nutritional transition, have contributed to the development of CVD, cancer and other non-comunicable diseases.

Since the Human Genome Project finished in April 2003, we have the information about the complete genome. However, we still unknown the role of the majority of genes involved in the development of CVD. For that reason, currently, considering diet as one of the most important environmental factor, the molecular nutrition begins with the approach to better understand the mechanism involved in the gene-diet interaction and to personalize the diet with the aim to prevent common diseases, among them, CVD. Since Human Genome Project finished, the classic candidate gene approach and the new genome-wide association studies have identified genetic variants that predispose people to CVD.

In this sense, it was shown that human genome is sensitive to nutritional environment in two ways: nutrients may regulate genes and genes also influence the effect of diet (Loktionov, 2003). Nutritional health is dependent on the interaction between the environmental aspects of dietary components and the genetically controlled aspects (Figure 1). The concept of gene-diet interaction describes the modulation of the effect of a dietary component on a specific phenotype (plasma lipid concentrations, obesity, etc.) by a genetic polymorphism (Ordovas & Corella, 2004). A better understanding of these interactions has the potential to support disease prevention and will lead to different requirements between individuals via modification of dietary recommendations. This research has led to the development of concepts that study the effect of genetic variation on the interaction between diet and specific phenotypes known as *nutrigenetics*.

The goal of nutrigenetics is to generate personalized recommendations regarding the genetic susceptibility of each individual. It is also known as *personalized nutrition*.

On the other hand, the study of the characterization of gene products and the physiological function and interactions of these products is known as *nutrigenomics* (Figure 1). The unifying term *"nutritional genomics"* refers to nutrigenomics and nutrigenetics (Ordovas & Corella, 2004). The term Nutrigenetics was named for the first time by Brennan in 1975 in his book "Nutrigenenetics: New concepts for Relieving Hypoglycemia", while nutrigenomics was used in 1999 by DellaPenna when he studied the plant genomics field. The new technology research together with the knowledge of the human genome sequence have led in the study of the new "omics" to better understand the molecular basis of the disease development. They are the disciplines known as:

- *Transcriptomic*: to quantify the level of gene expression by using techniques to analyse thousands of mRNA molecules at the same time by using a technique based on microarrays.
- *Proteomic*: large-scale study of proteins (particularly their structure and function) is possible to identify proteins that can diagnose disease or predict the evolution of it.
- *Metabolomics:* to study techniques dedicated to complete a system composed of a series of molecules that are metabolic intermediates, metabolites, hormones and other signal molecules, and secondary metabolites, which can be found in a biological system.
- *Systems Biology*: integration of proteomic data, genetic, metabolomics.
- *Bioinformatics*: to interpret the data to provide biological mechanisms to explain the experimental observations.

Following these new concepts, other related terms have emerged: *nutritranscriptomic* (the study of messenger RNA expression at the cellular level under some nutritional conditions), *nutriproteomic* (large-scale analysis of the structure and function of the protein, as well as protein-protein interactions in a cell to identify molecular targets of dietary components) or *nutrimetabolomic* (measuring all metabolites in response to stimuli nutritional body) (Panagiotou & Nielsen, 2009).

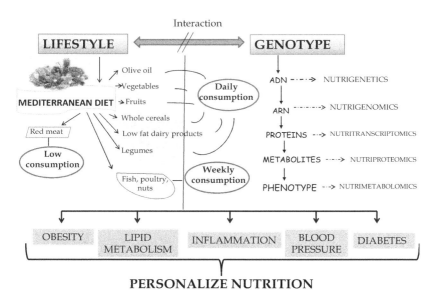

Fig. 1. Personalized Nutrition. As part of health determinants, lifestyle interacts with genetic susceptibility to modulate obesity risk, lipid metabolism, inflammation, blood pressure and diabetes. Among lifestyle factors, diet, and especifically, Mediterrranean diet, has an important role in gen-diet interactions. On the other hand, with the new technology research together with the knowledge of human genome sequence have led in the study of the nutrigenetics and nutrigenomics (nutritional genomics) to better understand the molecular basis of the disease development, they are the disciplines knows as: transcriptomic, proteomic, metabolomic that allow us to know phenotypes characteristics. These interactions between Mediterranean diet and genetic susceptibility will contribute to create personalized diets.

5. Gene-Mediterranean diet interaction in intermediate cardiovascular diseases phenotypes

In the following sections we are going to review some studies analyzing nutrigenetics and nutrigenomics effects on CVD.

5.1 Nutrigenetics in the prevention of cardiovascular diseases

In the last decades the eating pattern has changed considerably towards less healthy habits with excessive intake of calories and SFA. Considering this as a risk factor of CVD these changes are contributing to the increase of CVD. As a result, researchers are wondering which could be the best diet to prevent CVD and related phenotypes. Different opinions have emerged about the virtues of low-carbohydrate diets, low fat diets, high-protein diets or Mediterranean dietary pattern in the control of body weight and factors related to CVD (Shai et al., 2008, Larsen et al., 2010, Sacks et al., 2009).

Given the great diversity that exists with regard to dietary recommendations and their effects, several authors insist on the fact that there is no perfect diet. Diet will be different depending on individual characteristics. The response to the same diet has not the same effectiveness on different two people. While some people appear to have no response to dietary intervention (hiporesponders), others have a high response (hiperresponders) (Katan MB et al., 1986). It has been suggested that this inter-individual variability to dietary modification is determined by genetic factors, especially for phenotypes related to lipid metabolism (Loktionov, 2003).

Most of the studies carried out to determine whether genetic factors could explain these differences are based on the study of single nucleotide polymorphisms (SNPs) as well as dietary factors, particularly those that characterize Mediterranean Diet. The table 2 shows some studies conducted to assess genetic modulations according to different types of diets or macronutrients. In the following paragraphs we describe the results from intervention studies and observational studies that analyze gene-diet interactions on CVD.

Results from intervention studies

Intervention studies in which subjects receive a controlled dietary intake provide the most valuable information for the study of gene-nutrient-phenotype association. However, intervention studies have some limitations, such as the low number of participants. The sample size is important in nutrigenetic studies because otherwise, there is a lack of statistical power to assess the main associations. Something similar happens with the study of some genetic variants. Prevalence of certain polymorphisms is small and requires a large sample size to study these associations. Another limitation is the short duration of these interventions. A review conducted by Masson et al, (2003) concluded that there is evidence to suggest that variations in the *APOA1, APOA4, APOB* and *APOE* genes contribute to the heterogeneity of the lipid response to dietary interventions, and that these genes are directly or indirectly regulated by PPAR or other nuclear receptors. New examples that confirm the importance of gene-diet interaction in the field of nutrigenetics are the study of the perilipin gene (*PLIN*) (Corella D et al., 2005, Smith CE et al., 2010) and *SR-BI* (Perez-Martinez P et al., 2005).

Recently, some studies investigating the genetic modulation of the Mediterranean diet in PREDIMED study have been published. Thus, a study examining a polymorphism in the *FTO* gene (associated with obesity) shows that the A allele of the polymorphism rs9939609 in the FTO gene was not associated with baseline body weight, but after 3 years of nutritional intervention with Mediterranean diet carriers of A allele had a lower body weight gain than subjects with the ancestral allele (Razquin C et al., 2010 A).

Another example carried out in the PREDIMED study showed that CC subjects for the polymorphism-174G / C in the *IL-6* gene had a lower weight gain after three years only in those subjects who followed a Mediterranean diet supplemented with nuts and olive oil (Razquin et al., 2010 B)

Results from observational studies

Observational studies have the advantage of incorporating a large number of participants and the ability to estimate dietary habits. They also have the advantage that the distribution of genetic variants in the population is independent of eating behaviors by the principle of Mendelian randomization. Although nowadays the number of studies examining gene-diet interactions is increasing, few studies have investigated the interaction between SNPs in candidate genes and cardiovascular risk factors analyzing the consumption of Mediterranean diet or intake of MUFA, PUFA or SFA.

One of the most studied genes has been the Pro12Ala polymorphism in the *PPARG* gene and its interaction with MUFA intake. Obese subjects with the Ala12 allele have higher HOMA index when they eat low amounts of MUFA. Another example analyzing MUFA intake and body weight depending on variation in *APOA5* gene is one carried out in the Framingham study. They found a significant interaction between the promoter polymorphism -1131T>C in the *APOA5* gene and fat intake, particularly MUFA, regulating body weight (Corella D et al., 2007). The study of C677T polymorphism in the gene for methylenetetrahydrofolate reductase (*MTHFR*) is another example of modulation of LDL oxidation by the Mediterranean diet (Pitsavos et al., 2006). Recently, we published a significant gene-diet interaction in a variant of the promoter of *APOA2* gene. This study included 3462 volunteers from three different populations and it studied the interaction between the polymorphism-265T>C in the *APOA2* gene, food intake, and BMI. Carriers of the variant allele which had higher intake of SFA had a higher prevalence of obesity while this was not showed if the source of fat was MUFA or PUFA. These results were replicated for the first time in three independent populations (Corella et al., 2009). Subsequently, the authors replicated this interaction in Mediterranean and Chinese populations (Corella et al., 2011) confirming the importance of genetic modulation by dietary factors, and also the need to replicate gene-diet interactions to increase the scientific evidence and finally to contribute to personalize diet based on genetic susceptibility.

Author	Phenotype		Gene	Gen-diet interaction
Lopez-Miranda et al., 1994	Lipid metabolism	LDL-C	-75G>A APOA1	They studied the influence of the LDL-C postprandial response to MUFA intake. After high MUFA intake carriers of A allele had higher LDL-C but not the GG.
Jansen et al., 1997		LDL-C	Thr347Ser APOA4	347Ser carriers had lower LDL-C postprandial response when they switched from a diet rich in SFA to a diet based on NCEP.
Campos et al., 2001		VLDL, HDL-C	APOE	Higher VLDL and lower HDL-C in E2 with a high SFA intake.
Corella et al., 2001		LDL-C	APOE	E2 carriers had lower LDL-C in those with moderate alcohol consumption than in non-consumers. However, carriers of E4 allele that had a moderate alcohol consumption had higher LDL-C.
Brown et al., 2003		TC and LDL-C	T455C y T625 *APOC3*	In -45T and -625T homozygous subjects, SFA intake was associated with higher LDL-C.
Tai et al., 2005		TG and APOCIII	L162V *PPARA*	Carriers of 162V allele had higher TG concentrations and APOC3 levels only in that subjects with a low PUFA consumption.

Author	Phenotype		Gene	Gen-diet interaction
Robitaille et al., 2007		Lipids	Leu72Met Grelina	Interaction with fat intake modulating TG concentrations.
Ordovas, 2002		HDL-C	-514C>T *LIPC*	T alelle was associated with higher HDL-C in subjects that had an intake of fat < 30% of total energy.
Luan et al., 2001	Antropometric variables	BMI	Pro12Ala PPARG	AlaPPARG carriers had higher BMI than ProPPRG, but when the ratio PUFA:SFA was high, opposite results were shown.
Memisoglu et al., 2003		BMI	Pro12Ala PPARG	Among ProPro subjects, those with higher fat intake of had higher BMI compared to those with lower intake . No association was shown for 12Ala.
Robitaille et al., 2007		WC	Pro12Ala PPARA	Interaction Pro12Ala with the intake of fat modulating waist circunference.
Corella et al., 2009		BMI and Obesity	-265 T>C APOA2	C carriers that had high SFA intake had higher prevalence of obesity.
Corella et al., 2011		BMI and obesity	-265 T>C APOA2	Interaction of -265CC with SFA intake modulating risk of obesity.
Corella et al., 2010		BMI and obesity	rs9939609 FTO	Interacction of rs9939609 with educational level. A carriers had higher risk of obesity and BMI only in those without uneversity studies.
Razquin et al., 2010 (A)		Weight	rs9939609 FTO	A allele was associated with higher weight at the beginnung of the study. After three years of intervention with Mediterranean diet, A carriers had a lower weight gain.
Razquin et al., 2010 (C)		Weight	+45T/G, +276G/T Adiponectin	Genotype GG (+45T/G) was associated with higher weight gained during three years of intervention. TT (+276G/T) was associated with higher weight gain in men. Mediterranean diet suplemented with VOO and nuts reverted this effects.
Razquin et al., 2010 (B)		Weight	-174G/C IL-6	CC subjects that followed Mediterranean diet suplemented with VOO had lower weight gain after three years of intervention.

LDL-C: Low density lipoprotein cholesterol; VLDL: Very low density lipoprotein cholesterol
HDL: High density lipoprotein cholesterol; TC: Total cholesterol; BMI: Body mass index
WC: Waist circumference

Table 2. Nutrigenetics studies analysing gene-diet interactions.

5.2 Nutrigenomics in the prevention of cardiovascular diseases

As we explained in the previous section, there is increasing evidence that Mediterranean diet, whose emblematic component is virgin olive oil (VOO), has a beneficial effect on diseases associated with CVD and other diseases (neurodegenerative diseases, cancer).

VOO is a functional food containing high levels of MUFA and a number of minor components (bioactive components). These components are known as phenolic compounds. These phenolic compounds have a key role in plasma lipid concentrations and oxidative damage (that is related to CVD). It is believed that the benefits from the consumption of VOO are due to the interaction of its nutrients and minor components with genes. Several studies have shown changes in gene expression mediated by the consumption of VOO. In table 3 some studies analyzing changes in gene expression of some genes related to CVD by Mediterranean diet or its components are shown.

Autor	N /duración	Intervención	Cambios de expresión	Ruta implicada
Konstantinidou et al., 2010	N=90 (20-50 years) 3 months	1. MD +VOO 2. MD+ VOO 3. Control	INF-γ ARHGAP15 IL7R ADRB2 POLK	Inflammation Oxidative stress
Konstantinidou et al., 2009	N=6 Postprandial study (0-6h)	50 ml VOO (26082 genes)	USP48 OGT AKAP13 IL10 DCLRE1C POLK	Cellular process Inflammation DNA damage
Khymenets et al., 2009	N= 6 H(262-28 years; 4 M (20-44) 3 weeks	VOO (25 ml/day)	ADAM17, ALDH1A, BIRC1, ERCC5, LIAS, OGT,PPARBP, TNFSF10, USP48, XRCC5	Mechanism involved in atherosclerosis
Camargo et al., 2010	N=20 with MS (56 years, 9 H, 11 M) Postprandial state	Breakfast with VOO (40 ml).	EGR1 IL1B, IL6 CCL3 CXCL1 CXCL2 CXCL3 CXCR4 TRIB1, NFKBIA	Inflammation
Llorente-Cortes et al., 2009	N=48 (55-80 years)	MD+VOO MD+nuts Control group	COX-2 LRP1 MCP-1 CD36 TFPI	Inflammation, foam cell formation, thrombosis
De Mello VD et al., 2008	34overweight MS 33 weeks	Weight reduction (n=24) Control group (n=10)	TLR4 TLR2 CCL5 TNFRSF1A IKBKB	Related to insulin sensitivity
Crujeiras et al., 2008	12 Obese (37,7 years) 8 weeks	Hypocaloric diet	SIRT1 SIRT2 NDUFS2	

MD: Mediterranean diet; VOO: Virgin olive oil; MS: Metabolic Syndrome

Table 3. Nutrigenomics studies

6. Conclusions and future directions

Current results of the studies analyzing the effect of Mediterranean diet on CVD suggest that adherence to the Mediterranean dietary pattern was associated with lower CVD phenotypes. Mediterranean diet has a beneficial effect on abdominal obesity, lipids levels, glucose metabolism, blood pressure and inflammation. The antioxidant and anti-inflammatory effects of the Mediterranean diet as a whole, and also the effects of the individual components, specifically VOO, fruits, vegetables, whole grains and fish could offer an explanation for the aforementioned beneficial effects of the Mediterranean diet.

These results are of considerable public health importance because this dietary pattern can be easily adopted by all population groups and various cultures, and they cost effectively serve for the primary and secondary prevention of CVD.

On the other hand, the current evidence from nutrigenetics studies is not enough to begin implementing specific personalized information. However, there is a large number of examples of common SNPs modulating the individual response to Mediterranean diet and other components as proof of concept of how gene-diet interactions can influence lipid metabolism, BMI, or other disorders, and it is expected that in the near future we will be able to harness the information contained in our genomes by using the behavioural tools to achieve successful personalized nutrition. In order to achieve that, it is recommended that future advises on nutrition will be based on studies using the highest level of epidemiological evidence and supported by mechanistic studies within the Nutritional Genomics and Systems biology. However, we have to take into account that in order to forget successful results in personalized nutrition through genetic variation, health professionals need to be prepared to learn and interpret genetic knowledge about their patients.

7. References

Alvarez León, EE., Henríquez, P., & Serra-Majem, L. (2006). Mediterranean diet and metabolic syndrome: a cross-sectional study in the Canary Islands. *Public Health Nutr*; 9(8A):1089-98.

Ambring, A., Friberg, P., Axelsen, M., Laffrenzen, M., Taskinen, MR., & Basu, S. (2004). Effects of a Mediterranean-inspired diet on blood lipids, vascular function and oxidative stress in healthy subjects. *M Clin Sci*; 106(5):519-25.

Andreoli, A., Lauro, S., Di Daniele, N., Sorge, R., Celi, M., & Volpe, SL. (2008). Effect of a moderately hypoenergetic Mediterranean diet and exercise program on body cell mass and cardiovascular risk factors in obese women. *Eur J Clin Nutr*;62(7):892-7.

Athyros, VG., Kakafika, AI., Papageorgiou, AA., Tziomalos, K., Peletidou, A., Vosikis, C., Karagiannis, A., & Mikhailidis, DP. (2011). Effect of a plant stanol ester-containing spread, placebo spread, or Mediterranean diet on estimated cardiovascular risk and lipid, inflammatory and haemostatic factors. *Nutr Metab Cardiovasc Dis*;21(3):213-21.

Barzi, F., Woodward, M., Marfisi, RM., Tavazzi, L., Valagussa, F., & Marchioli, R. (2003). Mediterranean diet and all-causes mortality after myocardial infarction: results from the GISSI-Prevenzione trial. *Eur J Clin Nutr*; 57(4):604-11.

Bes-Rastrollo, M., Wedick, NM., Martinez-Gonzalez, MA., Li, TY., Sampson, L., & Hu, FB. (2009). Prospective study of nut consumption, long-term weight change, and obesity risk in women. *Am J Clin Nutr*; 89(6):1913-9.

Blum, S., Aviram, M., Ben-Amotz, A., & Levy, Y. (2006). Effect of a Mediterranean meal on postprandial carotenoids, paraoxonase activity and C-reactive protein levels. *Ann Nutr Metab*; 50(1):20-4.

Brennan, AM., Sweeney, LL., Liu, X., & Mantzoros, CS. (2010). Walnut consumption increases satiation but has no effect on insulin resistance or the metabolic profile over a 4-day period. *Obesity (Silver Spring)*;18(6):1176-82.

Brennan, RO. (1975) Nutrigenetics: new concepts for relieving hypoglycemia. New York: M. Evans and Co.

Brown, S., Ordovás, JM., Campos, H. (2003) Interaction between the APOC3 gene promoter polymorphisms, saturated fat intake and plasma lipoproteins. *Atherosclerosis*; 170(2):307-13.

Camargo, A., Ruano, J., Fernandez, JM., Parnell, LD., Jimenez, A., Santos-Gonzalez, M. et al. (2010). Gene expression changes in mononuclear cells in patients with metabolic syndrome after acute intake of phenol-rich virgin olive oil. *BMC Genomics*; 11:253.

Campos, H., D'Agostino, M., & Ordovás, JM. (2001). Gene-diet interactions and plasma lipoproteins: role of apolipoprotein E and habitual saturated fat intake. *Genet Epidemiol*; 20(1):117-128.

Castro, P., Miranda, JL., Gómez, P., Escalante, DM., Segura, FL., Martín, A., et al. (2000). Comparison of an oleic acid enriched-diet vs NCEP-I diet on LDL susceptibility to oxidative modifications. *Eur J Clin Nutr*; 54(1):61-7.

Chrysohoou, C., Panagiotakos, DB., Pitsavos, C., Das, UN., & Stefanadis, C. (2004). Adherence to the Mediterranean diet attenuates inflammation and coagulation process in healthy adults: The ATTICA Study. *J Am Coll Cardiol*; 44(1):152-8.

Corella, D., Carrasco, P., Sorlí, JV., Coltell, O., Ortega-Azorín, C., Guillén, M., et al. (2010). Education modulates the association of the FTO rs9939609 polymorphism with body mass index and obesity risk in the Mediterranean population. Nutr Metab Cardiovasc Dis. 2010 Dec 24. [Epub ahead of print]

Corella, D., Lai, CQ., Demissie, S., Cupples, LA., Manning, AK., Tucker, KL., & Ordovas, JM. (2007). APOA5 gene variation modulates the effects of dietary fat intake on body mass index and obesity risk in the Framingham Heart Study. *J Mol Med (Berl)*; 85(2):119-28.

Corella, D., & Ordovas, JM. (2005). Integration of environment and disease into 'omics' analysis. *Curr Opin Mol Ther*; 7(6):569-76.

Corella, D., Peloso, G., Arnett, DK., Demissie, S., Cupples, LA., Tucker, K., et al. (2009). APOA2, dietary fat, and body mass index: replication of a gene-diet interaction in 3 independent populations. *Arch Intern Med*; 169(20):1897-906.

Corella, D., Tai, ES., Sorlí, JV., Chew, SK., Coltell, O., Sotos-Prieto, M., et al. (2011). Association between the APOA2 promoter polymorphism and body weight in Mediterranean and Asian populations: replication of a gene-saturated fat interaction. *Int J Obes (Lond)*; 35(5):666-75.

Corella, D., Tucker, K., Lahoz, C., Coltell, O., Cupples, LA., Wilson, et al. (2001). Alcohol drinking determines the effect of the APOE locus on LDL-cholesterol concentrations in men: the Framingham Offspring Study. *Am J Clin Nutr*; 73(4):736-45.

Crujeiras, AB., Parra, D., Goyenechea, E., Abete, I., González-Muniesa, P., & Martínez, JA. (2008). Energy restriction in obese subjects impact differently two mitochondrial function markers. *J Physiol Biochem*; 64(3):211-9.

de Lorgeril, M., Renaud, S., Mamelle, N., Salen, P., Martin, JL., Monjaud, I., et al. (1994). Mediterranean alpha-linolenic acid-rich diet in secondary prevention of coronary heart disease. *Lancet*; 343(8911):1454-9.

de Lorgeril, M., Salen, P., Martin, JL., Monjaud, I., Delaye, J., & Mamelle, N. (1999). Mediterranean diet, traditional risk factors, and the rate of cardiovascular complications after myocardial infarction: final report of the Lyon Diet Heart Study. *Circulation*; 99(6):779-85.

de Mello, VD., Kolehmainen, M., Pulkkinen, L., Schwab, U., Mager, U., Laaksonen, DE., et al. (2008). Downregulation of genes involved in NFkappaB activation in peripheral blood mononuclear cells after weight loss is associated with the improvement of insulin sensitivity in individuals with the metabolic syndrome: the GENOBIN study. *Diabetologia*; 51(11):2060-7

DellaPenna, D. 1999. Nutricional genomics: manipulating plant micronutrients to improve human health. *Science*; 285:375-79

Elhayany, A., Lustman, A., Abel, R., Attal-Singer, J., & Vinker, S. (2010). A low carbohydrate Mediterranean diet improves cardiovascular risk factors and diabetes control among overweight patients with type 2 diabetes mellitus: a 1-year prospective randomized intervention study. Diabetes Obes Metab;12(3):204-9.

Esposito, K., Kastorini, CM., Panagiotakos, DB., & Giugliano, D. (2011). Mediterranean diet and weight loss: meta-analysis of randomized controlled trials . *Metab Syndr Relat Disord*; 9(1):1-12.

Esposito, K., Maiorino, MI., Di Palo, C., Giugliano, D., & Campanian. (2009). Postprandial Hyperglycemia Study Group. Adherence to a Mediterranean diet and glycaemic control in Type 2 diabetes mellitus. *Diabet Med*; 26(9):900-7.

Esposito, K., Marfella, R., Ciotola, M., Di Palo, C., Giugliano, F., Giugliano, G., et al. (2004) Effect of a mediterranean-style diet on endothelial dysfunction and markers of vascular inflammation in the metabolic syndrome: a randomized trial. *JAMA*; 292(12):1440-6.

Esposito, K., Pontillo, A., Di Palo, C., Giugliano, G., Masella, M., Marfella, R., & Giugliano, D. (2003). Effect of weight loss and lifestyle changes on vascular inflammatory markers in obese women: a randomized trial. *JAMA*; 289(14):1799-804.

Estruch, R., Martínez-González, MA., Corella, D., Salas-Salvadó, J., Ruiz-Gutiérrez, V., Covas, MI., et al, (2006). Effects of a Mediterranean-style diet on cardiovascular risk factors: a randomized trial. *Ann Intern Med*;145(1):1-11.

Fraser, GE., Bennett, HW., Jaceldo, KB., & Sabaté, J. (2002). Effect on body weight of a free 76 Kilojoule (320 calorie) daily supplement of almonds for six months. *J Am Coll Nut*; 21(3):275-83.

Fung, TT., McCullough, ML., Newby, PK., Manson, JE., Meigs, JB., Rifai, N., et al. (2005). Diet-quality scores and plasma concentrations of markers of inflammation and endothelial dysfunction. *Am J Clin Nutr*; 82(1):163-73.

Mediterranean Diet and Gene-Mediterranean Diet Interactions in Determining
Intermediate Cardiovascular Disease Phenotypes

201

García-Lorda, P., Megias Rangil, I., & Salas-Salvadó, J. (2003). Nut consumption, body weight and insulin resistance. *Eur J Clin Nutr*; 57 Suppl 1:S8-11.

Giuseppe, RD., Bonanni, A., Olivieri, M., Castelnuovo, AD., Donati, MB., Gaetano, GD., et al. (2008). Adherence to Mediterranena diet and anthropometric and metabolic parameters in an observational study in the "Alto Molise" region: The MOLI-SAL project. *Nutr Metab Cardiovasc Dis*; 18(6):415-21.

Goulet, J., Lamarche, B., Nadeau, G., & Lemieux, S. (2003). Effect of a nutritional intervention promoting the Mediterranean food pattern on plasma lipids, lipoproteins and body eight in healthy French-Canadian women. *Atherosclerosis*; 170(1):115-24.

Harris, RP., Helfand, M., Woolf, SH., Lohr, KN., Mulrow, CD., Teutsch, SM., et al. (2001). Third U.S. Preventive Services Task Force. Current methods of the U.S. Preventive Services Task Force: a review of the process. *Am J Prev Med*; 20(3S):21-35.

Haskell, WL. (2003). Cardiovascular disease prevention and lifestyle interventions: effectiveness and efficacy. *J Cardiovasc Nurs*; 18:245-55

Howard, BV., Van Horn, L., Hsia, J., Manson, JE., Stefanick, ML., Wassertheil-Smoller, S., Kuller, LH., et al. (2006). Low-fat dietary pattern and risk of cardiovascular disease: the Women's Health Initiative Randomized Controlled Dietary Modification Trial. *JAMA*; 295(6):655-66.

Jansen, S., Lopez-Miranda, J., Salas, J., Ordovas, JM., Castro, P., Marin, C., et al. (1997). Effect of 347-serine mutation in apoprotein A-IV on plasma LDL cholesterol response to dietary fat. Arterioscler *Thromb Vasc Biol*; 17(8):1532-8.

Kastorini, CM., Milionis, HJ., Esposito, K., Giugliano, D., Goudevenos, JA., & Panagiotakos, DB. (2011). The effect of Mediterranean diet on metabolic syndrome and its components: a meta-analysis of 50 studies and 534,906 individuals. *J Am Coll Cardiol*; 57(11):1299-313.

Katan MB, Beynen AC, de Vries JH, Nobels A. (1986). Existence of consistent hypo- and hyperresponders to dietary cholesterol in man. *Am J Epidemiol*; 123(2):221-34.

Keys, A. (1970). Coronary Heart Disease in Seven Countries. *Circulation*; 41(1):1-211.

Keys, A., Menotti, A., & Karoven, MI. (1986). The diet and the 15-year death rate in the Seven Countries Study. *Am J Epidemiol*; 124:903-915.

Khymenets, O., Fitó, M., Covas, MI., Farré, M., Pujadas, MA., Muñoz, D., Konstantinidou, V., & de la Torre, R. (2009). Mononuclear cell transcriptome response after sustained virgin olive oil consumption in humans: an exploratory nutrigenomics study. *OMICS*; 13(1):7-19

Knoops, KT., de Groot, LC., Kromhout, D., Perrin, AE., Moreiras-Varela, O., Menotti, A., et al. (2004). Mediterranean diet, lifestyle factors, and 10-year mortality in elderly European men and women: the HALE project. *JAMA*; 292(12):1433-9.

Konstantinidou, V., Covas, MI., Muñoz-Aguayo, D., Khymenets, O., de la Torre, R., Saez, G., et al. (2010). In vivo nutrigenomic effects of virgin olive oil polyphenols within the frame of the Mediterranean diet: a randomized controlled trial. *FASEB J*; 24(7):2546-57.

Konstantinidou, V., Khymenets, O., Fito, M., De La Torre, R., Anglada, R., Dopazo, A., & Covas, MI. (2009). Characterization of human gene expression changes after olive oil ingestion: an exploratory approach. *Folia Biol (Praha)*; 55(3):85-91

Krauss, RM., Eckel, RH., Howard, B., Appel, LJ., Daniels, SR., & Deckelbaum, RJ. (2000). AHA Dietary Guidelines: revision 2000: A statement for healthcare professionals from the Nutrition Committee of the American Heart Association. *Stroke*; 31(11):2751-66.

Lalonde, M. (1974). A new perspective on the health of canadians: a working document. Ottawa: Department of Health and Welfare.

Larsen, TM., Dalskov, SM., van Baak, M., Jebb, SA., Papadaki, A., Pfeiffer, AF., et al. (2010). Diet, Obesity, and Genes (Diogenes) Project. Diets with high or low protein content and glycemic index for weight-loss maintenance. *N Engl J Med*; 363(22):2102-13.

Li, Z., Song, R., Nguyen, C., Zerlin, A., Karp, H., Naowamondhol, K., et al. (2010). Pistachio nuts reduce triglycerides and body weight by comparison to refined carbohydrate snack in obese subjects on a 12-week weight loss program. *J Am Coll Nutr*; 29(3):198-203.

Lichtenstein, AH., Ausman, LM., Jalbert, SM., Vilella-Bach, M., Jauhiainen, M., McGladdery, S., et al. (2002). Efficacy of a Therapeutic Lifestyle Change/Step 2 diet in moderately hypercholesterolemic middle-aged and elderly female and male subjects. *J Lipid Res*;43(2):264-73.

Linton MF, Fazio S, National Cholesterol Education Program (NCEP)- the third Adult Treatment Panel (ATP III). (2003). A practical approach to risk assessment to prevent coronary artery disease and its complications. *Am J Cardiol*; 92(1A):19i-26i.

Llorente-Cortés V, Estruch R, Mena MP, Ros E, González MA, Fitó M, et al. (2010). Effect of Mediterranean diet on the expression of pro-atherogenic genes in a population at high cardiovascular risk. . *Atherosclerosis*; 208(2):442-50

Loktionov, A. (2003) Common gene polymorphisms and nutrition: emerging links with pathogenesis of multifactorial chronic diseases (review). *J Nutr Biochem*;14(8):426-51.

Lopez-Miranda J, Ordovas JM, Mata P, Lichtenstein AH, Clevidence B, Judd JT, Schaefer EJ. (1994). Effect of apolipoprotein E phenotype on diet-induced lowering of plasma low density lipoprotein cholesterol. *J Lipid Res*; 35(11):1965-75.

Luan, J., Browne, PO., Harding, AH., Halsall, DJ., O'Rahilly, S., Chatterjee, VK., & Wareham NJ. (2001). Evidence for gene-nutrient interaction at the PPARgamma locus. *Diabetes*; 50(3):686-9.

Martínez-González, MA., & Bes-Rastrollo, M. (2011). Nut consumption, weight gain and obesity: Epidemiological evidence. *Nutr Metab Cardiovasc Dis*;21 Suppl 1:S40-5.

Martínez-González, MA., Fuente-Arrillaga, CD., Nunez-Cordoba, JM., Basterra-Gortari, FJ., Beunza, JJ., Vazquez, Z., et al. (2008). Adherence to Mediterranean diet and risk of developing diabetes: prospective cohort study. *BMJ*; 336(7657):1348-51.

Masala, G., Bendinelli, B., Versari, D., Saieva, C., Ceroti, M., Santagiuliana, F., et al. (2008). Anthropometric and dietary determinants of blood pressure in over 7000 Mediterranean women: the European Prospective Investigation into Cancer and Nutrition-Florence cohort. *J Hypertens*; 26(11):2112-20.

Masson, LF., McNeill, G., & Avenell, A. (2003). Genetic variation and the lipid response to dietary intervention: a systematic review. *Am J Clin Nutr*; 77(5):1098-111.

Memisoglu, A., Hu, FB., Hankinson, SE., Manson, JE., De Vivo, I., Willett, WC., & Hunter, DJ. (2003). Interaction between a peroxisome proliferator-activated receptor gamma

Mediterranean Diet and Gene-Mediterranean Diet Interactions in Determining
Intermediate Cardiovascular Disease Phenotypes

203

gene polymorphism and dietary fat intake in relation to body mass. *Hum Mol Genet*; 12(22):2923-9.

Michalsen, A., Lehmann, N., Pithan, C., Knoblauch, NT., Moebus, S., Kannenberg, F., et al. (2006). Mediterranean diet has no effect on markers of inflammation and metabolic risk factors in patients with coronary artery disease. *Eur J Clin Nutr*; 60(4):478-85.

Müller-Nordhorn, J., Rossnagel, K., Mey, W., & Willich, SN. (2004). Regional variation and time trends in mortality from ischaemic heart disease: East and West Germany 10 years after reunification. *J Epidemiol Community Health*; 58:481–485.

Núñez-Córdoba, JM., Valencia-Serrano, F., Toledo, E., Alonso, A., & Martínez-González, MA. (2009). The Mediterranean diet and incidence of hypertension: the Seguimiento Universidad de Navarra (SUN) Study. *Am J Epidemiol*; 169(3):339-46.

Obarzanek, E., Sacks, FM., Vollmer, WM., Bray, GA., Miller, ER3rd., Lin, PH., et al. DASH Research Group. (2001). Effects on blood lipids of a blood pressure-lowering diet: the Dietary Approaches to Stop Hypertension (DASH) Trial. *Am J Clin Nutr*; 74(1):80-9.

Ordovas, JM., Corella, D., Demissie, S., Cupples, LA., Couture, P., Coltell, O., et al. (2001). Dietary fat intake determines the effect of a common polymorphism in the hepatic lipase gene promoter on high-density lipoprotein metabolism: evidence of a strong dose effect in this gene-nutrient interaction in the Framingham Study. *Circulation*;106(18):2315-21.

Ordovas, JM., & Corella, D. (2004). Nutritional genomics. *Annu Rev Genomics Hum Genet*; 5:71-118

Ordovas JM, Mooser V. (2004). Nutrigenomics and nutrigenetics. *Curr Opin Lipidol*; 15(2):101-8.

Panagiotakos, DB., Pitsavos, C., Arvaniti, F., & Stefanadis, C. (2007). Adherence to the Mediterranean food pattern predicts the prevalence of hypertension, hypercholesterolemia, diabetes and obesity, among healthy adults; the accuracy of the MedDietScore. *Prev Med*; 44(4):335-40.

Panagiotakos, DB., Pitsavos, C., & Stefanadis, C. (2006). Dietary patterns: a Mediterranean diet score and its relation to clinical and biological markers of cardiovascular disease risk. *Nutr Metab Cardiovasc Dis*; 16(8):559-68.

Panagiotakos, DB., Tzima, N., Pitsavos, C., Chrysohoou, C., Zampelas, A., Toussoulis, D., et al. (2007). The association between adherence to the Mediterranean diet and fasting indices of glucose homoeostasis: the ATTICA Study. *J Am Coll Nutr*; 26(1):32-8.

Panagiotou, G., Nielsen J. (2009). Nutritional systems biology: definitions and approaches. *Annu Rev Nutr*; 29:329-39.

Papadaki, A., Scott JA. (2008). Follow-up of a web-based tailored intervention promoting the Mediterranean diet in Scotland. *Patient Educ Couns*; 73(2):256-63.

Pérez-Martínez, P., Pérez-Jiménez, F., Bellido, C., Ordovás, JM., Moreno, JA., Marín, C., et al. (2005). A polymorphism exon 1 variant at the locus of the scavenger receptor class B type I (SCARB1) gene is associated with differences in insulin sensitivity in healthy people during the consumption of an olive oil-rich diet. *J Clin Endocrinol Metab*; 90(4):2297-300.

Pitsavos, C., Panagiotakos, D., Trichopoulou, A., Chrysohoou, C., Dedoussis, G., Chloptsios, Y., et al. (2006). Interaction between Mediterranean diet and methylenetetrahydrofolate reductase C677T mutation on oxidized low density lipoprotein concentrations: the ATTICA study. *Nutr Metab Cardiovasc Dis*; 16(2):91-9.

Pitsavos, C., Panagiotakos, DB., Chrysohoou, C., & Stefanadis, C. (2003). Epidemiology of cardiovascular risk factors in Greece: aims, design and baseline characteristics of the ATTICA study. *BMC Public Health*; 3:32-40.

Pitsavos, C., Panagiotakos, DB., Tzima, N., Lentzas, Y., Chrysohoou, C., Das, UN-, et al. (2007). Diet, exercise, and C-reactive protein levels in people with abdominal obesity: the ATTICA epidemiological study. *Angiology*;58(2):225-33.

Polychronopoulos, E., Panagiotakos, DB., Polystipioti. (2005). A.Diet, lifestyle factors and hypercholesterolemia in elderly men and women from Cyprus. *Lipids Health Dis*; 6;4:17

Posner, BM., Cobb, JL., Belanger, AJ., et al. (1991). Dietary lipid predictors of coronary heart disease in men. The Framingham Study. *Arch Intern Med*; 151:1181-7.

Psaltopoulou, T., Naska, A., Orfanos, P., Trichopoulos, D., Mountokalakis, T., Trichopoulou, A. (2004). Olive oil, the Mediterranean diet, and arterial blood pressure: the Greek European Prospective Investigation into Cancer and Nutrition (EPIC) study. *Am J Clin Nutr*;80(4):1012-8.

Rajaram, S., & Sabaté, J. Nuts, body weight and insulin resistance. Br J Nutr. 2006;96 Suppl 2:S79-86.

Razquin, C., Martinez, JA., Martinez-Gonzalez, MA., Bes-Rastrollo, M., Fernández-Crehuet, & J., Marti, A. (2010 A). A 3-year intervention with a Mediterranean diet modified the association between the rs9939609 gene variant in FTO and body weight changes. *Int J Obes (Lond)*; 34(2):266-72.

Razquin, C., Martinez, JA., Martinez-Gonzalez, MA., Fernández-Crehuet, J., Santos, JM., & Marti, A. (2010 B). A Mediterranean diet rich in virgin olive oil may reverse the effects of the -174G/C IL6 gene variant on 3-year body weight change. *Mol Nutr Food Res*;54 Suppl 1:S75-82.

Razquin, C., Martínez, JA., Martínez-González, MA., Salas-Salvadó. J-, Estruch, R., & Marti, A. (2010 C). A 3-year Mediterranean-style dietary intervention may modulate the association between adiponectin gene variants and body weight change. *Eur J Nutr*; 49(5):311-9.

Robitaille, J., Pérusse, L., Bouchard, C., & Vohl, MC. (2007). Genes, fat intake, and cardiovascular disease risk factors in the Quebec Family Study. *Obesity (Silver Spring)*;15(9):2336-47.

Romaguera, D., Norat, T., Vergnaud, AC., Mouw, T., May, AM., Agudo, A., et al. (2010). Mediterranean dietary patterns and prospective weight change in participants of the EPIC-PANACEA project. *Am J Clin Nutr*; 92(4):912-21.

Ros, E., Núñez, I., Pérez-Heras, A., Serra, M., Gilabert, R., Casals, E., et al. (2004). A walnut diet improves endothelial function in hypercholesterolemic subjects: a randomized crossover trial. *Circulation*; 109(13):1609-14.

Sabaté, J., Oda, K., & Ros, E. (2010). Nut consumption and blood lipid levels: a pooled analysis of 25 intervention trials. *Arch Intern Med*; 170(9):821-7.

Sacks, FM., Bray, GA., Carey, VJ., Smith, SR., Ryan, DH., Anton, SD., et al. (2009). Comparison of weight-loss diets with different compositions of fat, protein, and carbohydrates. *N Engl J Med*; 360(9):859-73.

Mediterranean Diet and Gene-Mediterranean Diet Interactions in Determining
Intermediate Cardiovascular Disease Phenotypes

205

Salas-Salvadó, J., Bulló, M., Babio, N., Martínez-González, MÁ., Ibarrola-Jurado, N., Basora, J., et al. PREDIMED Study Investigators. (2011). Reduction in the incidence of type 2 diabetes with the Mediterranean diet: results of the PREDIMED-Reus nutrition intervention randomized trial. *Diabetes Care*; 34(1):14-9.

Salas-Salvadó, J., Garcia-Arellano, A., Estruch, R., Marquez-Sandovalm F., Corellam D., Fiol, M., et al. (2008). Components of the mediterranean-type food pattern and serum inflammatory markers among patients at high risk for cardiovascular disease. *Eur J Clin Nutr*, 62(5):651-9.

Sans, S., Kesteloot, H., & Kromhout, D. (1997). The burden of cardiovascular diseases mortality in Europe. Task Force of the European Society of Cardiology on Cardiovascular Mortality and Morbidity Statistics in Europe. *Eur Heart J*; 18:1231–1248.

Schröder, H., Marrugat, J., Vila, J., Covas, MI., & Elosua, R. (2004). Adherence to the traditional mediterranean diet is inversely associated with body mass index and obesity in a Spanish population. *J Nutr*; 134(12):3355-61.

Schröder H. (2007). Protective mechanisms of the Mediterranean diet in obesity and type 2 diabetes. *J Nutr Biochem*; 18(3):149-60.

Serra-Majem, L., Trichopoulou, A., Ngo de la Cruz, J., Cervera, P., García Alvarez, A., La Vecchia, C., et al. (2004). Does the definition of the Mediterranean diet need to be updated? *Public Health Nutr*; 7(7):927-9.

Serrano-Martínez M, Martínez-González MA. (2007). Effects of Mediterranean diets on plasma biomarkers of inflammation. *Eur J Clin Nutr*; 61(8):1035-6; author reply 1036.

Shai, I., Schwarzfuchs, D., Henkin, Y., Shahar, DR., Witkow, S., & Greenberg, I.; Dietary Intervention Randomized Controlled Trial (DIRECT) Group. (2008). Weight loss with a low-carbohydrate, Mediterranean, or low-fat diet. *N Engl J Med*; 359(3):229-41.

Singh, RB., Dubnov, G., Niaz, MA., Ghosh, S., Singh, R., Rastogi, SS., et al. (2002). Effect of an Indo-Mediterranean diet on progression of coronary artery disease in high risk patients (Indo-Mediterranean Diet Heart Study): a randomised single-blind trial. *The Lancet*; 360(9344):1455-61.

Slimani, N., Kaaks, R., Ferrari, P., Casagrande, C., Clavel-Chapelon, F., Lotze, G., et al. (2002). European Prospective Investigation into Cancer and Nutrition (EPIC) calibration study: rationale, design and population characteristics. *Public Health Nutr*; 5(6B):1125-45.

Smith, CE., Arnett, DK., Corella, D., Tsai, MY., Lai, CQ., Parnell, LD., et al. (2010). Perilipin polymorphism interacts with saturated fat and carbohydrates to modulate insulin resistance. *Nutr Metab Cardiovasc Dis*. 2010 Dec 30. [Epub ahead of print].

Sotos-Prieto, M., Zulet, MA., & Corella, D. (2010). Scientific evidence of the mediterranean diet effects in determining intermediate and final cardiovascular disease phenotypes. *Med Clin (Barc)*;134(1):22-9

Tai, ES., Collins, D., Robins, SJ., O'Connor, JJ., Bloomfield, HE., Ordovas, JM., et al. (2006). The L162V polymorphism at the peroxisome proliferator activated receptor alpha locus modulates the risk of cardiovascular events associated with insulin resistance and diabetes mellitus: the Veterans Affairs HDL Intervention Trial (VA-HIT). *Atherosclerosis*; 187(1):153-60.

Trichopoulou, A., Costacou, T., Bamia, C., & Trichopoulous, D. (2003). Adherente to a Mediterranean diet and survival in a Greek population. *N Eng J Med*; 348:2599-2608.

Tzima, N., Pitsavos, C., Panagiotakos, DB., Skoumas, J., Zampelas, A., Chrysohoou, C., et al. (2007). Mediterranean diet and insulin sensitivity, lipid profile and blood pressure levels, in overweight and obese people; the Attica study. *Lipids Health Dis*; 6:22.

Vincent-Baudry, S., Defoort, C., Gerber, M., Bernard, MC., Verger, P., Helal, O., et al. (2005). The Medi-RIVAGE study: reduction of cardiovascular disease risk factors after a 3-mo intervention with a Mediterranean-type diet or a low-fat diet. *Am J Clin Nutr*; 82(5):964-71.

Permissions

The contributors of this book come from diverse backgrounds, making this book a truly international effort. This book will bring forth new frontiers with its revolutionizing research information and detailed analysis of the nascent developments around the world.

We would like to thank Dr. Mehnaz Atiq, for lending her expertise to make the book truly unique. She has played a crucial role in the development of this book. Without her invaluable contribution this book wouldn't have been possible. She has made vital efforts to compile up to date information on the varied aspects of this subject to make this book a valuable addition to the collection of many professionals and students.

This book was conceptualized with the vision of imparting up-to-date information and advanced data in this field. To ensure the same, a matchless editorial board was set up. Every individual on the board went through rigorous rounds of assessment to prove their worth. After which they invested a large part of their time researching and compiling the most relevant data for our readers. Conferences and sessions were held from time to time between the editorial board and the contributing authors to present the data in the most comprehensible form. The editorial team has worked tirelessly to provide valuable and valid information to help people across the globe.

Every chapter published in this book has been scrutinized by our experts. Their significance has been extensively debated. The topics covered herein carry significant findings which will fuel the growth of the discipline. They may even be implemented as practical applications or may be referred to as a beginning point for another development. Chapters in this book were first published by InTech; hereby published with permission under the Creative Commons Attribution License or equivalent.

The editorial board has been involved in producing this book since its inception. They have spent rigorous hours researching and exploring the diverse topics which have resulted in the successful publishing of this book. They have passed on their knowledge of decades through this book. To expedite this challenging task, the publisher supported the team at every step. A small team of assistant editors was also appointed to further simplify the editing procedure and attain best results for the readers.

Our editorial team has been hand-picked from every corner of the world. Their multi-ethnicity adds dynamic inputs to the discussions which result in innovative outcomes. These outcomes are then further discussed with the researchers and contributors who give their valuable feedback and opinion regarding the same. The feedback is then collaborated with the researches and they are edited in a comprehensive manner to aid the understanding of the subject.

Apart from the editorial board, the designing team has also invested a significant amount of their time in understanding the subject and creating the most relevant covers. They scrutinized every image to scout for the most suitable representation of the subject and create an appropriate cover for the book.

The publishing team has been involved in this book since its early stages. They were actively engaged in every process, be it collecting the data, connecting with the contributors or procuring relevant information. The team has been an ardent support to the editorial, designing and production team. Their endless efforts to recruit the best for this project, has resulted in the accomplishment of this book. They are a veteran in the field of academics and their pool of knowledge is as vast as their experience in printing. Their expertise and guidance has proved useful at every step. Their uncompromising quality standards have made this book an exceptional effort. Their encouragement from time to time has been an inspiration for everyone.

The publisher and the editorial board hope that this book will prove to be a valuable piece of knowledge for researchers, students, practitioners and scholars across the globe.

List of Contributors

Takeshi Otsuki and Yasuko Okuda
Ryutsu Keizai University & Hiroshima Bunka Gakuen University, Japan

Edita Stokić and Dragana Tomić-Naglić
Department of Endocrinology, Institute of Internal Disease, Clinical Centre Vojvodina, Novi Sad, Serbia

Biljana Srdić
Department of Anatomy, Medical Faculty, Novi Sad, Medical Faculty Novi Sad, Serbia

Vladimir Brtka
Technical Faculty "Mihajlo Pupin" Zrenjanin, Serbia

Aida Pilav
Federal Ministry of Health, Faculty of Health Studies, University of Sarajevo, Bosnia and Herzegovina

Asija Začiragić
Department of Physiology, School of Medicine, University of Sarajevo, Bosnia and Herzegovina

Fumiko Furukawa
School of Nursing, University of Shizuoka, Japan

Tatsuya Morimoto
School of Pharmaceutical Sciences, University of Shizuoka, Japan

Marco A.A. Torquato Jr., Bruno P.F. de Souza, Dan V. Iosifescu and Renerio Fraguas
University of São Paulo, Institute of Psychiatry, Brazil

María Dueñas, Alejandro Salazar, Begoña Ojeda and Inmaculada Failde
Preventive Medicine and Public Health Department, University of Cádiz, Spain

Sara Arranz and Ramón Estruch
Department of Internal Medicine, Hospital Clinic, Institut d.'Investigacions Biomédiques August Pi i Sunyer (IDIBAPS), University of Barcelona, Barcelona, Spain
CIBEROBN Fisiopatología de la Obesidad y la Nutrición and RETIC RD06/0045 Alimentación Saludable en la Prevención Primaria de Enfermedades Crónicas: la Red Predimed, Instituto de Salud Carlos III, Spain

Alex Medina-Remón and Rosa M. Lamuela-Raventós
CIBEROBN Fisiopatología de la Obesidad y la Nutrición and RETIC RD06/0045 Alimentación Saludable en la Prevención Primaria de Enfermedades Crónicas: la Red Predimed, Instituto de Salud Carlos III, Spain
Nutrition and Food Science Department, CeRTA, INSA, Pharmacy School, University of Barcelona, Barcelona, Spain

Mario Ciampolini
Università di Firenze, Italy

Mercedes Sotos Prieto
University of Valencia, Department of Preventive Medicine and Public Health and CIBER Fisiopatología de la Obesidad y Nutrición, Spain

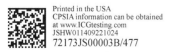

Printed in the USA
CPSIA information can be obtained
at www.ICGtesting.com
JSHW011409221024
72173JS00003B/477